Limbic Seizures in Children

Fondazione Pierfranco e Luisa Mariani ONLUS
viale Bianca Maria 28
20129 Milan, Italy

Telephone: +39 02 795458
Fax: + 39 02 76009582
e-mail: info@fondazione-mariani.org
www.fondazione-mariani.org

Limbic Seizures in Children

Edited by
Giuliano Avanzini, Anne Beaumanoir & Laura Mira

Dedicated to

Claudio Munari

Mariani Foundation Paediatric Neurology Series: 8
Series Editor: Maria Majno

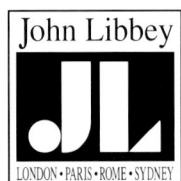

British Library Cataloguing in Publication Data

Limbic seizures in children – Mariani Foundation paediatric neurology series: vol. 8
  1. Convulsions in children   2. Spasms   3. Epilepsy in children
  I. Avanzini, G.   II. Beaumanoir, A. (Anne)   III. Mira, L.

  618.9' 2853
  ISSN: 0969-0301
  ISBN: 0 86196 595 7

Cover illustration: Costanza Magnocavallo

Published by

John Libbey & Company Ltd, PO Box 276, Eastleigh, SO50 5YS, England.
Telephone: +44 (0)23 8065 0208: Fax +44 (0)23 8065 0259

© 2001 John Libbey & Company Ltd. All rights reserved.
Unauthorized duplication contravenes applicable laws.

Printed in Malaysia by Kum-Vivar Printing, 48000 Rawang, Selangor Darul Ehsan.

Contents

Chapter 1	Historical notes: from psychomotor to limbic seizures *Anne Beaumanoir and Joseph Roger*	1
Chapter 2	The limbic system: anatomical structures and embryologic development *Flavio Villani, Rita Garbelli, Barbara Cipelletti and Roberto Spreafico*	11
Chapter 3	Functional organization of the limbic system *Giuliano Avanzini*	21
Chapter 4	Propagation of limbic seizures: experimental studies *Nicolas Chevassus-au-Louis, Roustem Khazipov and Yezekiel Ben-Ari*	33
Chapter 5	Mesial temporal sclerosis: electroclinical and pathological correlations and applications to limbic epilepsy in childhood *Susan S. Spencer, Edward Novotny, Nihal de Lanerolle and Jung Kim*	41
Chapter 6	Loss of contact and impairment of consciousness *Roberto Mai, Stefano Francione, Francesco Cardinale, Giorgio Lo Russo and Claudio Munari*	55
Chapter 7	Neuro-vegetative manifestations in temporo-limbic seizures *Dominique Broglin*	61
Chapter 8	Language and speech disturbances in patients with limbic epilepsy *Hans O. Lüders*	79
Chapter 9	Motor automatisms in limbic seizures *Arnaud Biraben, Delphine Taussig, Serge Belliard, Eric Seigneuret and Jean-Marie Scarabin*	89
Chapter 10	Postural disturbances and changes in facial expression during temporo-limbic seizures in children *Elisabeth Landré, Baris Turak, Francine Chassoux, Dominique Chagot, Jean-Paul Gagnepain and Jean-Paul Chodkiewicz*	105
Chapter 11	Perisylvian cortex involvement in seizures affecting the temporal lobe *Philippe Kahane, Jean-Claude Huot, Dominique Hoffmann, Giorgio Lo Russo, Alim Louis Benabid and Claudio Munari*	115
Chapter 12	Mesio-temporal seizures *Jean Isnard*	129

Chapter 13	Symptoms differentiating 'temporal' and 'frontal' complex partial seizures *Claudio Munari, Roberto Mai, Laura Tassi, Stefano Francione, Giorgio Lo Russo, Lorella Minotti and Philippe Kahane*	137
Chapter 14	Limbic seizures in children *Christian E. Elger and Guillén Fernández*	147
Chapter 15	Temporal lobe epilepsy in childhood *Christa Pachatz, Raffaella Cusmai and Federico Vigevano*	151
Chapter 16	Aetiological role of febrile convulsive attacks in limbic epilepsy *Andrea Van Lierde and Laura Mira*	159
Chapter 17	Memory disturbances in early hippocampal pathology *Daria Riva, Veronica Saletti, Sara Bulgheroni, Irene Bagnasco and Francesca Nichelli*	167
Chapter 18	Psychic alterations in temporal lobe seizures in children *Charlotte Dravet and Michelle Bureau*	175
Chapter 19	Perceptual and intellectual disturbances *Heinz Gregor Wieser*	187
Chapter 20	Ictal EEG during limbic seizures in children *Laura Tassi, Giorgio Lo Russo and Claudio Munari*	201
Chapter 21	Focal seizures in infancy. Do ictal and interictal features suggest limbic involvement? *Silvana Franceschetti, Tiziana Granata, Simona Binelli, Laura Canafoglia, Marina Casazza, Elena Freri, Annalisa Pozzi and Giuliano Avanzini*	211
Chapter 22	Ictal SPECT in temporal lobe seizures in children *Catherine Chiron, Pierre Véra, Andreas Hollo, Anna Kaminska, Cécile Cieuta, Dorothé Ville, Jean Louis Stiévenart, Isabelle Gardin, Perrine Plouin, Martin Fohlen, Olivier Delalande, Claude Jalin and Olivier Dulac*	217
Chapter 23	MRI in limbic structures in the epileptic and non-epileptic child *Ludovico D'Incerti*	225
Chapter 24	The medical therapy of limbic seizures in children *Paola Costa, Andrea Van Lierde and Laura Mira*	231
Chapter 25	Surgical treatment of 'limbic' seizures in children: methodological aspects and strategies *Claudio Munari, Lorella Minotti, Giorgio Lo Russo, Laura Tassi, Roberto Mai, Stefano Francione, Emilia Berta, Dominique Hoffmann, Francesco Cardinale, Massimo Cossu and Philippe Kahane*	237
Chapter 26	Is there a benign limbic epilepsy in children? *Bernardo Dalla Bernardina, Francesca Darra, Elena Fontana and Anne Beaumanoir*	241
Chapter 27	Synopsis *Giuliano Avanzini*	249
	Index	255

Chapter 1

Historical notes: from psychomotor to limbic seizures

Anne Beaumanoir and Joseph Roger[*]

Fondazione Pierfranco e Luisa Mariani, Viale Bianca Maria 28, 20129 Milan, Italy
[*]*Centre Saint Paul, 300 Boulevard Saint Marguerite, 13009 Marseille, France*

Summary

The history of limbic seizures starts in the last century with H. Jackson's clinical observations and with the studies which led to the anatomo-histological identification of rhinencephalic structures. In the 1950s a relevant number of clinical and experimental studies led to the description of the limbic lobe as functionally distinct from temporal neocortical structures. Limbic seizures have been termed under different labels: psychomotor seizures, temporal seizures, focal seizures with diffuse expression, rhinencephalic seizures ..., before they were classified as complex partial seizures (CPC). Recently, the temporal lobe epileptic syndromes have been subdivided into several groups, among which is 'mesial temporal lobe epilepsy' (MTLE), characterized by complex partial seizures considered to be the consequence of glial lesions of the mesial limbic lobe, including the Ammon's horn. Similar glial hippocampal lesions had been described since 1825 by Bouchet & Cazauvieihl and studied at that time by several authors. A century later, in 1951, Sholz considered them as the consequence of repeated convulsive seizures in infancy. Despite the fact that this hypothesis has been confirmed by other authors, so far few studies have been concerned with children's limbic seizures, even if many question are still open: the papers collected in this volume try to give answers to these questions.

The history of limbic seizures tells us how from Jackson's first description of seizures with 'intellectual aura' and 'dreamy state' in 1888 and 1898, a century later complex partial seizures (CPS) were differentiated from other seizures. It also tells us how in the last 20 years the simple 19th century anatomo-physiologists' 'olfactory' hippocampus has become the 'fetish' object of all epilepsy researchers.

In 1941 Penfield & Erickson, on the basis of data obtained by stimulation during neurosurgical procedures, proposed the term of '*temporal lobe epilepsy*' to label epilepsy characterized by

EEG temporal spikes (S) or slow waves (SW) and seizures with automatisms and 'some signs which can not be classified from a physiopathogenetic viewpoint'.

Pointing out that his term *'psychic variant seizures'* did not entail the motor symptoms (automatisms, wandering) presented by epileptic patients, in 1937 Gibbs & Gibbs together with Lennox proposed to replace it by that of *'psychomotor seizures'*. Ten years later Gibbs, Gibbs & Furster (1948) showed that the critical symptomatology of patients with intercritical evidence of a focus in the anterior temporal region essentially consisted of automatisms. They adopted the term *'automatic seizures'* to differentiate them from other psychomotor seizures. Thereafter a terminological controversy arose, to which, besides the Montreal school (Jasper *et al.*, 1951; Jasper & Rassmussen, 1958), Bailey & Van Bonin (1951), Gibbs (1951), Lennox (1951), Gastaut (1953), Symonds (1954), De Jong (1957) and Beaumanoir *et al.* (1982) participated, as well as others including MacNaughton, who in his proposed classification of epilepsies of 1952 acknowledged the difficulty of classifying focal temporal seizures and stated that the term 'psychomotor seizures' was the most appropriate.

EEG recording of 'psychomotor' seizures showed that they differentiated from other focal seizures because of slow theta activity quickly spreading over the corresponding hemiscalp and sometimes over the contralateral hemisphere. This feature led Gastaut *et al.* (1958) to suggest calling them *'partial seizures with diffuse (EEG) expression'*. Other authors, making reference to anatomical data, adopted the term *temporal lobe seizures* or *rhinencephalic seizures*. The observation of 'temporal' seizures recorded by EEG or stereoencephalography showed that in some cases they were accompanied by consciousness disturbances. They were then classified as *'complex partial seizures'*, in a great number of cases pointing to involvement of the basal limbic system. Therefore temporal lobe epilepsy further fractionated into multiple syndromes, including epilepsy consequent to glial lesions of the mesial limbic lobe, i.e. Spencer's (1998) *'medial temporal lobe epilepsy (MTLE)'*.

Before the technique of stereoencephalography allowed the location of critical epileptic discharges in human cortical as well as subcortical structures in a large number of cases, animal physiologists had been interested in the issue of *'psychomotor epilepsy'*. From 1950 to 1960 a wealth of studies exploring the temporal lobe, the amygdaloid nuclei, the hippocampus and the cingulum, such as those by Lennox *et al.* (1950), Pribam *et al.* (1950, 1953, 1954), MacLean (1952, 1955), Kaada (1951, 1953, 1954, 1960), Liberson with Cadilhac & Ackert (1953, 1955), Gloor (1955), Green & Adey (1956), Green & Arduini (1954), Green & Shimamoto (1956), Creutzfeld (1956), Gastaut & colleagues (from 1950 to 1958) brought out data which proved essential to the understanding of the electroclinical symptomatology of *'psychomotor seizures manifesting on human scalp by intercritical temporal discharges and critical more diffuse discharges'*.

The anatomists of the first half of the century demonstrated that the rhinencephalon, i.e. the olfactory brain of macrosomatics, undergoes atrophy in primates, leaving only its limbic portion, rearranged by the development of the corpus callosum. They also studied how in the course of species evolution the neocortex comes to envelop the hippocampal and piriform allocortex and the underlying paleo- and neocortical structure: the amygdaloid complex. On the basis of phylogenetic, ontogenetic, architectonic and vascular data, they separated the temporal lobe into two portions: a neocortical one, including the proper temporal cortex and the posterior temporal cortex, and a paleocortical one, including the temporopolar region and the rhinencephalon or limbic lobe according to Broca's terminology (1878). Given architectonic similarities confirmed by functional identities, in 1951 Bailey & Von Bonin included the posterior orbital cortex, the anterior insula and the pole of the temporal lobe as well as the amygdaloid complex as components of the limbic lobe.

Data accrued from studies of lesion, stimulation, degeneration and ionophoresis of these structures demonstrated their role in vegetative, motor, emotional and cognitive functions. In 1949 and 1952 MacLean identified the limbic lobe with the *'visceral brain'* involved in vegetative activities and related somatomotor responses. According to Kaada (1951) the term was appropriate only to indicate the rostral portion of the limbic lobe, inclusive of the anterior cingular area, the orbito-insulo-temporal polar region and the amygdala, but exclusive of the hippocampus and the posterior cingulum. In 1954 Pribam & Kruger distinguished two rhinencephalic systems, the first corresponding to Kaada's and the other (hippocampus–fornix–cingulum) as part of a closed circuit, anterior thalamus/cingular gyrus/cingulum/hippocampus/fimbria/fornix/mammillary bodies and back to the anterior thalamus, i.e. the *'affective brain'* identified by Papez in 1937, who related it to emotions.

In 1938 Jung & Kormuller, confirmed by Liberson & Ackert in 1955, showed that the Ammon's horn, an histologically distinctive structure, was also characterized by specific electrophysiological features, stressing its typical theta rhythm in response to sensory stimulation in every modality. They started a series of studies on this paradoxical response which in the 1960s led to the hypothesis of the hippocampal role in memory processes (Penfield & Milner, 1958). The study of the effects of sodium amytal intracarotid injection emphasized the role of the *'medial temporal lobe'* (MTL) in short-term memory processing.

In 1949 Jung and then Liberson & Cadilhac (1953) showed that the hippocampus, the amygdala and the piriform cortex had a very low epileptic threshold. On the other hand some authors explained the wide and quick discharge spreading by an ephaptic propagation to the whole hippocampal field.

The epileptic discharge in the rhinencephalon was studied by means of the technique of afterdischarge to electrical stimulation and by resorting to semi-chronic and chronic models, which in the 1950s and 1960s implied the creation of an epileptogenic focus by injection of aluminum cream. Gastaut's school should be credited with the observation that in the cat the electroencephalographic responses to amygdala stimulation with a given intensity seemed to vary in latency in different structures. They were accompanied by clinical signs related to after-discharge in structures connected to the amygdaloid nuclei: orbitary, insular, temporal, cingular, hypothalamic regions.

Taking these animal results into account, Gastaut & A. Roger (1955) explained the complexity of psychomotor seizures in man by the simultaneous or time-scattered onset of critical discharges in different cortical and/or subcortical structures.

We believed (Roger, 1955) that the psychomotor seizure corresponded to the overlapping of 'erratic' self-progressing seizures.

The chronic focal epilepsy model by aluminum cream injection allowed the description of a focal epilepsy in the cat with amygdala-periamygdala lesions in which the critical symptomatology started with an 'arrest reaction' (staring?) followed by licking and lapping automatisms, vegetative signs (piloerection, salivation, occasionally mydriasis), fear reactions with flight or sometimes aggression. Seizure recording allowed the electroclinical study of symptoms which especially demonstrated that the amygdala discharge could produce a flattening of EEG activity.

The intercritical EEG suggested two relevant observations which nowadays appear to be straightforward:

1. An isolated lesion generates multiple perilesional foci;

2. In the chronic animal, after spontaneous seizures occurring over many months, '*mirror foci*' appear in the contralateral amygdala, a phenomenon already reported in extralimbic regions by Pope *et al.* (1947) which we interpreted as '*the functional mark in the contralateral cortex that has acquired epileptogenic potentiality through bombing*' (Gastaut & Roger, 1955). This epileptogenic transfer from one structure to another was studied by Morrell (1960) who starting from 1973 interpreted his results in the light of those yielded by the kindling effect (Morrell, 1973).

In fact the discovery of the kindling effect by Goddard *et al.* in 1969 renewed interest in studying the diffusion of amygdalo-hippocampal discharges. Among the results achieved from 1970 to 1985 by this technique developed by Wada and others (Wada, 1976, 1978), at least two still deserve our consideration:

1. Within the amygdalo-hippocampal complex, the amygdala requires weaker stimulations than the hippocampus to obtain a kindling, while the latter one has a markedly lower threshold for after-discharge.

2. The kindling varies according to the phylogenetic development and especially according to the animal proneness to convulsion, as Wada *et al.* (1978) showed. Therefore generalized seizures could not be produced in *macacus rhesus* but they were easily obtained in the baboon *papio papio* genetically fit to convulsions.

These first experimental data and consequent speculations opened the way to the studies of the limbic lobe epileptogenicity, pioneered by Yamamoto and McIlwain in 1966, using *in vitro* models on hippocampus slices and *in vivo* models by injection of a glutammic analogue, the kainic acid, directly into the hippocampus or the amygdala. These studies, started by Meldrum & Brierley (1973), acquired their full relevance through the work of Ben Ari in the 1980s.

Since 1981, thanks to Watkins & Evans, the different types of kainate and NMDA receptors have been identified in different limbic structures and particularly in the hippocampus. This led to studies on the pathophysiology of the epileptogenic focus in the limbic lobe which are still under way.

As far as man is concerned, the improvement of the techniques of identification of sites to explore, brought about by the Paris school with Bancaud in the 1960s, has produced (1965, 1966, and later in 1987) many arguments to differentiate the cortical seizures of the convexity from those of the inferior portion of the temporal lobe, seizures which were labelled 'primary rhinencephalic'.

The regions involved by the critical discharge of psychomotor epilepsy have long been shown to be damaged in epilepsies. Bouchet & Cazauvieilh's observations about the '*Ammon's horn sclerosis*' did not draw much interest in 1825, probably because at that time epilepsy was still considered a mental illness. Only at the end of the 19th century did Chaslin (1889) in France and Bratz (1889) in Germany wonder about the histological changes displayed by epileptics, which Sommer (1880) had shown to disarrange the pyramidal cells bands while sparing all the other layers of the hippocampus. Chaslin pointed out that the sclerosis is not strictly limited to Ammon's horn, although this is its preferential site. Bratz demonstrated that a sclerosis of

Sommer's sector can be identified in other neurological conditions beside epilepsy provided that the patient suffered convulsive seizures. However, he stated that these lesions are congenital. The discussion about the meaning, i.e. cause or effect, of Ammon's horn sclerosis in epilepsy had been opened.

The morphology and topography of these lesions were better defined by Spielmayer (1927) and later by Scholz (1951, 1954), who regarded them as the consequence of repeated convulsive seizures. These authors did not wonder about a possible relationship between these lesions and a peculiar clinical type of epilepsy, as Stauder did in 1935.

Only after the neurosurgery experiences proved that these anatomical lesions were present in patients cured of epilepsy after temporal lobe ablation was it finally acknowledged that ammonic and peri-insular damage was not the consequence but the cause of psychomotor epilepsy (Earle et al., 1953; Sano & Malamud, 1953; Gastaut et al., 1958, 1959; Cavanagh et al., 1958; Meyer et al., 1954; Falconer, 1971, 1974). In his 1988 exhaustive study of 249 temporal lobe surgical specimens, Bruton demonstrated that even if the lesions are somewhat diffuse in the limbic structures, they are markedly prevalent (122 cases, i.e. 50 per cent) within the Ammon's horn. When the lesion is ammonic, this is often the only histoanatomical abnormality (107 cases out of 122).

In a short time the issue of the pathogenesis of structural changes of the basal limbic system (neuronal degeneration and reactive gliosis) was set. In 1953 Earle et al. regarded them as the consequence of hippocampal herniation occurring at the time of delivery. Gastaut & A. Roger (1955) as well as Norman (1956, 1958) emphasized the sensitivity to hypoxia of the uncus, the Ammon's horn and the amygdala to explain temporal lobe seizures. In Gastaut's opinion the lesions of the internal portion of the temporal lobe, the amygdaloid nucleus and the hippocampus were linked by the sequence of cerebral oedema, temporal engagement and consequent vascular compression. According to Gastaut and to Sano & Malamud (1953) the starting step was often represented by a febrile unilateral status epilepticus.

Since the time of identification of psychomotor epilepsy, all authors have emphasized early onset of seizures in this kind of epilepsy. Only in 1953 did A. Roger (1954) and J. Roger (1954), followed by Glaser et al. and Glaser alone (1956, 1967) and later by Deonna et al. (1986), Holmes (1986) and Yamamoto et al. (1987) take an interest in possible electroclinical peculiarities of children's psychomotor epilepsy. According to these studies, children's and adults' temporal lobe seizures do not differ semiologically to any significant degree. In children, automatisms are simple in most cases, conscious symptoms are especially epigastric or represented by ill defined unpleasant sensations and fear; vegetative symptoms, particularly vomiting, are more frequent than in adults. In 1989 Dravet et al., and later Yamamoto et al. (1987), Duchowy (1987) and Blume (1989) were interested in semiological peculiarities in infants of less than 4 years of age, whereas Dalla Bernardina et al. (1985), tried to identify a group characterized by a favourable prognosis, possibly corresponding to an idiopathic temporal epilepsy.

Unfortunately, for the time being no result can be taken as conclusive. As a matter of fact all these studies are flawed with gaps (lack of long term follow-up; no studies on the relationship between clinical data, EEG and imaging in a significant number of cases).

On the other hand, most of these studies dealt with partial complex seizures in the lines of the wrong equation: partial complex seizure = temporal lobe seizure, while a relevant number of them are frontal lobe seizures or parieto-occipital seizures spreading to the limbic system.

Systematic use of current investigation techniques, in particular neuroimaging, should yield answers to still unresolved issues, such as: what is the cause and what is the semiology of the initial events deemed responsible of the Ammon's horn lesions? at what time do they appear? are these lesions evolutive?

The crucial question can be posed as follows: can a clinico-electro-anatomical syndrome be identified to allow an early evolutive diagnosis? The answer to this question is even more important when one considers that all the available data prove that in drug resistant limbic epilepsy surgical treatment is often appropriate and that good clinical results, including psycho-affective development, depend on early surgery.

References

Bailey, P. & Von Bonin, N. (1951): *The isocortex in man*, pp. 1–301. Illinois: University of Illinois Press.

Baldwin, M. & Bailey, P. (1948): *Temporal lobe epilepsy*, pp. 1–580. Springfield, IL: Charles C. Thomas.

Bancaud, J. (1987): Sémiologie clinique des crises epileptiques d'origine temporale. *Rev. Neurol.* **5**, 392–400.

Bancaud, J., Talairach, J., Bonis, A., Shaub, C., Morel, P. & Bordas-Ferrer, M. (1965): *La stéréoencéphalographie dans l'épilepsie*, pp. 1–315. Paris: Masson.

Bancaud, J., Talairach, J., Morel, P. & Bresson, M. (1966): La corne d'Ammon et le noyau amygdalien: effets cliniques et électriques de la stimulation chez l'homme. *Rev. Neurol.* **115**, 329–352.

Beaumanoir, A., Naquet, R. & Vigouroux, R. (1982): Temporal lobe epilepsy: experimental reproduction. In: *Gastaut and the Marseilles school's contribution in the Neurosciences,* pp. 159–170. EEG Clin. Neurophysiol. Suppl.

Ben Ari, Y., Tremblay, E. & Ottersen, O. (1980): Injections of kainic acid into the amygdaloid complex of the rat: an electrographic, clinical and histological study in relation to the pathology of epilepsy. *Neuroscience* **5**, 515–528.

Blume, W.T. (1989): Medical profile of partial seizures beginning at less than four years of age. *Epilepsia* **30**, 813–819.

Bouchet, C. & Cazauvieihl, L. (1825): De l'épilepsie considérée dans ses rapports avec l'aliénation mentale. *Arch. gen. Médecine* **9**, 510–542.

Bratz, E. (1889): Ammons Horn Befunde bei Epileptischen. *Arch. Psychiatr. Nervenkr.* **31**, 820–836.

Broca, P. (1878): Description élémentaire des circonvolutions cérébrales de l'homme d'après le cerveau schématique. *Rev. d'Anthroplogie* 25ème Série, Ch VI.

Bruton, C.J. (1988): *The neuropathology of temporal lobe epilepsy*, pp. 1–128. Oxford: Oxford University Press.

Cavanagh, J.B. & Meyer, A. (1956): Aetiological aspects of Ammon Horn sclerosis associated with temporal lobe epilepsy. *BMJ* **2**, 1403–1407.

Cavanagh, J.B., Falconer, M.A. & Meyer, A. (1958): Somes pathogenic problems of temporal lobe epilepsy. In: *Temporal lobe epilepsy*, eds. Baldwin & Bailey, pp. 140–148. Springfield, IL: Charles C. Thomas.

Chao, D., Sexton, J.A. & Santos-Pardo, L. (1962): Temporal lobe epilepsy in children. *J. Pediatr.* **60**, 686–693.

Chaslin, H. (1889): Note sur l'anatomie pathologique de l'épilepsie essentielle: la sclérose névroglique. *C. R. Soc. Biol.* **1**, 169–171.

Creutzfeld, O. (1956): Die Krampfausbreitung in temporallappen der Katze. *Schweiz. Archiv. fur Neurol. u. Psychiat.* **77**, 163–194.

Dalla Bernardina, B., Chiamenti, C., Capovilla, G., Trevisan, E. & Tassinari, C.A. (1985): Benign partial epilepsy with affective symptoms (Benign psychomotor epilepsy). In: *Epileptic syndromes in infancy, childhood and adolescence*, eds. J. Roger, Ch. Dravet, M. Bureau *et al.*, pp. 171–175. London: John Libbey.

De Jong, R.N. (1957): 'Psychomotor' or 'Temporal Lobe' epilepsy. A review of the development of our present concept. *Neurology* **7**, 1–14.

Deonna, T., Ziegler, A.L., Desplant, P.A. & Van Melle, G. (1986): Partial epilepsy in neurologically normal children. *Epilepsia* **27**, 241–247.

Dravet, C., Catani, C., Bureau, M. & Roger, J. (1989): Partial epilepsies in infancy: a study of 40 cases. *Epilepsia* **30**, 807–812.

Duchowy, M.S. (1987): Complex partial seizures in infancy. *Arch. Neurol.* **44**, 911–914.

Earle, K., Baldwin, M. & Penfield, W. (1953): Incisural sclerosis and temporal lobe seizures produced by hippocampal herniation at birth. *Arch. Neurol. Psych.*. **69**, 27–41.

Falconer, M.A. (1971): Genetic and related aetiological factors in temporal lobe epilepsy. *Epilepsia* **12**, 13–31.

Falconer, M.A. (1974): Mesial temporal (Ammon' horn) sclerosis as a common cause of epilepsy. *Lancet* **2**, 767–770.

Gastaut, H. (1952): Corrélations entre le système nerveux végétatif et le système de la vie de relation dans le rhinencéphale. *J. Physiol.* **44**, 431–470.

Gastaut, H. (1953): So called 'psychomotor'and 'temporal' epilepsy: a critical study. *Epilepsia* **3**, 59–76.

Gastaut, H. & Roger, A. (1955): Origine et propagation des décharges épileptiques temporales provoquées. In: *Les grandes activités du lobe temporal,* ed. Th. Alajouanine, pp. 83–113. Paris: Masson.

Gastaut, H., Naquet, R. & Roger, A. (1952): Comportements émotionnels divers par stimulation rhinencéphalique chez le chat avec électrodes à demeure. *Rev. Neurol.* **86**, 319–326.

Gastaut, H., Naquet, R., Roger, A. *et al.* (1953): Etude électroencéphalographique chez l'homme et chez l'animal des décharges épileptiques dites 'psychomotrices'. *Rev. Neurol.* **88**, 310–354.

Gastaut, H., Vigouroux, M. & Fisher-Williams M. (1958): Electroclinical correlations in 500 cases of psychomotor seizures In: *Temporal lobe epilepsy,* eds. E. Baldwin & P. Bailey, pp. 118–128. Springfield, IL: Charles C. Thomas.

Gastaut, H., Toga, M., Roger, J. *et al.* (1959): A correlation of clinical, electroencephalographic and anatomical findings in nine autopsied cases of temporal lobe epilepsy. *Epilepsia* **1**, 56–85.

Gibbs, F.A. (1951): Ictal and non ictal psychiatric disorders in temporal lobe epilepsy. *J. Nerv. Ment. Dis.* **113**, 522–528.

Gibbs, F.A., Gibbs, E.L. & Lennox, W.G. (1937): Epilepsy: a paroxysmal dysrhythmia. *Brain* **60**, 377–382.

Gibbs, E.L., Gibbs, F.A. & Furster, B. (1948): Psychomotor epilepsy. *Arch. Neurol. Psych.* **60**, 331–339.

Glaser, G.H. (1967): Limbic epilepsy in childhood. *J. Nerv. Dis.* **114**, 391–397.

Glaser, G.H. & Dixon, M.S. (1956): Psychomotor seizures in childhood, a clinical study. *Neurology* **6**, 646–655.

Glaser, G.H. & Gollub, L.M. (1956): The electroencephalogram of psychomotor seizures in childhood. *Electroencephal. Clin. Neurophysiol.* **7**, 329–340.

Gloor, P. (1955): Electrophysiological studies on the connections of the amygdaloid nucleus in the cat: (1) the neuronal organization of the amygdaloid projections system; (2) the electrophysiological properties of the amygdaloid projections systems. *Electroencephal. Clin. Neurophysiol.* **7**, 223–242.

Gloor, P. (1960): Amygdala. In: *Handbook of physiology,* vol. II, pp. 1395–1419. Baltimore, MD: American Physiological Society.

Goddard, G.V., Mc Intyre, D.C. & Leech, C.K. (1969): A permanent change in brain function resulting from daily electrical stimulation. *Exp. Neurol.* **25**, 295–330.

Green, J.D. & Adey, W.R. (1956): Electrophysiological studies of hippocampal connections and excitability. *EEG Clin. Neurophysiol.* **8**, 245–262.

Green, J.D. & Arduini, A.A. (1954): Hippocampal electrical activity in arousal. *J. Neurophysiol.* **17**, 533–557.

Green, J.D & Shimamoto, T. (1956). Hippocampal seizures and their propagation. *Arch. Neurol. Psych.* **70**, 687–702.

Holmes, G.H. (1986): Partial seizures in children. *Pediatrics* **77**, 725–731.

Jackson, J.H. (1888): On a particular variety of epilepsy ('intellectual aura'). One case with symptoms of organic brain disease. *Brain* **11**, 179–207.

Jackson, J.H. & Collman, W.S. (1898): Case of epilepsy with tasting movements and 'dreamy state' and very small patch of softening in the left uncinate gyrus. *Brain* **21**, 580–590.

Jasper, H.H. (1958): Functional subdivisions of temporal regions in relation to seizure patterns and subcortical connections. In: *Temporal lobe epilepsy,* eds. E. Baldwin & P. Bailey, pp. 40–58. Springfield, IL: Charles C. Thomas.

Jasper, H.H. & Rassmussen, T. (1958): Study of clinical and electrical responses to deep-temporal in man and some considerations of functional anatomy. *Ass. Res. Nerv. Ment. Dis. Proc.* **36**, 316–334.

Jasper, H.H., Pertuiset, B. & Flaniging, H. (1951): EEG and cortical electroencephalograms in patients with temporal lobe seizures. *Arch. Neurol. Psych.* **65**, 267–290.

Jung, R. (1949): Hirnelektrische Untersuchungen über den Elektrokrampf; die Errengungsläufe in corticalen und sub-corticalen Hirnregionen bei Katze und Hund. *Arch. Psychiat. und Zeitsch. Neurol.* **183**, 206–244.

Jung, R. & Kormuller, A.E. (1938): Eine Methodik der ableitung lokalisirter Potentialschankungen aus subcorticalen Hirngebieten. *Arch. Psych. Nervenkr.* **109**, 1–30.

Kaada, B.R. (1951): Somato-motor-autonomic and electrocorticographic responses to electrical stimulation of 'rhinencephalic' and other structures in primates, cat and dog. *Acta Physiol. Scand.* **24** (Suppl. 83), 1–285.

Kaada, B.R. (1960): Cingulate, posterior orbital, anterior insular and temporal pole cortex. In: *Handbook of physiology*, vol. ii, pp. 1345–1372. Baltimore, MD: American Physiological Society.

Kaada, B.R., Jansen, J. & Andersen, P. (1953): Stimulation of the hippocampus and medial cortical areas in unanesthetized cats. *Neurology* **3**, 844–857.

Kaada, B.R., Andersen, P. & Jansen, J. (1954): Stimulation of the amygdaloid nuclear complex in unanesthetized cats. *Neurology* **4**, 48–64.

Lennox, M.A., Dunsmore, R.H., Eostein, J.A. & Pribaam, C.K. (1950): Electrographic effects of stimulation of posterior orbital, temporal and cingular areas in Macaca Mulatta. *J. Neurophsiol.* **13**, 383–388.

Lennox, W.G. (1951): Phenomena and correlates of psychomotor Triad. *Neurology* **1**, 357–371.

Liberson, W.T. & Akert, T. (1955): Hippocampal seizure states in guinea pigs. *Electroencephal. Clin. Neurophysiol.* **7**, 211–222.

Liberson, W.T. & Cadilhac, J.C. (1953): Electroshock and rhinencephalic seizure state. *Conf. Neurol.* **13**, 278–286.

MacLean, P. (1949): Psychosomatic disease and the 'visceral brain'. Recents developments bearing on the Papez theory of emotion. *Psychosom. Med.* **2**, 338–351.

MacLean, P. (1952): Some psychiatric implications of physiological studies on fronto-temporal portion of the limbic system ('visceral Brain'). *Electroencephal. Clin. Neurophysiol.* **4**, 407–418.

MacLean, P. (1955): The limbic system and its hippocampal formation. Studies in animal and their possible application to man. *Arch. Neurol. Psych.* **73**, 130–164.

MacNaughton, F.L. (1952): The classification of the epilepsies. *Epilepsia* **1**, 7–12.

Meldrum, B.S. & Brierley, R.W. (1973): Prolonged epileptic seizures in primates ischemic cells changes and its relation to ictal physiological events. *Arch. Neurol.* **28**, 10–17.

Morrell, F. (1960): Secondary epileptogenic lesions. *Epilepsia* **1**, 538–569.

Morrell, F. (1973): Goddard kindling phenomenon: a new model of the 'mirror focus'. In: *Chemical modulation of brain function*, ed. H.C. Sabell, pp. 207–223. New York: Raven Press.

Meyer, A., Falconer, M.A. & Beck, E. (1954): Pathological findings in temporal lobe epilepsy. *J. Neurol. Neurosurg. Psychiat.* **18**, 24–33.

Norman, R. (1956): La sclérose lobaire dans l'épilepsie et l'encéphalopathie de la naissance. *Acta Neurol. Belgica* **2**, 89–102.

Norman, R. (1958): The pathogenesis of amygdaloid lesions in early life. In: *Temporal lobe epilepsy,* eds. E. Baldwin & P. Bailey, pp. 203–219. Springfield, IL: Charles C. Thomas.

Papez (1937): A proposal for the mechanism of emotions. *Arch. Neurol.* **38**, 725–743.

Penfield, W. & Erickson, T.C. (1941): *Epilepsy and cerebral localizations.* Springfield, IL: Charles C. Thomas.

Penfield, W. & Milner, B. (1958): Memory deficits by bilateral lesions in the hippocampal zones. *Arch. Neurol. Psych.* **79**, 475–497.

Pribam, K.H. & Kruger, S. (1954): Functions of the olfactory brain. *Ann. NY Acad. Sci.* **58**, 109–138.

Pribam, K.H. & MacLean, P.D. (1953): Neuronographic analysis of medial and basal cerebral cortex in cat. *J. Neurophysiol.* **16**, 312–323.

Pribam, K.H., Lennox, W. & Dunsmore, R.H. (1950): Some connections of the orbito-frontal, temporal, limbic and hippocampal areas of Macaca Mulatta. *J. Neurophysiol.* **12**, 127–135.

Pope, A., Morris, A., Jasper, H. *et al.* (1947): Histochemical and action potentials studies on epileptogenic area of cerebral cortex in man and the monkey. *Res. Nerv. Ment. Dis. Proc.* **21**, 218–233.

Roger, A. (1954): Etude EEG de l'épilepsie psychomotrice de l'enfant. *Rev. Neuropsych. Infantile* **1**, 23–37.

Roger, J. (1954): Etude clinique de l'épilepsie psychomotrice de l'enfant. *Rev. Neuropsych. Infantile* **1**, 15–21.

Roger, A.R. (1955): Contribution à l'étude expérimentale de l'épilepsie partielle. Thése Médecine Fac. Aix-Marseille, pp. 1–60. Laval, Barneoud Imp.

Sano, K. & Malamud, N. (1953): Clinical significance of sclerosis of the Cornu Ammonis. *Arch. Neurol. Psych.* **70**, 40–53.

Scholz, W. (1951): *Des Krampfschadigungen des Gehirns*. Berlin: Springer Verlag.

Scholz, W. (1954): Les lésions cérébrales rencontrées chez les épileptiques. Précisions sur la sclérose de la corne d'Ammon. *Acta Neurol. Belgica* **61**, 43–60.

Sommer, W. (1880): Erkrankung des Ammonhornes als aetiologisches Moment der Epilepsie. *Arch. Psychiat.* **10**, 631–674.

Spencer, S.S. (1998): Substrates of localization-related epilepsies: biological implications of localizing findings in humans. *Epilepsia* **39**, 114–123.

Spielmeyer, W. (1927): Die pathogenese des epileptichen Krampfes. *Ztschr. Ges Neurol. u Psychiat.* **109**, 501–520.

Stauder, K.H. (1935): Epilepsis und Schläfenlappen. *Arch. Psych.* **104**, 181–212.

Symonds, Ch. (1954): Classification of the epilepsies with particular reference to psychomotor seizures. *Arch. Neurol. Psychiat.* **72**, 631.

Wada, J.A. (1976): *Kindling*, pp. 1–260. New York: Raven Press.

Wada, J.A., Mizoguchi, T. & Osawa, T. (1978): Secondarily generalized convulsive seizures induced by daily stimulation in rhesus monkey. *Neurology* **47**, 1026–1036.

Watkins, J.C. & Evans, R.H. (1981): Excitatory amino acid neurotransmitters. *Ann. Rev. Pharm. Toxicol.* **21**, 165–204.

Yamamoto, C. & MacIlwain, H. (1966): Electrical activities in thin sections from the mammalian brain maintained in chemically defined media *in vitro*. *J. Neurochem.* **13**, 1333–1343.

Yamamoto, N., Watanabe, K., Negoro, T. *et al.* (1987): Complex partial seizures in children: ictal manifestations and their relations to clinical outcome. *Neurology* **37**, 1379–1382.

Chapter 2

The limbic system: anatomical structures and embryologic development

Flavio Villani, Rita Garbelli, Barbara Cipelletti and Roberto Spreafico

Divisione di Neurofisiologia, Istituto Nazionale Neurologico 'C. Besta', via Celoria, 11, 20133 Milan, Italy

Summary

The ill-defined term of 'limbic system' has identified since the 1800s an anatomical entity constituted by a heterogeneous group of cerebral structures mainly located in the mesial portion of the brain. Its widest anatomical boundaries may be anatomically and embryologically grossly delineated among temporal, extratemporal, cortical and subcortical structures. The amygdala, septal nuclei, substantia innominata, bed nucleus of the stria terminalis, thalamus, and hypothalamus, are the main subcortical structures involved in the system. The cortical structures are differentiated on the basis of their laminar structure. The isocortex, allocortex (or atypical cortex), and mesocortex, all concur to the limbic system. The hippocampal formation is the central core of the system and represents the major allocortical structure of the brain.

Although the limbic system is observed in all mammals, the evolution of the brain regions involved in the limbic circuitry of different animal species explains the various odhological and functional properties of the system. In mammals, along with the evolutionary increase of the isocortex, the limbic system has progressively shifted from a structure primarily associated to the olfactory function to a system heavily interconnected to the associative cortices.

During the early embryonic development all neurons are generated at sites different from their final positions in the adult brain. The migration rate is different for each part of the limbic system, with the migrating cells reaching their final destination with different delays. The rate of migration influences the degree of differentiation of the neurons at the time of their arrival at the final site and, as a consequence, the formation of the neural pathways. Different rates of migration, the differentiation of neurons, and the formation of well defined neural pathways may have pathophysiological implications in the limbic system.

Anatomical aspects

Almost one hundred years ago Pierce Paul Broca (1878) observed a peculiar region of the nervous system located in the mesial portion of the hemispheres at the borders of the neocortex and named it *'le grand lobe de l'ourlet'*. Subsequently, the same author renamed it *'le grand lobe limbique'*, using the term 'limbique' (limbic) to mean 'the border' or 'the limit' (of the cortex). Later on, this area was named 'rhinencephalon', since it was assumed that the structures forming the limbic system were somehow involved in the olfactory sense. Although the olfactory tract is the only primary sensory structure directly connected to the limbic ring, it was observed that the olfactory system is not the only major input to the limbic system, since it is also widely connected to the association cortices. The old term of 'limbic system' was therefore resumed and in 1937 James Papez proposed a new concept of limbic system, considering it as the major anatomical substrate for the elaboration of emotion and behaviour. Since then, many investigations have been performed to study and better define the structures involved in the odhology of this system.

Although numerous studies have been performed, it is still very difficult to provide a universally acceptable definition of the limbic system, this having changed over time depending on the preference of the individual authors. At different times the investigators have, sometimes arbitrarily, added or excluded from this system various anatomical structures.

Nowadays, the term 'limbic system' defines only an anatomical entity (and not functional properties) that for the sake of simplicity can be considered as formed by cortical and subcortical groups of anatomically and embryologically different structures. Its widest anatomical boundaries may be grossly delineated among temporal, extratemporal, cortical and subcortical structures (Table 1).

Table 1. Schematic representation of the main cortical and subcortical structures composing the limbic system.

```
                                    isocortex
                                                    proisocortex
                                    mesocortex
                                                    periallocortex
              cortical structures
                                                    piriform cortex
                                    allocortex
                                                    hippocampus
LIMBIC SYSTEM
                                    thalamus
                                    septal nuclei
              subcortical structures  preoptic area
                                    amygdala
                                    n. accumbens
```

The amygdala together with the septal nuclei, part of the substantia innominata, the bed nucleus of the stria terminalis, some thalamic nuclei, the hypothalamus, the anteroventromedial striatum and the ventral pallidum are the main subcortical structures involved in the system.

Like the subcortical structures, also the cortical areas are histologically and odhologically heterogeneous. The cortical structures are differentiated on the basis of their laminar structure.

The neocortex, also defined **isocortex,** is formed by six clearly defined layers, whereas in the **allocortex** (or atypical cortex) the six layers are not present despite its laminar structure. In between these two cortices an intermediate cortex, the **mesocortex,** is present.

Since the structures involved in the limbic system are particularly numerous, it is not possible to give in the present paper morphological, odhological, and functional details of all of them. Thus, for the main anatomo-functional aspects some general reviews are suggested (Gloor, 1997; Lopes da Silva et al., 1990).

In the present report we will focus on some areas of the temporal lobe for two main reasons: first, many of the most important structures involved in the limbic system are located within the temporal lobe; second, these temporal structures are frequently involved in the epileptogenesis.

Among the cerebral lobes, the temporal is the most heterogeneous one, since it comprises the isocortex, allocortex and mesocortex, along with the nucleus of the amygdala.

The primate amygdaloid body is a relatively large conglomerate of gray substance lying in the depth of the antero-medial part of the temporal lobe. Although it would be considered as a single structure, the amygdala is actually an heterogeneous area involved in the modulation of neuroendocrine functions, visceral mechanisms and complex patterns of integrated behaviour (Pitkänen et al., 1997; Swanson & Petrovich, 1998).

The neocortical mantle (isocortex), visible from the outer aspect of the temporal lobe, covers the mesial structures formed by the amygdala and by other types of cortices.

The transition between the iso- and allocortex is not abrupt, being mediated by the mesocortex; the borders between the iso- and mesocortex, named proisocortex, are characterized by the presence of a limited number of granular cells. The perirhinal cortex and the parahippocampal gyrus, encompassing the entorhinal cortex, the parasubiculum, the presubiculum and the parahippocampal proisocortex, constitute the mesocortical belt surrounding the hippocampal formation. Among the mesocortical structures, the most typical component is the entorhinal cortex. This is clearly recognizable in all mammals for the presence of two large superficial and deep layers, separated by a useful landmark, the *lamina dissecans*, corresponding to the fourth isocortical layer.

The **hippocampal formation** is the central core of the system and represents the major allocortical structure of the brain. The term 'hippocampal formation' is usually applied to a group of cytoarchitectonically distinct fields associated with the hippocampus. The different areas contributing to the hippocampal formation vary depending on different authors and may include the subiculum, the hippocampus proper (the Ammon's horn), and the dentate gyrus (see Table 2).

The hippocampus is a very peculiar anatomical structure characterized in all mammals by a convoluted profile clearly visible in a section perpendicular to its major axis. When the section includes the adjacent mesocortical regions the transition from a six- to a three-layered cortex is easily observed (Fig. 1).

According to Lorente de Nó (1934) the hippocampus proper can be divided into three fields named Cornu Ammonis (CA) 1, 2, and 3. The CA3 field borders the hilus of the dentate gyrus (DG) where it terminates in a complex fashion. The DG is a C-shaped structure ventrally separated from the CA1 field and the subiculum by the fused hippocampal fissure.

Table 2. Scheme depicting the cytoarchitectonic organization of the limbic system in relation with the different cortical areas according to Brodman.

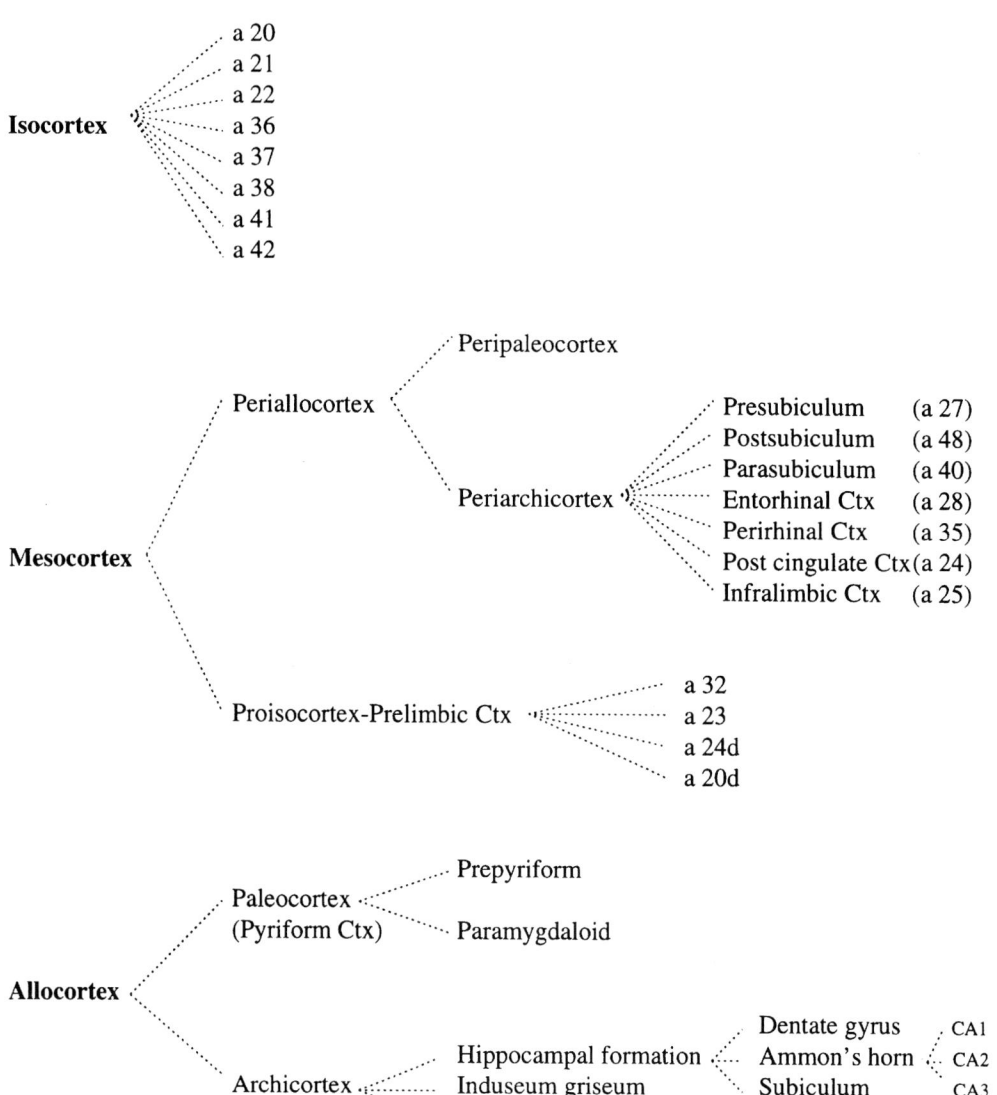

Within the hippocampal formation a progressive thickening of the superficial layer is observed; this layer, characterized by few scattered cells and by the apical dendrites of the pyramidal cells, corresponds to the molecular layer (layer I) of the isocortex. In the allocortex of the hippocampus proper, layer I is classically subdivided into other sublayers, named from the depth *stratum radiatum*, *stratum lucidum*, and *stratum lacunosum-moleculare*. The second layer is composed of packed pyramidal neurons in the CA1, CA2 and CA3 fields, and by a concentration of granular cells in the DG. This layer is just above a polymorphic layer named *stratum oriens* formed by scattered neurons and basal dendrites of the pyramidal cells.

Chapter 2 The limbic system: anatomical structures and embryologic development

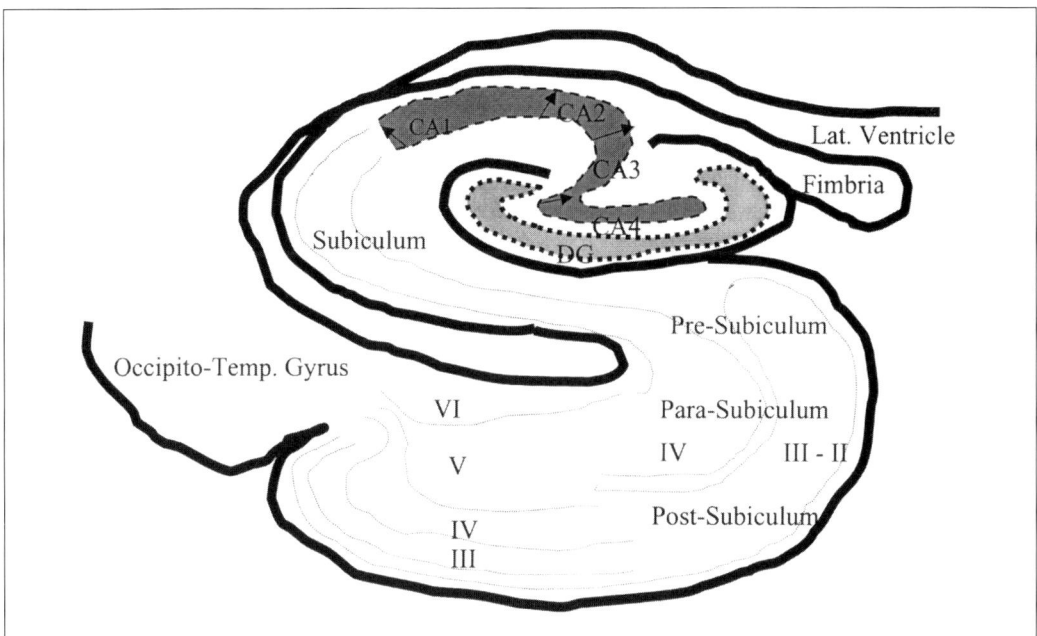

Fig. 1. Schematic drawing of the hippocampal formation.

This simple tri-layered structure of the hippocampus is found in all of its segments, except where it enters the hilus of the dentate gyrus; here the pyramidal neurons are more dispersed and are not aligned parallel to one another. The deepest hippocampal cell layer rests on a thin subependymal sheet of myelinated fibres on the ventricular wall, called *alveus*.

Depending on the number and complexity of the anatomical structures involved in the limbic system, the connectivity between them is clearly very complex. The core of the limbic system is constituted by the reentrant transhippocampal loop; it starts in the entorhinal cortex and passes through the dentate gyrus, sectors CA3, CA2, CA1 of the hippocampus, and the subiculum, before returning to the entorhinal cortex (Fig. 2). This loop indirectly connects the hippocampus to widespread isocortical association areas of the temporal, parietal and frontal lobes.

The entorhinal cortex receives afferents from vast cortical areas, including the olfactory allocortex (the only primary sensory cortex directly connected), the mesocortex, and the multimodal association cortex from temporal, parietal, frontal, insular, and cingulate territories, and from subcortical structures like the amygdala, the claustrum, the medial septal nuclei, the nucleus of the diagonal band of Broca (1878), the nucleus basalis of Meynart, and thalamic, hypothalamic and brainstem nuclei. The input from unimodal sensory association cortices enters the entorhinal cortex only relaying in the perirhinal and parahippocampal areas (Fig. 3). Signals enter in the entorhinal cortex through layers II and III (external principal stratum), from which originates the perforant path (temporo-ammonic path). The perforant path originates from the large stellate neurons of layer II and from the pyramidal neurons of layer III of the entorhinal cortex. Its terminals relay on the granule cells of the DG, this being the first relay of a trisynaptic intrahippocampal circuit. The second step of this circuit is the synapse between the DG's mossy fibres and the pyramidal CA3 neurons. The mossy fibres are well demonstrated by the Timm's stain for zinc. The third relay station is the one between the CA3 Schaffer collaterals and the

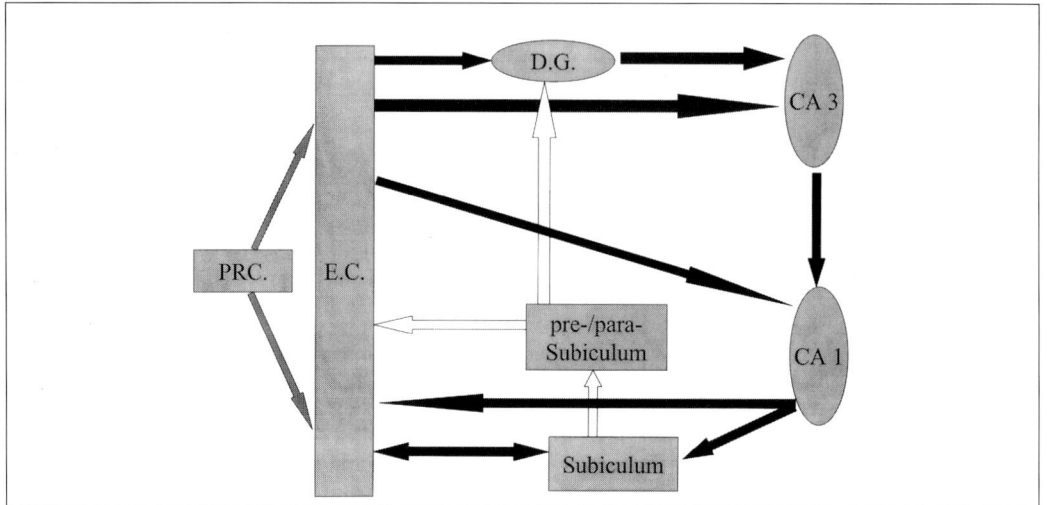

Fig. 2. Diagram depicting the reentrant trans-hippocampal loop. Starting in the entorhinal cortex (EC), it passes through the DG, and the CA sectors of the hippocampus.

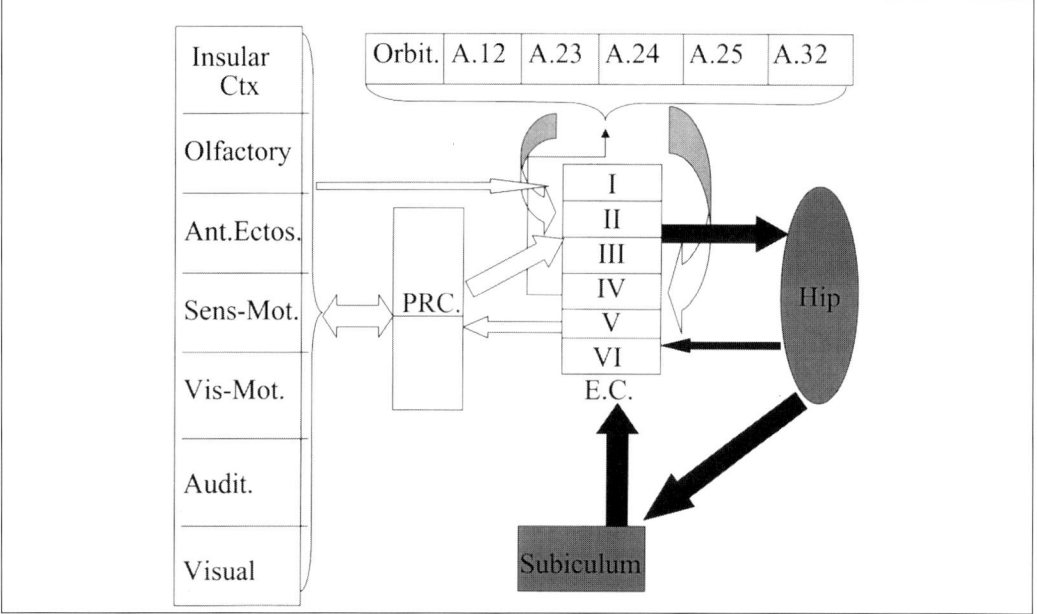

Fig. 3. Diagram showing the widespread connections of the hippocampal formation with the association cortices.

CA2 and CA1 neurons. Some perforant path fibres bypass the circuit, directly connecting with all hippocampal sectors, the hilus of the DG, and the subiculum. Other fibre systems originating from the entorhinal cortex reach the subiculum and the contralateral hippocampal formation respectively through the alvear path and the crossed temporo-ammonic path.

The output of the hippocampus to the cerebral cortex is as restricted as the input; it is mostly directed to the subicular complex, which is the last segment of the hippocampal formation along the transhippocampal loop. Although its main cortical projection is the one directed to the entorhinal cortex (layers IV–VI), the subicular complex has also major projections to other cortical and subcortical areas. In the monkey almost to the entire medial mesocortical ring (the frontal cortex swinging around the genu and the rostrum of the corpus callosum, the gyrus rectus, the orbitofrontal cortex, and the retrosplenial cortex) and various subcortical structures (nucleus accumbens, lateral septum, thalamus, mamillary nuclei, basolateral amygdala, hypothalamus) receive afferents from the subicular complex.

The entorhinal, perirhinal, and parahippocampal cortices constitute the last steps of the hippocampal-cortical output; through them the signals are reciprocally projected to widespread association cortical areas, from which the hippocampal formation receives its input afferents. In rats virtually all areas of the cerebral isocortex receive afferents from the entorhinal cortex. A moderately dense projection has been described to the orbitofrontal, insular (including auditory cortex), visual (areas 17 and 18) cortices; a more sparse projection has been described to the motor and somatosensory cortices. The allo- and mesocortical regions receive heavy projections from the entorhinal cortex as well.

In primates the entorhinal projections are well demonstrated to the temporo-polar regions, to portions of the first temporal gyrus (including Wernicke's area), to the basal temporal cortex (including the perirhinal and parahippocampal regions), and to medial frontal, orbitofrontal, anterior cingulate, insular, and inferior peristriate cortices.

Phylogenetic aspects

The cytoarchitectonic differences observed in different areas of the limbic system reflect the peculiar odhologic and functional properties of each structure. These properties undergo important modifications during phylogenesis.

Although the limbic system is observed in all mammals, the evolution of the brain regions involved in the limbic circuitry of different animal species explains the various odhological and functional properties of the system (Fig. 4). In rodents, for example, a large and well-developed olfactory bulb represents the major input to the limbic system. During phylogeny the olfactory system progressively shrinks, becoming in primates very small; the olfactory projection to the core of the limbic system (i.e. the hippocampal formation) loses progressively its predominance, being partly substituted by a newly developed isocortical associative input. During the phylogenesis of mammals, the neocortex (particularly the associative cortices) progressively gains importance and dimension (Fig. 4). Along with the evolutionary process, the limbic system progressively shifts from a structure primarily associated to the olfactory system to a system heavily interconnected to the associative cortices.

Ontogenesis

During the early embryonic development all neurons are generated at sites different from their final positions in the adult brain.

At first the neural tube is constituted by the proliferative ventricular zone (VZ), followed shortly after by the so-called marginal zone and, in the second month of embryonic development, by the intermediate zone. At the third month of embryonic development the transient cortical plate is observed beneath the marginal zone. At the fourth month from the pial surface inward, the marginal zone, the cortical plate and subplate, the intermediate zone, the subventricular zone,

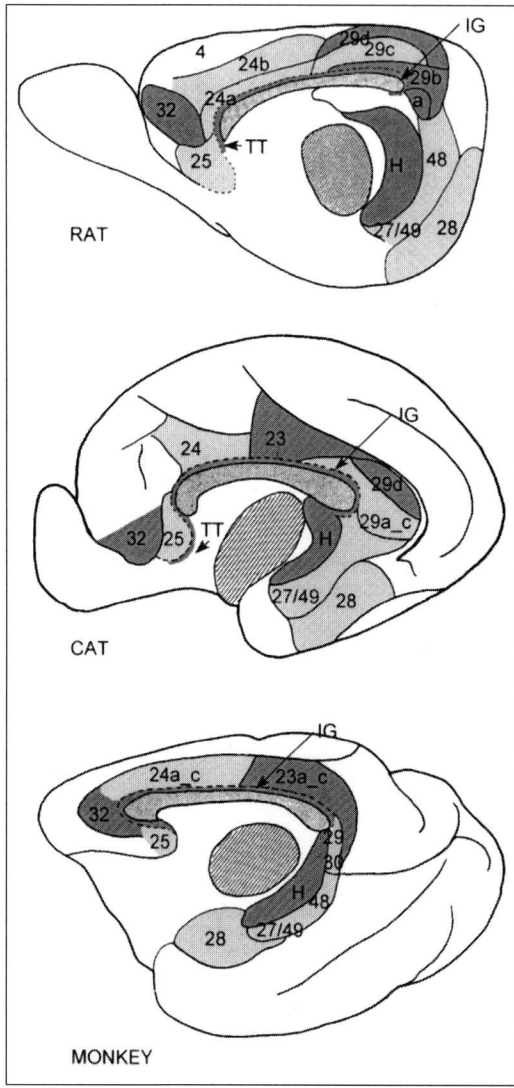

Fig. 4. Schematic drawing showing the evolution of the brain regions involved in the limbic system, in different animal species.

and the ventricular zone are well recognizable. The cortical plate represents the anlage of the cortical laminae with the exception of layer I, which originates from the marginal zone.

Neuronal migration comprises the time interval between the departure of the postmitotic neuroblast from the proliferative zone and the arrival to the final destination. In the rhesus monkey isocortex, the migration time is different from that of the hippocampal formation allocortex: the isocortex and the entorhinal cortex precursor neurons migrate quickly, reaching, with a speed of migration of about 100 mm/day, the developing cortical plate within three days after their final mitosis; the hippocampal precursors speed of migration is about 15 mm/day. Different rates of migration may be due to local factors in the microenvironment of the intermediate zone.

Neurons of the hippocampal formation are generated in all animal species during a characteristic prenatal period; in primates the neurogenesis starts in a restricted period of time in all subdivisions of the hippocampal formation. Thus, the duration of migration is different for each portion of the limbic system, with the migrating cells reaching their final destination with different delays (Fig. 5). At least two gradients of cell generation are present: the rhino-dentate gradient (the closest cells to the rhinal sulcus are generated earlier than those more distant from the sulcus) and the antero-posterior gradient (neurons of the anterior entorhinal cortex are generated earlier than those of the posterior portion). The duration of the proliferative period varies in different parts of the hippocampal formation (Fig. 5).

In the subiculum the generating period is shorter than in other areas, presumably reflecting the philogenetic processes. In fact subicular and presubicular neurons constitute the most important afferent input to the hypothalamus, which is considered one of the oldest pathways present in all vertebrates. By contrast, granular cells of the dentate gyrus have a very long proliferative period spanning, in rodents, up to the third postnatal week. In monkeys the 80 per cent of neurons of the dentate gyrus are generated almost until the end of the gestation. Due to these delays, it is clear that the entorhinal fibres reach the dentate gyrus before granule cells are completely generated; they therefore must wait the final positioning of their targeted neurons.

Like in the isocortex some transient structures are observed also in the hippocampal formation during the ontogenesis. Of particular interest are the VZ and the subventricular zone (SV). This latter appears later than the VZ and in general is thicker in the most recent phylogenetic areas. This is involved in the proliferative process of both neuronal and glial lineage soon after the functional end of the VZ. In some areas of the hippocampal formation, however, like in the hippocampal proper and subiculum, the proliferative SV is absent. As a consequence, in these regions, most of the gliogenesis occurs in the VZ or *in situ*, after the migration of glial precursors.

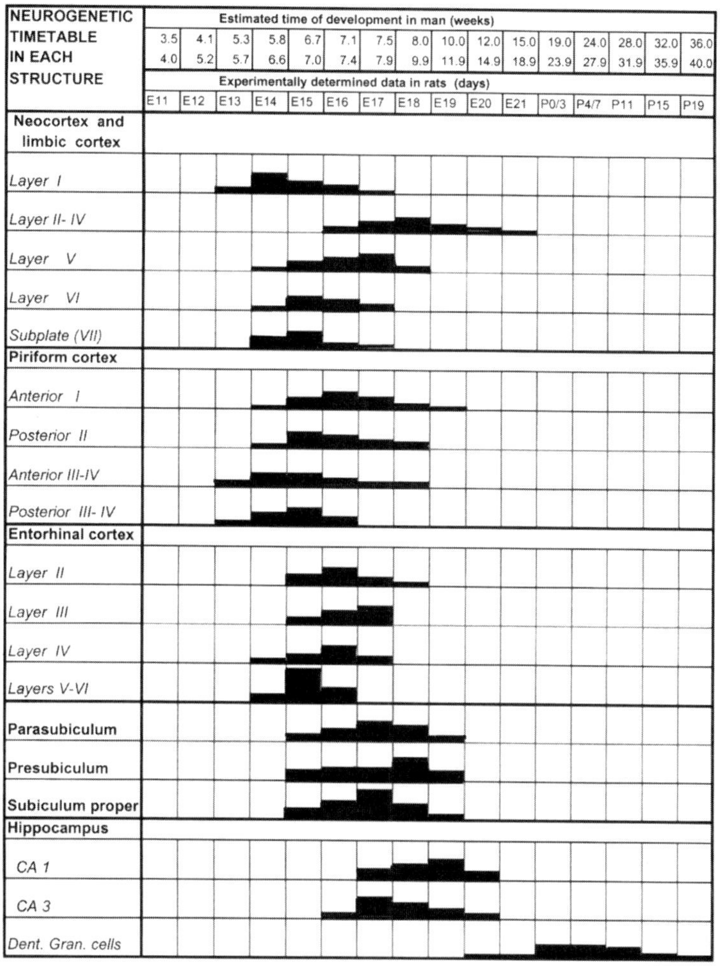

Fig. 5. Diagram showing the timetable of the neurogenesis for the different structures involved in the limbic system (modified from Bayer et al. (1993).

In DG neurons arrive from two distinct areas: the VZ and the hilar region. This structure does not follow the general inside-out rule of other cortical regions, since the first granular cells are present below the molecular layer and the youngest neurons are progressively added in the deep layers thus forming an outside-in gradient.

In summary three different processes are present:

1. inside-out: in neocortex, parahippocampal region, subiculum, CA1, CA2, CA3;
2. outside-in: granular layer of DG;
3. supragranular-infragranular: in DG.

It should be noticed that also in the entorhinal cortex the inside-out gradient is modified and called 'sandwich' since the neurons of layers II and IV are generated earlier than those of layer III.

Considering all these variants, the complex morphology of the structure, and that most of the granular cells of DG are generated also in the hilar region, it is clear that the neuroblasts must travel through different, long, and tortuous pathways before reaching their final position. The neuroblasts directed to CA3 and DG follow a longer and more complex pathway than those directed to CA1 and CA2. The degree of differentiation of the hippocampal neuroblasts during the migratory processes is therefore higher than that of the neocortical cells.

If we consider that hippocampal pyramidal cells are homologous to the neocortical pyramidal neurons of layers V and VI, and that the subventricular zone is absent in the hippocampal region, we can deduce the following:

- The deep layer originates from VZ;

- The intermediate layer originates from VZ and SV;

- The superficial layer originates from SV.

In the projecting system the projection from the entorhinal cortex to the DG, the perforant path, deserves some mention. This is a massive pathway in the adult but it is also evident during the embryonic life after the maturation of the entorhinal neurons. During development there is another massive projection toward CA1; this projection shrinks progressively during maturation and almost disappears in the adult. This bundle is considered to subserve the maturative processes of the Ammon horn and thus its progressive reduction parallels the maturation of these areas.

The rate of migration influences the degree of differentiation of the neurons at the time of their arrival at the final site and, as a consequence, the formation of the neural pathways.

Different rates of migration, the differentiation of neurons, and the formation of well defined neural pathways may have pathophysiological implications in the limbic system.

Acknowledgements: The authors wish to thank Ms. Marina Denegri for editorial support. This work is supported by the Mariani Foundation for Pediatric Neurology.

References

Bayer, S.A., Altman, J., Russo R.J. & Zhang X. (1993): Timetables of neurogenesis in the human brain based on experimentally determined patterns in the rat. *Neurotoxicology* **14**, 83–144.

Broca, P. (1878): Anatomie comparée des circonvolutions cérébrales. Le grand lobe limbique et la scissure dans la série des mammiféres. *Rev. Anthropol. Paris* **2**, 285–498.

Gloor, P. (1997): *The temporal lobe and limbic system*. New York, Oxford: Oxford University Press.

Lopes da Silva, F.H., Witter, M.P., Boeijinga, P.H. & Lohman, A.H.M. (1990): Anatomic organization and physiology of the limbic cortex. *Physiol. Rev.* **70**, 453–511.

Lorente de Nó, R. (1934): Studies on the structure of the cerebral cortex. II. Continuation of the study of the ammonic system. *J. Psychol. Neurol.* **46**, 114–177.

Papez, J.W. (1937): A proposed mechanism of emotion. *Arch. Neurol. Psychiat.* **38**, 725–743.

Pitkänen, A., Savander, V. & LeDoux, J.E. (1997): Organization of intra-amygdaloid circuitries in the rat: an emerging framework for understanding functions of the amygdala. *Trends Neurosci.* **20**, 517–523.

Swanson, L.W. & Petrovich, G.D. (1998): What is the amygdala? *Trends Neurosci.* **21**, 323–331.

Chapter 3

Functional organization of the limbic system

Giuliano Avanzini

Servizio di Neurofisiopatologia, Istituto Nazionale Neurologico Carlo Besta, Via Celoria 11, 20133 Milan, Italy

Summary

The series of structures located at the edge of the cerebral mantle and surrounding the hilus of the hemisphere was first called the limbic lobe (*grand lobe limbique*) by Broca (1878), but the term *limbus* (fringe or border) had already been used by Willis in his anatomical treatise (Willis, 1664). Subsequently, Papez (1937) and then MacLean (1952) extended the definition to include all of the structures involved in integrating the emotions and autonomic functions: the subcallosal, cingulate and parahippocampal circumvolutions, the hippocampus and dentate gyrus, the hypothalamus, the anterior thalamic nuclei, the septal nuclei, the preoptic area, the amygdala and the nucleus accumbens. The margins and the concept itself of the limbic system have been and still are the subject of discussion (Blessing, 1997a; 1997b; Spyer, 1997; Herbert, 1997), with some authors restricting the definition to the cingulate and deep temporal structures, and others who extend it to the point that it becomes practically meaningless.

We shall here limit ourselves to reviewing the experimental data and clinical observations relating to our understanding of the function of the limbic structures involved in some types of epileptic seizures.

Anatomo-functional organization

Hippocampus and parahippocampal cortex

The hippocampus is the main part of the archicortical component of the oligostratified cortex or archicortex. A cross-section (Fig.1) shows the *fascia dentata* and the four divisions of Ammon's horn (CA) known as CA4 (or the hippocampal hilus), CA3, CA2 and CA1, which passes directly into the subiculum (itself a part of the archicortex), presubiculum, parasubiculum, the entorhinal cortex and the adjacent part of the perirhinal cortex corresponding to the fifth temporal circumvolution. The entorhinal cortex and subiculum are considered fundamental stations of the pathways entering and leaving the hippocampus. As shown in the figure taken from Witter & Groenewegen (1990), the entorhinal cortex, which receives olfactory input from the pyriform cortex, projects to the *fascia dentata* through the perforant fibres making up the first part of the trisynaptic pathway terminating in the cells of area 1 of Ammon's horn (CA1). The exit is essentially represented by the axons of the CA1

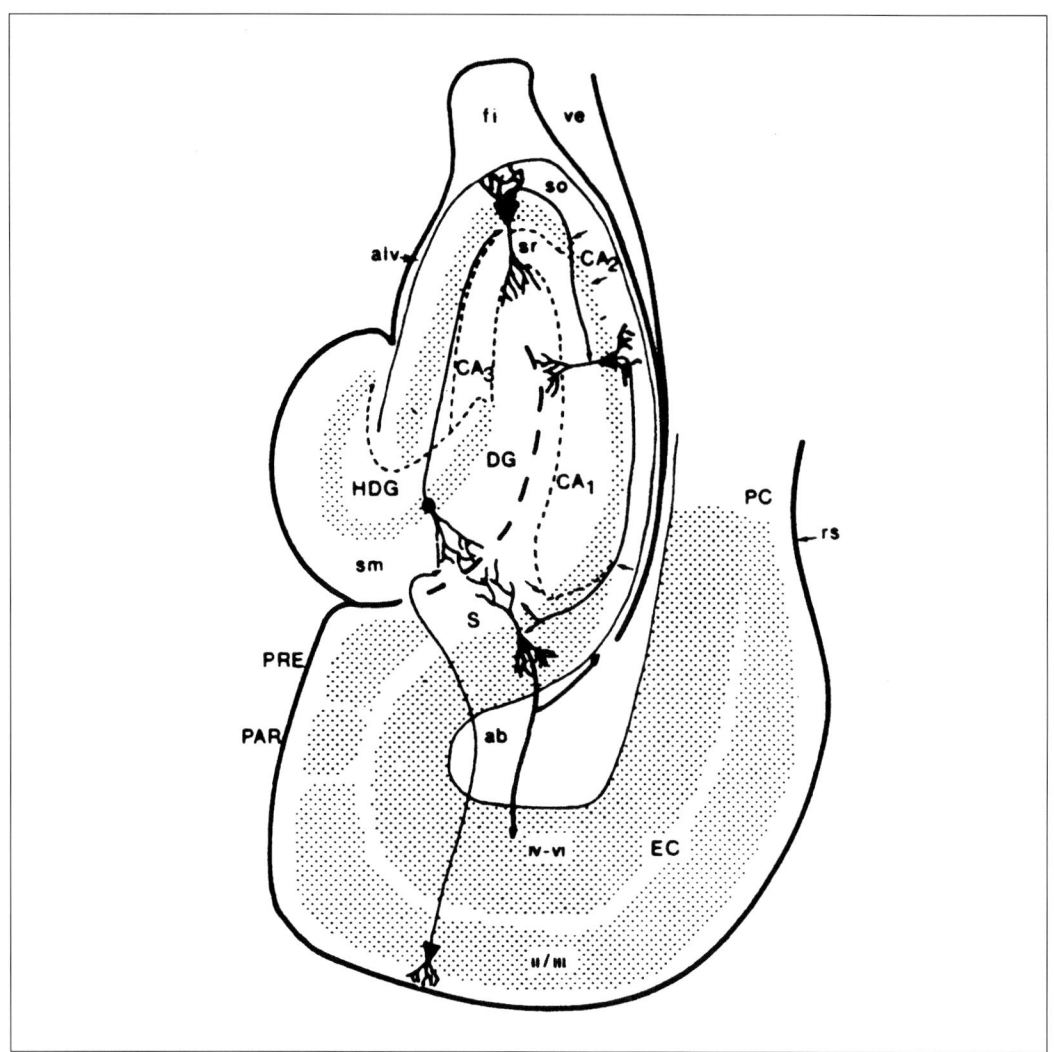

*Fig. 1. Schematic representation of the multisynaptic hippocampo-parahippocampal circuit.
rs: rhinal sulcus; PC: perirhinal cortex; EC: entorhinal cortex (strata II / III; IV–VI); PAR: parasubiculum; PRE: presubiculum; ab: angular bundle; sm: stratum moleculare; CA1, CA2, CA3: Ammon's horn areas 1, 2, 3; HDG: hilus of the dentate gyrus (corresponding to CA4, as better specified in the text); DG: dentate gyrus (or fascia dentata); fi: fimbria; alv: alveus; so: stratum oriens; sr: stratum radiatum; ve: lateral ventricle. For further information concerning the organization of the circuit, see text (from Witter & Groenewegen, 1990). [In: Progress in Brain Research **83**, 47–58, with permission from Elsevier Science.]*

cells that terminate in the subiculum (and the pre- and parasubiculum). The physiology of this multisynaptic system has been the subject of a striking number of research studies, and it is here necessary to stress two important points: (1) the entorhinal cortex does not only receive olfactory information, but is the place where all sensory modalities converge; (2) the entorhinal cortex and subicular complex also have reciprocal connections that are independent of those mediated by the hippocampal structures.

In addition to the Na$^+$ and K$^+$ conductances responsible for action potentials, both the granule cells making up the principal population of the *fascia dentata* and the pyramidal cells of Ammon's horn also possess a broad repertoire of Ca^{2+} and K$^+$ conductances (including Ca^{2+}-dependent K$^+$ conductances) that contribute towards modulating their firing properties. In particular, the Ca^{2+} conductance is responsible for generating the depolarizing after potential (DAP) that follows the action potential, whereas the Ca^{2+}-dependent K$^+$ conductances are essentially responsible for the pronounced after hyperpolarizing potential (AHP) that follows individual or repetitive (burst) action potentials. The CA3 pyramidal cells have a marked DAP, which keeps the membrane depolarized and determines burst discharges with a much greater degree of probability than that observed in CA1. On the contrary, the granule cells have much shorter DAPs and, under physiological conditions, rarely produce burst discharges. They are, therefore, particularly suited to the production of graduated activities that are linearly correlated with the intensity of the stimulus, whereas the CA3 cells can act as amplifiers capable of having a secondary effect on the CA1 cells through Schaeffer's collateral projection that makes up the exit stage of the circuit. Both the *fascia dentata* and Ammon's horn contain GABAergic interneurons that are activated directly by the fibres in arrival (feed forward inhibition) as well as by the axonal collaterals of the principal cells (feedback inhibition).

The set of physiological properties of the cells belonging to the various stages of the hippocampal circuit form the basis of the integrative processes that the different types of input mediated by the entorhinal cortex undergo inside the hippocampus. Some information concerning the significance of integrative hippocampal activities has come from studies of the correlations between cell activities and behaviour. Above all, these have demonstrated a fundamental relationship between the discharging properties of hippocampal cells and arousal, the most important finding being the modifications created during the acquisition of conditioned responses (Thompson, 1988). These modifications are thought to be based on the synaptic plasticity discovered by Bliss & Lømo (1973) in the connections between rabbit entorhinal cortex and the dentate gyrus (perforant fibres). They observed that high-frequency stimuli of the entorhinal cortex increased the effectiveness of synaptic transmission to granule cells, which continued for hours or days and led to what they called 'long-term potentiation' (LTP). Subsequent observations documented the occurrence of LTP (but also long-term depression: LTD) in other intra- and extra-hippocampal districts, thus demonstrating that synaptic plasticity is particularly pronounced in the limbic system and plays a fundamental role in the mechanisms of integration occurring in the hippocampus (Lopes da Silva *et al.*, 1990). Thanks to these properties, the limbic (and particularly hippocampal) circuits are capable of recording and storing traces of information originating from the various sensory systems (see above) by constructing a cognitive map that is continuously updated on the basis of experience (O'Keefe & Nadel, 1978). These observations are clearly of interest in relation to the memory functions attributed to the hippocampus (Scoville & Milner, 1957; Jones-Gotman, 1991).

Over the last few years, a large number of research studies have been dedicated to the possible involvement of the synaptic plasticity of hippocampal circuits in the pathophysiology of temporal lobe epilepsies. These started with the classical experiment of amygdaloid kindling (Goddard, 1967), which demonstrated the gradual development of epilepsy with repeated spontaneous seizures in animals subjected to daily amygdala stimulation for many days. The phenomenon of kindling was subsequently observed in other limbic districts and associated with a synaptic rearrangement that was particularly evident in the perforant pathway connecting the entorhinal cortex with the *fascia dentata* (see above).Taking advantage of the elective positivity of granule cells and their axons for zinc-staining methods, it has been possible to document the new formation (or *sprouting*) of granule axon collaterals (Cavazos et al., 1991), and the presence of sprouting has been confirmed in other experimental models (Tauck & Nadler, 1985), the pilocarpine model (Mello et al., 1993) and in human tissue taken from patients undergoing temporal lobectomy because of intractable epilepsy (in whom it is accompanied by neuronal degeneration mainly involving Ammon's horn: see below).

The interpretation of the results of a selective entorhinal cortex lesion is complicated by the need to take into account its indirect consequences on the function of the deafferented hippocampus. Animals bearing selective lesions of the parahippocampal cortex generally fail at tasks involving memories acquired before the lesion, as well as in the acquisition of new tasks. In primates, Moss et al. (1981), and Murray & Mishkin (1986), observed defects in the execution of tasks learned before parahippocampal lesions when these involved the ability to discriminate different objects visually.

The selective involvement of the parahippocampal cortex probably contributes significantly to the integrative defects observed in Alzheimer's disease (Hyman et al., 1984). In this sense, it is interesting to note Serby's observation (Serby, 1986) that Alzheimer patients show a much more marked inability to recognise olfactory stimuli than patients with other forms of dementia.

The close interaction between the parahippocampal cortex and the hippocampus generally makes it difficult to evaluate the specific responsibility of the former in determining the symptoms due to lesions or the discharges involving it.

Amygdala

The amygdaloid complex includes various nuclei whose classification has been recently reviewed by Pitkänen et al. (1997). The classical distinction considered an internal nuclear group whose activation favours aggressive behaviour, sexual impulses and the feeding instinct, and an external group that exercises a moderating effect on the same functions (N'Guyen et al., 1906). These effects were essentially attributed to the involvement of the ventral hypothalamus upon which the two components exert an antagonistic action mediated by amygdala fibres respectively running in the ventral pathway and the terminal stria (Gloor, 1976). The reactions evoked by a stimulation of the excitatory component, or a lesion of the inhibitory component, include dilated pupils, piloerection, an increased heart rate and aggressiveness, and are reminiscent of the picture of the 'sham rage' known to be abolished by hypothalamus ablation observed by Bard (1928) in hypothalamic animals. In freely moving animals, a low intensity of amygdala stimulation leads to an arrest of ongoing movements that is often associated with the orientation reaction (Kaada, 1951, 1972; Gastaut et al., 1952). Increasing the intensity of the stimulation transforms the alert into the alarm and defence reaction described above (Gastaut et al., 1952). Wurtz & Olds ((1963) observed that rats chronically implanted with amygdala-stimulating electrodes tend to avoid self-stimulation of the basolateral portion and to seek avidly that of the dorso-medial region, thus suggesting that the first activates avoidance behaviour and the second a system of gratification probably connected with feeding and sexual functions. The value of this observation is limited by the possible interference of aspecific effects associated with the spread of the stimulus and the influence of environmental factors associated with laboratory syndrome. In a series of experiments involving captured cercopiths subsequently returned to their natural environment after bilateral amygdala ablation, Kling (1972) did not observe the dramatic picture of 'psychic blindness' reported by Klüver & Bucy (1937, 1938, 1939), but did note that the animals could not reintegrate themselves in their social context because of their inability to interpret the motivational significance of social stimuli. These behavioural alterations were so great that the amygdalectomized monkeys failed to survive in their natural habitat.

The work of Kling (1972) underlines the need to consider the results of the old lesion and stimulation experiments done on caged laboratory animals with caution. The modern approach to amygdala research is based on a complete redefinition of the amygdaloid nuclei and their connections that distinguishes two nuclear groups: (1) superficial (only partially corresponding to the previous definition of external nuclei); and (2) deep (partially corresponding to the internal nuclear group) to which has been added (3) a third grouping that includes topographically non-homogeneous nuclei (Pitkänen et al., 1997). Sensory information reaches the amygdala through the lateral nucleus and is then distributed in parallel to the various other nuclei by means of a system of highly organized intra-amygdaloid circuits. The most recent data (see review in Pitkänen et al., 1997) confirm the role of the amygdaloid nuclei in integrative activities connected with associations of emotional and neutral stimuli, with the control of homeostasis and the participation of current and memorized experiences. The hierarchical organization of the various amygdaloid nuclei and their specific functional role seem to be clear from the studies that are currently being developed on the basis of this new definition.

Bearing in mind the interpretative limitations mentioned above, it seems that there is some correlation between the results of experimental studies and the unmotivated fear described in man during the course of discharges involving the amygdala, or as a result of electrical stimulation of the amygdaloid or peri-amygdaloid region (Penfield & Jasper, 1954; Gloor, 1972). However, in general, emotional expressions of anger and aggressiveness are rarely observed in man during amygdala discharges, the most frequent expression of which are oral/feeding automatisms (chewing movements) sometimes accompanied by salivation (Munari et al., 1979).

Cingulate gyrus

The cingulate region appears to be involved in conditioned responses presumably connected with the acquisition of avoidance reactions. In rabbits trained to avoid a painful stimulus associated with a conditioned acoustic stimulus, Gabriel et al. (1980) observed a modification in the activity of the cells of the anterior cingulate cortex that coincided with the acquisition of the conditioned response. In another study of rabbits, Buchanan & Powell (1982) observed that the conditioned response to the auditory stimulus was attenuated after cingulectomy, thus confirming the role of the anterior cingulate cortex in the associative processes underlying the conditioning. In these experiments, the unconditioned stimulus was always a painful shock in accordance with the idea that the anterior cingulate cortex plays a specific role in the acquisition of avoidance responses. This function is probably based on the efferent projections from the intralaminar thalamic nuclei and midline (a relay of the paleospinothalamic pathway) and the projections afferent to the periaqueductal grey matter, an essential structure of the descendent pain inhibition system.

In line with this hypothesis are the characteristics of the vegetative (changes in arterial blood pressure, heart rate, respiratory rate and pupil diameter; piloerection) and somatomotor responses (changes in muscle tone and vocalizations) evoked by the stimulation of the anterior cingulate cortex in primates and carnivores (Kaada, 1951). The stimulation of the anterior cingulate cortex in man (Brodmann's area 24 (Brodmann, 1909)) evokes emotional, vegetative and motor responses that are similar to, although less severe than those observed during discharges originating from this region: terror, screams, aggressive verbal expressions, complex gestural automatisms, vegetative disturbances, and visual hallucinations associated with only partial alterations in consciousness (Talairach *et al.*, 1973; Bancaud & Talairach, 1992; Veilleux *et al.*, 1992). The basis underlying the motor expression of the responses are the connections between this region and the caudate nucleus, the ventral pontine nuclei, the ventral part of the periaqueductal grey matter, and the deep strata of the superior colliculus (Villani *et al.*, 2001).

The posterior or retrosplenial cingulate region seems to be particularly involved in the processes of spatial discrimination associated with visual information.

Specific modifications in the responses of individual cingulate cells have been observed by Niki & Watanabe (1976) during the establishment of conditioned reflexes to visual stimulation. Bilateral cingulate infarction in man leads to asomatognosia and selective deficiency in visual attention (Barris & Schuman, 1953; La Plane *et al.*, 1981).

Neurotransmitter systems and epileptogenesis

The excitatory aminoacids (EAAs), glutammate and aspartate, are the main neurotransmitters involved in the limbic circuits, together with gamma-aminobutyric acid (GABA) as far as the local inhibitory circuits are concerned. Observations made in man during temporal lobe seizures have demonstrated a considerable increase in glutamate and aspartate, but also in GABA and taurin (which is involved in gylycinergic transmission) (Wilson *et al.*, 1996).

Another neurotransmitter system that may be involved in limbic epileptogenesis is the cholinergic system. The cholinergic pathways originate from the basal nucleus of Meinert and the interpeduncular nucleus, from where they spread to the majority of the cortex but particularly to the septal structures, which in their turn project into the hippocampus. Recordings made by Bernardo & Prince (1982) have shown that the application of acetylcholine causes persistent membrane depolarization, with very frequent discharges and epileptic-type potentials. This effect seems to be particularly important for the passage from the inter-seizure to the seizure phase, rather than for the generation of inter-seizure potentials.

From the physiological point of view, the cholinergic system is involved in memory and learning processes: the cholinergic fibres originating from the septum have to do with learning, whereas those originating in the nucleus of Meinert seem to be mainly involved in memory (Nicoll, 1985).

The noradrenergic fibres originating from the locus ceruleus spread widely to the structures of the limbic lobe, whereas the dopaminergic fibres originating in the brain stem structures (particularly the locus niger) mainly terminate in the hippocampus with a topography that is sufficiently specific to suggest that this projection plays a role in the physiology and physiopatholoby of the limbic structures (Baulac *et al.*, 1986).

Finally, the serotoninergic pathways widely innervate the amygdala and may play a specific role in amygdaloid function and its involvement in epileptogenic processes.

In general, any condition favouring excitatory over inhibitory synaptic influences can give rise to a state of hyperexcitability of epileptogenic significance.

A classical experiment is to perfuse an *in vitro* incubated slice of hippocampus with GABA-antagonists (bicucullin or penicillin). During the perfusion, a micro-electrode inserted into a pyramidal cell of Ammon's horn makes it possible to follow a progressive reduction in post-synaptic inhibitory potentials that is accompanied by a gradual transformation of the simple post-synaptic responses into the long-lasting complex excitatory potentials characteristic of epileptic activities (Schwarzkroin & Prince, 1980). It was therefore originally hypothesized that

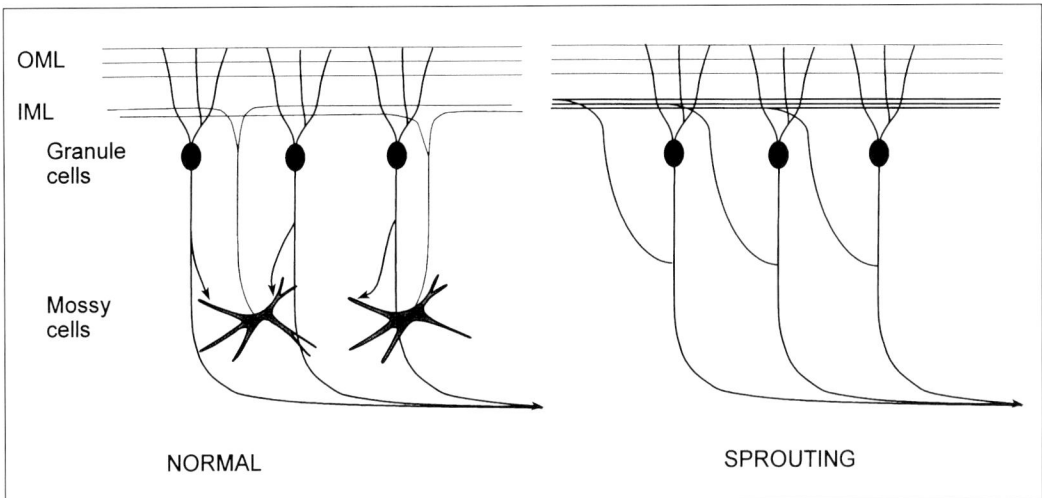

Fig. 2. Schematic representation of the connections of granule cells under normal conditions (left) and in an experimental model of epilepsy that leads to the anomalous regeneration of axonal collaterals (sprouting). OML: outer molecular layer occupied by afferent fibres (in much of the entorhinal cortex); IML: inner molecular layer occupied (left) by mossy cell axons. Right: the degeneration of the mossy cells frees the inner molecular layer that is re-occupied by newly-formed collaterals of the granule axons. For further information, see text.

the selective degeneration of GABAergic neurons may be the cause of temporal epilepsy in man, but this hypothesis has not been confirmed by the analysis of autoptic and bioptic material, which has rather documented the existence of complex circuit alterations of possible pathogenetic significance (Liu et al., 1995).

The interpretation of these alterations, which is based on the comparison of experimental models and tissues removed during the course of epileptic surgery, can be summarized as follows. By means of an excitotoxic mechanism, prolonged epileptic seizures (such as febrile convulsions in children or those experimentally induced in animals by kainic acid or biculculine) cause the degeneration of Ammon's horn neurons, particularly in area 4 (CA4) or the hilus. The mossy cells of the hilus, which project to the granule cells of the *fascia dentata*, are particularly susceptible to excitotoxic agents (Fig. 2). The result is a depopulation of the dendrite endings of granule cells that is compensated for by the regeneration of the cells' axonal collaterals, which reoccupy the depopulated zone and create a glutamatergic and aspartatergic-mediated excitatory circuit (Tauck & Nadler, 1985; Babb et al., 1988; Sutula et al., 1988). This re-excitation amplifies the excitatory events in the granule cells by generating paroxystic potentials that are transmitted to CA3 by means of the dentate-hippocampal pathway, and then to CA1 and the entorhinal cortex. The hyperexcitability of the granule cells is further potentiated by the deafferentation of the GABAergic inhibitory interneurons of the *fascia dentata* which, although not showing any signs of degeneration, become hypoactive because they are deprived of the input from the mossy cells (Sloviter, 1994).

This interpretation explains how degenerative phenomena (electively involving the CA4 region) can be translated into a synaptic rearrangement that determines the hyperactivity of EEA-mediated transmission and the hypoactivity of GABAergic circuits. The fact that this chain of events can be set in motion by prolonged seizures justifies the processual characteristics of temporal lobe epilepsies, which often evolve towards a condition of resistance to pharmacological therapy. Early treatment with drugs that potentiate GABAergic transmission, inhibit glutamatergic transmission or reduce the intrinsic excitable properties of nerve cells, can partially prevent the worsening evolution of temporal lobe epilepsies. Less is known about pharmacological manipulations of serotoninergic, catecholaminergic or cholinergic transmission, which could also be involved in the epileptogenesis of limbic structures. There is also preliminary evidence that the phenomena of pathological epileptogenic plasticity studied in the hippocampal and para-hippocampal circuits may also occur in other districts of the limbic system.

Conclusions

Without entering into the discussion concerning the concept of the limbic system, there is no doubt that there are close anatomical and functional interrelationships between the cingulate cortex, the amygdaloid nuclei, the hippocampus and the parahippocampal cortex.

The common basis underlying the integrative processes they carry out is the availability of multimodal (particularly visual, olfactory and nociceptive) information that is significant at a behavioural level. The functional property characterizing all of the considered structures is their synaptic plasticity, which allows continuous updating of associative responses within the context of the spatio-temporal coordinates which form the physiological basis for conditioning processes. The responses of the neurons of the limbic structures express selected previous experiences in relation to their motivational value. On the basis of memorized information, they control autonomic functions and behavioural models aimed at maintaining homeostasis, individual survival (avoidance, flight, defence, attack and feeding behaviour) and survival of the species (sexual behaviour).

It is therefore logical to expect that seizure-related discharges generated in the limbic structures can manifest themselves as vegetative, olfactory and somatomotor symptoms representing more or less stereotyped fragments of complex behavioural models. However, it is still very difficult to establish a precise correlation between the symptomatology of epileptic seizures and the site of the generating discharges inside the limbic system.

It is worth giving particular consideration to the relationship between the limbic structures and memory, the existence of which is supported by many of the physiological and pathophysiological observations described above. Phenomena such as LTP and LTD certainly indicate the aptitude of hippocampal circuits to modify themselves in a plastic manner to preserve permanent traces of appropriate stimuli. The entorhinal cortex-*fascia dentata*-CA3-CA1-subiculum-entorhinal circuit is organized in such a way as to compare a stimulus that is expected (on the basis of previous experience) with the stimulus that actually arrives.

Furthermore, the onset of memory disturbances following hippocampal lesions, and the dysmnesic symptoms (*déja veçu, jamais veçu*) observable during the course of temporal lobe seizures, support the role of the hippocampus in memory processes.

Of course, this does not mean that a complex function such as memory can be reduced to the elementary physiology of a circuit, but information coming from research studies of synaptic plasticity opens up the possibility of significant correlations between neuropsychology and neurophysiology, the value of which needs to be further explored.

References

Babb, T.L., Kupfer, W.R. & Pretorius, J.K. (1988): Synaptic reorganization of mossy fibers into inner molecular layer in human epileptic *fascia dentata*. *Neurosci. Abstr.* **14,** 881.

Bancaud, J. & Talairach, J. (1992): Clinical semiology of frontal lobe seizures. In: *Frontal lobe seizures and epilepsies. Advances in Neurology*, vol. 57, eds. P. Chauvel, A.V. Delgado Escueta, E. Halgren & J. Bancaud, pp. 3–58. New York: Raven Press.

Bard, P. (1928): A diencephalic mechanism for the expression of rage with special reference to the sympathetic nervous system. *Am. J. Physiol.* **84,** 490–515.

Barris, R.W. & Schuman, H.R. (1953): Bilateral anterior cingulate gyrus lesions. Syndrome of the anterior cingulate gyri. *Neurology* **3,** 44–52.

Baulac, M., Verney, C. & Berger, B. (1986): Innervation dopaminergique des régions para-hippocampiques et hippocampique du rat. *Rev. Neurol.* **142,** 895–905.

Bernardo, L.S. & Prince, D.A. (1982): Ionic mechanisms of cholinergic excitation in mammalian hippocampal pyramidal cells. *Brain Res.* **249,** 333–334.

Blessing, W.W. (1997a) Inadequate frameworks for understandig bodily homeostasis. *Trends Neurosci.* **20,** 235–239.

Blessing, W.W. (1997b): Reply. *Trends Neurosci.* **20,** 509.

Bliss, T.V.P. & Lømo, T. (1973): Long lasting potentiation of synaptic transmission in the dentate area of the unanesthetized rabbit following stimulation of the perforant path. *J. Physiol. Lond.* **232,** 331–356.

Broca, P. (1878): Anatomie comparée des circonvolutions cérébrales. Le grand lobe limbique et la scissure dans la série des mammifères. *Rev. Anthropol. Paris* **2,** 285–498.

Brodmann, K. (1909): *Vergleichende Lokalisationslehre der Grosshirnrinde in ihren Prinzipien dargestellt auf Grund des Zellenbaues*, no. 82. Leipzig, Germany: Barth.

Buchanan, S.L. & Powell, D.A. (1982): Cingulate cortex: its role in Pavlovian conditioning. *J. Comp. Physiol. Psychol.* **96,** 755–774.

Cavazos, J.E., Golarai, G. & Sutula, T.P. (1991): Mossy fiber synaptic reorganization induced by kindling: time course of development, progression and permanence. *J. Neurosci.* **11,** 2795–2803.

Gabriel, M., Foster, K., Orona, E., Stalwick, S.E. & Stanton, M. (1980): Neuronal activity of cingulate cortex, anteroventral thalamus, and hippocampal formation in discriminative conditioning: encoding and extraction of the significance of conditioned stimuli. In: *Progress in psychobiology and physiological psychology*, vol. 9, eds. J.M. Sprague & A.N. Epstein, pp. 125–231. New York: Academic Press.

Gastaut, H., Vigoroux, R. & Naquet, R. (1952): Comportement posturaux et cinétiques provoqués par stimulation sous-corticale chez le chat non-anesthésié. Leur relation avec 'réflexe d'orientation'. *J. Psych. Norm. Pathol.* **45,** 257–271.

Gloor, P. (1972): Temporal lobe epilepsy: its possible contribution to the understanding of the functional significance of the amygdala and of its interaction with neocortical-temporal mechanisms. In: *The neurobiology of the amygdala*, ed. B.E. Eleftheriou, pp. 423–457. New York: Plenum Press.

Gloor, P. (1976): Physiology of the limbic system. In: *Advances in neurology: complex partial seizures and their treatment*, vol. II, eds. J.K. Penry & D.D. Daly, pp. 27–55. Amsterdam: Excerpta Medica.

Goddard, G.V. (1967): Development of epileptic seizures through brain stimulation at low intensity. *Nature* **214,** 1020–1023.

Herbert, J. (1997): Do we need a limbic system? *Trends Neurosci.* **20,** 508–509.

Hyman, B.T., van Hoesen, G.W., Damasio, A.R. & Barnes, C.L. (1984): Alzheimer's disease: cell-specific pathology isolates the hippocampal formation. *Science* **225,** 1168–1170.

Jones-Gotman, M. (1991): Localization of lesions by neuropsychological testing. *Epilepsia* **32,** S41–S52.

Kaada, B.R. (1951): Somato-motor, autonomic and electrocorticographic responses to electrical stimulation of rhinencephalic and other structures in primates, cat and dog. *Acta Physiol. Scand.* **24** (Suppl. 83), 1–285.

Kaada, B.R. (1972): Stimulation and regional ablation of the amygdaloid complex with reference to functional representations. In: *The neurobiology of the amygdala*, ed. B.E. Eleftheriou, pp. 205–281. New York: Plenum Press.

Kling, A. (1972): Effects of amygdalectomy on social-affective behavior in non-human primates. In: *The neurobiology of the amygdala*, ed. B.E. Eleftheriou, pp. 511–536. New York: Plenum Press.

Klüver, H. & Bucy, P. (1937): 'Psychic blindness' and other symptoms following temporal lobectomy in Rhesus monkey. *Am. J. Physiol.* **119**, 352–353.

Klüver, H. & Bucy, P. (1938): An analysis of certain effects of bilateral temporal lobectomy in the Rhesus monkey with special reference to 'psychic blindness'. *J. Psychol.* **5**, 33–54.

Klüver, H. & Bucy, P. (1939): Preliminary analysis of functions of the temporal lobes in monkeys. *Arch. Neurol. Psychiat.* **42**, 979–1000.

La Plane, D., Degos, J.D., Baulac, M. & Gray, F. (1981): Bilateral infarction of the anterior cingulate gyri and of the fornices. *J. Neurol. Sci.* **51**, 289–300.

Liu, Z., Mikati, M. & Holmes, G.L. (1995): Mesial temporal sclerosis: pathogenesis and significance. *Pediatr. Neurol.* **12**, 5–16.

Lopes da Silva, F.H., Witter, M.P., Boeijinga, P.H. & Lohman, A.H. (1990): Anatomic organization and physiology of the limbic cortex. *Physiol. Rev.* **70**, 453–511.

Maclean, P.D. (1952): Some psychiatric implications of physiological studies on frontotemporal portion of limbic sistem. *Electroencephalogr. Clin. Neurophysiol.* **4**, 407–418.

Mello, L.E.A.M., Cavalheiro, E.A., Tan, A.M., Kupfer, W.R., Pretorius, J.K., Babb, T.L. & Finch, D.M. (1993): Circuit mechanisms of seizures in the pilocarpine model of chronic epilepsy: cell loss and mossy fiber sprouting. *Epilepsia* **39**, 985–995.

Moss, M., Mahut, H. & Zola-Morgan, S, (1981): Concurrent discrimination learning of monkey after hippocampal, entorhinal, or fornix lesons. *J. Neurosci.* **1**, 227–240.

Munari, C., Bancaud, J., Bonis, A. et al. (1979): Rôle du noyau amygdalien dans la survenue de manifestations oroalimentaires au cours des crises épileptiques chez l'homme. *Rev. EEG Neurophysiol.* **9** (3), 236–240.

Munckenbeck, K.E. & Schwark, W.S. (1982): Serotoninergic mechanisms in amygdaloid kindled seizures in the rat. *Exp. Neurol.* **76**, 246–253.

Murray, E.A. & Mishkin, M. (1986): Visual recognition in monkeys following rhinal cortical ablation combined with either amygdalectomy or hippocampectomy. *J. Neurosci.* **6**, 1991–2003.

N'Guyen, J.P., Kéravel, Y. & Poirier, J. (1906): Vues anatomiques commentées du rhinencéphale. *Encycl. Méd.-Chir. (Paris, France) Neurologie*, 17001 R[10], 4–12–06, 22 p.

Nicoll, R.A. (1985): The septo-hippocampal projection: a model cholinergic pathway. *Trends Neurosci.* **8**, 533–536.

Niki, H. & Watanabe, M. (1976): Cingulate unit activity and delayed response. *Brain Res.* **110**, 381–386.

O'Keefe, J. & Nadel, L. (1978): *The hippocampus as a cognitive map*. Oxford: Oxford University Press.

Papez, J.W. (1937): A proposed mechanism of emotion. *Arch. Neurol. Psychiat.* **38**, 725–743.

Penfield, W. & Jasper, H.H. (1954): *Epilepsy and functional anatomy of the human brain*. Boston: Little Brown.

Pitkänen, A., Savander, V. & LeDoux, J.E. (1997): Organization of intra-amygdaloid circuitries in the rat: an emerging framework for understanding functions of the amygdala. *Trends Neurosci.* **20**, 517–523.

Schwarzkroin, P.A. & Prince, D.A. (1980): Changes in excitatory and inhibitory synaptic potentials leading to epileptogenic activity. *Brain Res.* **183**, 61–79.

Scoville, W.B. & Milner, B. (1957): Loss of recent memory after bilateral hippocampal lesions. *J. Neurol. Neurosurg. Psychiat.* **20**, 11–21.

Serby, M. (1986): Olfaction in Alzheimer's disease. *Prog. Neuro-Psychogharmacol. Biol. Psychiat.* **10**, 579–586.

Sloviter, R.S. (1994): The functional organization of the hippocampal dentate gyrus and its relevance to the pathogenesis of temporal lobe epilepsy. *Ann. Neurol.* **35,** 640–654.

Spyer, K.M. (1997): Do we need a limbic system? *Trends Neurosci.* **20,** 508.

Sutula, T., He, X.-X., Cavazos, J. & Scott, G. (1988): Synaptic reorganization in the hippocampus induced by abnormal functional activity. *Science* **239,** 1147–1150.

Talairach, J., Bancaud, J., Geier, S. *et al.* (1973): The cingulate gyrus and human behavior. *Electrocephalogr. Clin. Neurophysiol.* **34,** 45–52.

Tauck, D.L. & Nadler, J.V. (1985): Evidence of functional mossy fiber sprouting in hippocampal formation of kainic acid-treated rats. *J. Neuroci.* **5,** 1016–1022.

Thompson, R.F. (1988): The neural basis of associate learning of discrete behavioral responses. *Trends Neurosci.* **11,** 152–155.

Veilleux, F., Saint-Hilaire, J.M., Giard, N. *et al.* (1992): Seizures of the human medial frontal lobe. In: *Advances in neurology: frontal lobe seizures and epilepsies,* vol. 57, eds. P. Chauvel, A.V. Delado Escueta, E. Halgren & J. Bancaud, pp. 245–255. New York: Raven Press.

Villani, F., Garbelli, R., Cipelletti, B. & Spreafico, R. (2001): The limbic system: anatomical structures and embryologic development. In: *Limbic seizures in children*, eds. G. Avanzini, A. Beaumanoir & L. Mira, pp. 11–20. London: John Libbey.

Willis, T. (1664): *Cerebri anatome: cui accessit nervorum descriptio et usus*. London: J. Flesher.

Wilson, C.L., Maidment, N.T., Shomer, M.H. Behnke, E.J., Ackerson, L., Fried, I. & Engel, J. Jr. (1996): Comparison of seizure related amino acid release in human epileptic hippocampus versus a chronic kainate rat model of hippocampal epilepsy. *Epilepsy Res.* **26,** 245–254.

Witter, M.P. & Groenewegen, H.J. (1990): The subiculum: cytoarchitectonically a simple structure, but hodologically complex. In: *Progress in brain research*, vol 83, eds. J. Storm-Mathisen, J. Zimmer & O.P. Oftersen, pp. 47–58. Amsterdam: Elsevier Science Publishers BV.

Wurtz, R.H. & Olds, J. (1963): Amygdaloid stimulation and operant reinforcement in the rat. *J. Comp. Physiol. Psychol.* **56,** 941–949.

Chapter 4

Propagation of limbic seizures: experimental studies

Nicolas Chevassus-au-Louis, Roustem Khazipov and Yezekiel Ben-Ari

INSERM U29, Avenue de Luminy, BP 13, 13273 Marseille Cedex 09, France

Summary

Although there are numerous studies on the mechanisms of seizure initiation in the hippocampus, few studies have addressed the issue of the propagation of hippocampal paroxysmal activity either within the limbic system or to the neocortex. Using a novel preparation that allows *in vitro* recordings of interconnected limbic structures in immature rats, we have shown that the expression and propagation of kainic acid (KA) induced hippocampal seizures are age-dependent. At P2, KA generates brief sequences of interictal bursts that propagate to the septum but not to the entorhinal cortex. By contrast, at P6, KA generates ictal episodes that propagate to both the septum and the entorhinal cortex and have long-term effects. In an other set of experiments, we have investigated the role of intrahippocampal cortical heterotopias on the propagation of hippocampal seizure activity. We have shown that heterotopias form a bridge between the hippocampus and the neocortex that allows the direct propagation of hippocampal seizure activity to the neocortex. Therefore, intrahippocampal heterotopias can contribute to the generalization of hippocampal focal paroxysmal activity.

One of the earliest and strongest pieces of evidence supporting the limbic system concept is that limbic afterdischarges spread within the anatomically defined limbic circuitry (*see Chapter 2, this volume*) and produce a stereotyped pattern of behavioural alterations. This phenomenon is well illustrated by this quote from MacLean (1992):

> *Somewhat like stampeding cattle within a corral, the propagating nerve impulses stay within the confines of limbic circuitry. If the nerve impulse 'jumps the fence' and invades the neocortex, it usually results in a generalized seizure.*

Therefore, there are two distinct modes of propagation of limbic seizures: (i) propagation within the limbic system, that is responsible for the variety of behavioural limbic symptomatology; (ii) propagation out of the limbic system to the neocortical mantle, that is responsible for the generalization of seizures.

Although there have been numerous studies dealing with the mechanisms of seizure initiation in the limbic system and especially in the hippocampus, few experimental studies have addressed the issue of the mechanisms of seizure propagation within and out of the limbic system. In the present chapter, we will review results from our laboratory on the ontogenesis of intra-limbic propagation and on the facilitation of generalization of limbic seizures by cortical malformations.

Ontogenesis of hippocampal seizure propagation

Ontogenesis of kainate-induced seizures: *in vivo* data

In adult rats, it is well-established that injection of the glutamate agonist kainic acid (KA) produces the following sequence of correlated behavioural and electrographical abnormalities (reviewed in Ben-Ari, 1985): (i) staring with localized paroxysmal discharge in the hippocampus; (ii) individual recurrent limbic seizures with paroxysmal discharges extended to other limbic structures, especially the amygdala; (iii) full status epilepticus with generalization of paroxysmal activity to non-limbic structures. This sequence of events was also described using functional mapping with 2-deoxyglucose (2 DG) autoradiography (Ben-Ari *et al.*, 1981; White & Price, 1993) and *fos* immunostaining (Popovici *et al.*, 1990).

By contrast, in immature rats, parenteral KA injection induces tonic or tonico-clonic convulsions but not limbic motor signs (Cherubini *et al.*, 1983; Stafstrom *et al.*, 1992; Okada *et al.*, 1984). Limbic motor seizures are first observed from the end of the third week. The shift from tonico-clonic to limbic seizures is sudden with almost no intermediate stages. Functional mapping has shown that the rise in 2 DG labelling induced by KA is exclusively restricted to the hippocampal CA3 region and to the connected lateral septum (Tremblay *et al.*, 1984).

Therefore, *in vivo* data suggest that the intra-limbic propagation of hippocampal seizure activity is different in immature and adult rats, and depends on the functional maturation of the limbic circuitry.

The limbic system in a dish: *ex vivo* data

To further investigate the functional ontogenesis of the limbic circuitry, we took advantage of the recently developed intact limbic structures preparation that allows *ex vivo* recording of the whole and interconnected immature hippocampi, septum and entorhinal cortex (Khalilov *et al.*, 1997).

We first studied the ontogenesis of kainate-induced seizures in isolated whole hippocampi. In postnatal day 0 (P0), kainate did not generate paroxysmal activity even at high doses, which is in agreement with the absence of high affinity KA receptors at this age (Berger *et al.*, 1984). Starting from P2–P3, kainate generated a brief sequence of interictal bursts that were synchronous in field and whole cell recordings. In P4–P8 hippocampi, KA generated ictal episodes with tonic and clonic phases followed by post-ictal depression. Interestingly, repeated (3–8) applications of KA induced long-lasting transformations of the hippocampal activity manifested by spontaneous recurrent ictal discharges. This epileptic activity replaced network driven giant depolarizing potentials (Leinekugel *et al.*, 1997) that are a characteristic physiological pattern of activity in the developing hippocampus.

To analyse the propagation of KA-induced epileptiform activity, we extended the intact hippocampus preparation to include the two hippocampi, septum and entorhinal cortex with conserved connections. In a P2 reconstructed limbic system, KA-induced hippocampal discharges propagated to the contralateral hippocampus and to the septum, but not to the entorhinal cortex. After cutting the septohippocampal fibre tract, epileptiform activity was no longer observed in the septum suggesting the propagation of seizure activity from the hippocampus to the neocortex. At P6, hippocampal epileptiform activity propagated to the septum and to the entorhinal cortex, the propagation being suppressed by transection of the fibre tract connecting these structures with the hippocampus.

Therefore, in keeping with *in vivo* data, the hippocampus is the primary site of KA-induced seizure initiation in the immature rat brain. The propagation of hippocampal epileptiform activity to other limbic structures (and hence the behavioural manifestations) is clearly age-dependent.

Facilitation of neocortical propagation of hippocampal seizure activity by cortical heterotopias

Cortical malformations in epilepsy

The development of modern imaging techniques has revealed the high frequency of cortical malformations in symptomatic epilepsy, especially in children. These malformations can be either diffuse and affect the whole cortex (lissencephaly, hemimegalencephaly ...) or focal. One example of focal or mutifocal malformation are the subcortical heterotopias (Barkovich & Kjos, 1992; Barkovich, 1996). Heterotopias appear as nodules or bands of cortical grey matter in the subcortical white matter of all lobes, including the temporal lobe. Patients with cortical heterotopias have usually normal intelligence but suffer epilepsy, with seizure onset in the second decade (Dubeau *et al.*, 1995; Eksioglu *et al.*, 1996; Battaglia *et al.*, 1997). The seizures are partial with secondary generalization, and are frequently therapy resistant (Raymond *et al.*, 1994; Smith *et al.*, 1988; Li *et al.*, 1997). Yet little is known on the pathophysiological mechanisms of these epilepsies, which prompted us to develop an animal model.

Intahippocampal cortical heterotopias can form a bridge between the hippocampus and the neocortex

A useful animal model for epileptogenic cortical malformation consists in prenatal treatment with the antimitotic agent methylazoxymethanol (MAM) (reviewed in Cattabeni & Di Luca, 1997). The offsets, the so-called MAM rats have microcephaly, cortical disorganization (Dambska *et al.*, 1982; Yurkewicz *et al.*, 1984) and cortical heterotopias in the white matter as well as in the CA1 region of the hippocampus (Chevassus-au-Louis *et al.*, 1998c; Colacitti *et al.*, 1998). Although they do not seem to suffer from spontaneous seizures, MAM rats have an increased sensitivity to various convulsing agents (Germano *et al.*, 1996; Baraban & Schwartzkroin, 1996; reviewed in Chevassus-au-Louis *et al.* (1999) and thus appear to be seizure-prone.

We recently characterized an abnormal cortical network involving the intrahippocampal cortical heterotopias with dramatic functional consequences (Chevassus-au-Louis *et al.*, 1998b). As discussed earlier, heterotopic masses of neocortex are consistently observed in the hippocampus of MAM-treated rats. Using electrophysiological recordings, we demonstrated that heterotopic neurones have bidirectional connections with the adjacent neocortex, while receiving an excitatory monosynaptic input from hippocampal fibres. A functional consequence of these aberrant connections is that bicuculline-induced paroxysmal activity triggered in the hippocampus can spread directly to the neocortex (Fig. 1.).

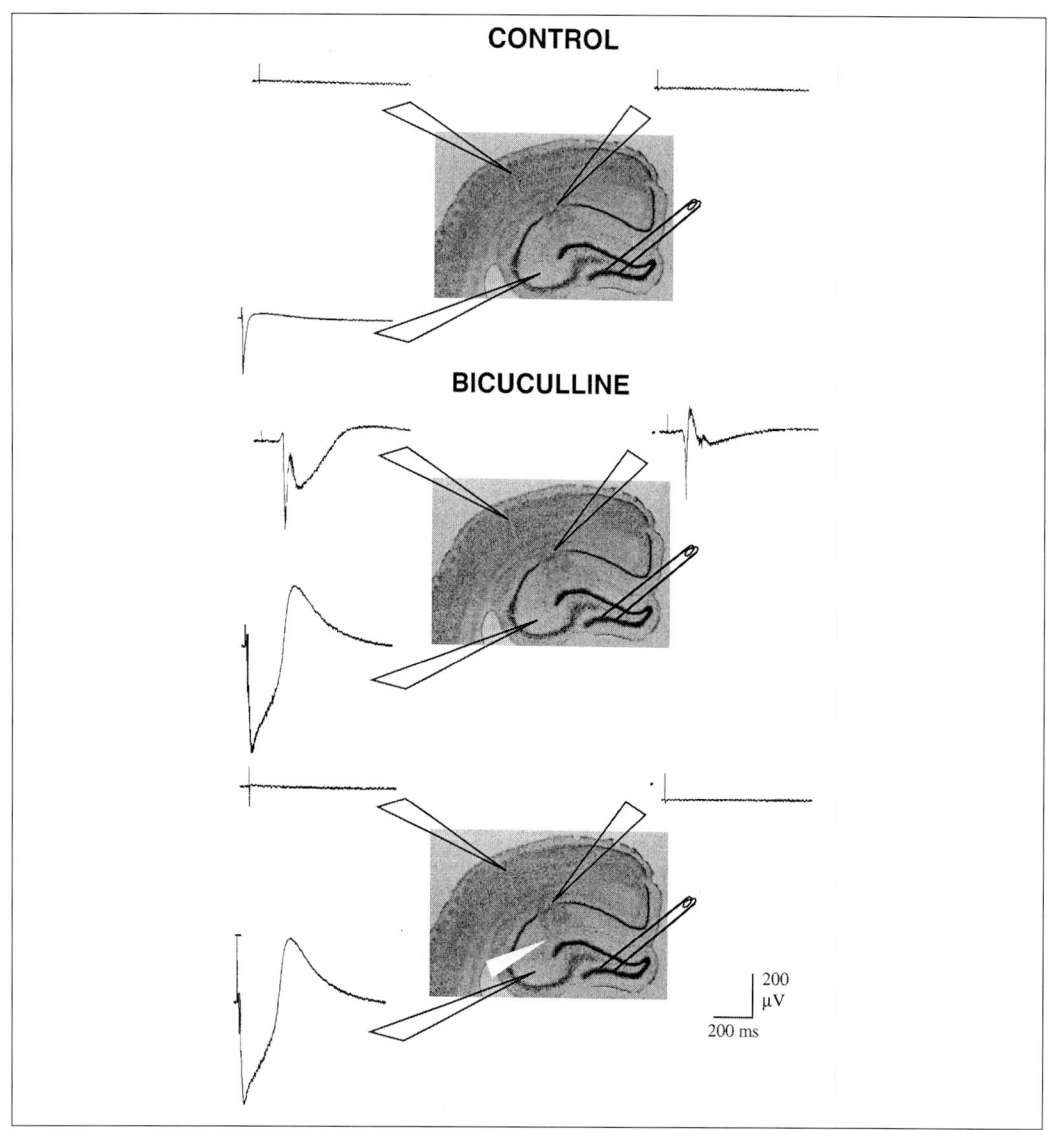

Fig. 1. Heterotopias allow the propagation of hippocampal paroxysmal activity to the neocortex.
In control conditions (top traces), electrical stimulation of the dentate gyrus evoked a negative field EPSP in CA3 region, but neither in the heterotopia nor in neocortex.
When bicuculline was bath applied (middle traces), the same stimulation evoked an epileptiform discharge in the CA3 region, followed by an epileptiform discharge in the heterotopia and neocortex. Since it was difficult to determine the onset of the epileptiform discharge in the heterotopia, we can only estimate the delay between the epileptiform discharges recorded in the CA3 region and heterotopia (this delay ranges from 8 to 15 ms, with a mean of 7.8 ± 2 ms, $n = 6$). Except in one case, it was impossible to determine the delay between the epileptiform discharges recorded in the heterotopia and neocortex for the same reason. In this case the delay was 2 ms.
When the CA3 and CA1 regions were disconnected by a knife cut of the Schaffer collaterals (bottom traces), the same stimulation only evoked an epileptiform discharge in the CA3 region with no synaptic response in the heterotopia and neocortex.

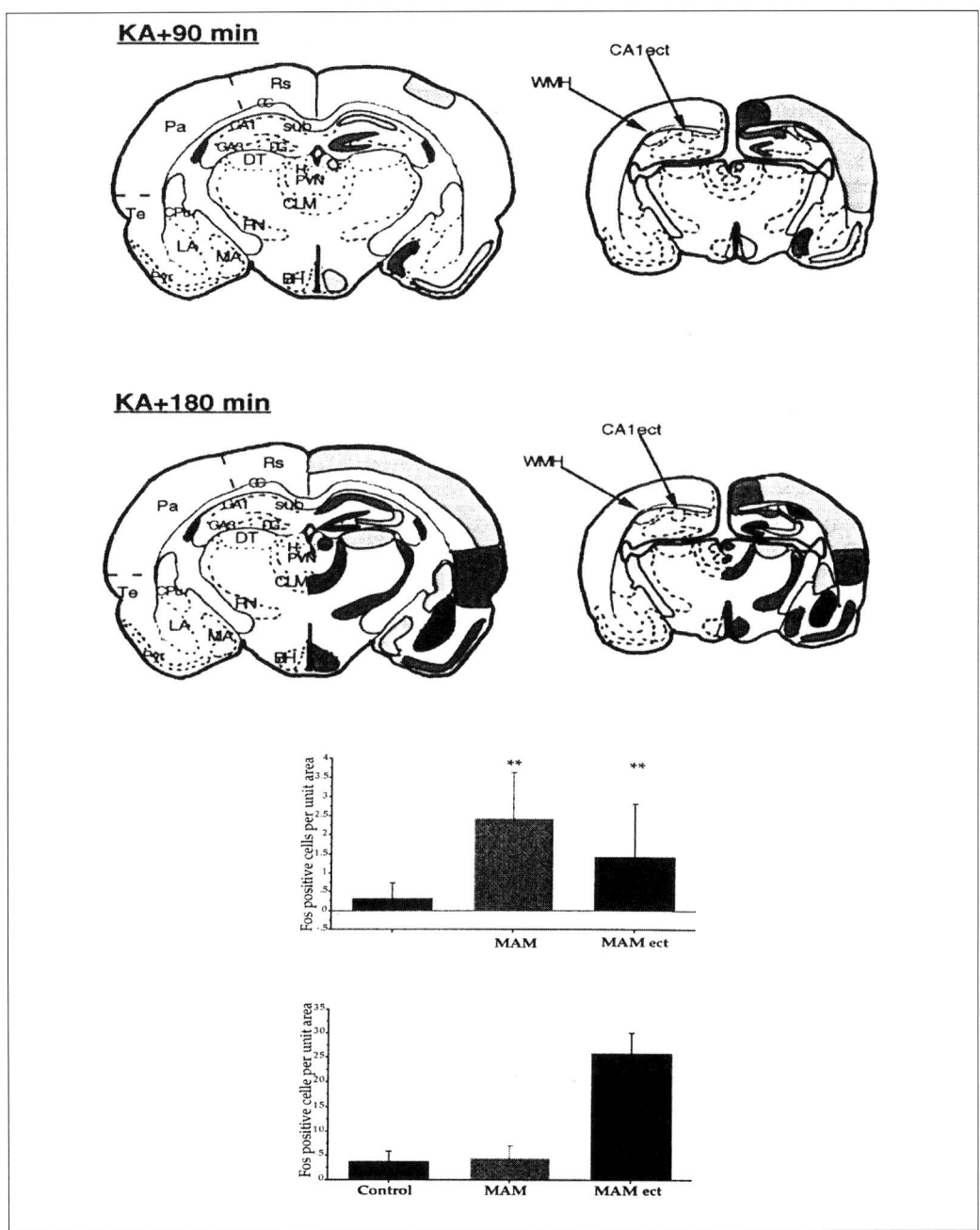

Fig. 2. Early fos expression in the neocortex of MAM rats during kainate-induced seizures.
The illustration depicts the semi-quantitative analysis of fos positive cells (a biochemical marker of metabolic activity) in the brain of control and MAM rats after parenteral kainate injection. The density of fos positive cells in the normotopic and ectopic neocortex of MAM rats as well as in control is depicted in the right part of the figure (different scale in 90 min and 180 min). Note the early fos expression in the neocortex of MAM rats and the high density of fos-positive cells in cortical ectopias during status epilepticus.

Along the same lines, two *in vivo* evidences have been obtained that support the existence of a bridge between the hippocampus and the neocortex in MAM rats. First, focal hippocampal seizure activity induced *in vivo* by electrical stimulation propagates more frequently to the frontal neocortex in MAM-treated rats that in control (Chevassus-au-Louis *et al.*, 1998a). Second, the increased sensitivity of MAM rats to KA-induced seizures (De Feo *et al.*, 1995; Germano *et al.*, 1996) has been shown to be associated with a more rapid generalization of seizure activity monitored by *fos* immunostaining to the neocortex (Fig. 2.). Therefore, it would appear that heterotopic neurones are integrated into both hippocampal and neocortical circuitry, allowing the rapid generalization of hippocampal paroxysmal activity to the neocortex (Chevassus-au-Louis *et al.*, 1998b). These results demonstrate, for the first time, that heterotopic regions can support hyperexcitability by forming an abnormal bridge between normally unconnected structures.

References

Baraban, S.C. & Schwartzkroin, P.A. (1996): Flurothyl seizure susceptibility in rats following prenatal methylazoxymethanol treatment. *Epilepsy Res.* **23**, 189–194.

Barkovich, A.J. (1996): Subcortical heterotopia: a distinct clinicoradiologic entity. *Am. J. Neuroradiol.* **17**, 1315–1322.

Barkovich, A.J. & Kjos, B.O. (1992): Gray matter heterotopias: MR characteristics and correlation with developmental and neurological manifestations. *Radiology* **182**, 493–499.

Battaglia, G., Granata, T., Farina, L., D'Incerti, L., Franceschetti, S. & Avanzini, G. (1997): Periventricular nodular heterotopia: epileptogenic findings. *Epilepsia* **38**, 1173–1182.

Ben-Ari, Y. (1985): Limbic seizures and brain damage produced by kainic acid: mechanisms and relevance to human temporal lobe epilepsy. *Neuroscience* **14**, 375–403.

Ben-Ari, Y., Tremblay, E., Riche, D., Ghilini, G. & Naquet, R. (1981): Electrographic, clinical and pathological alterations following systemic administration of kainic acid, bicuculline or pentetrazole: metabolic mapping using the deoxyglucose method with special reference to the pathology of epilepsy. *Neuroscience* **6**, 1361–1391.

Berger, M.L., Tremblay, E., Nitecka, L. & Ben-Ari, Y. (1984): Maturation of kainic acid seizure brain-damage syndrome in the rat. III: Postnatal development of kainic acid binding sites in the limbic system. *Neuroscience* **13**, 1095–1104.

Cattabeni, F. & Di Luca, M. (1997): Developmental models of brain dysfunctions induced by targeted cellular ablations with methylazoxymethanol. *Phys. Rev.* **77**, 199–215.

Cherubini, E., De Feo, M.R., Mecarelli, O. & Ricci, G.F. (1983): Behavioral and electrographic patterns induced by systemic administration of kainc acid in developing rats. *Dev. Brain Res.* **9**, 69–77.

Chevassus-au-Louis, N., Baraban, S.C., Gaiarsa, J-L. & Ben-Ari, Y. (1999): Cortical malformations and epilepsy: new insights from animal models. *Epilepsia* **40**, 811–821.

Chevassus-au-Louis, N., Ben-Ari, Y. & Vergnes, M. (1998a): Decreased seizure threshold and more rapid kindling in rats with prenatal treatment with methylzoxymethanol. *Brain Res.* **812**, 252–255.

Chevassus-au-Louis, N., Congar, P., Represa, A., Ben-Ari, Y. & Gaiarsa, J-L. (1998b): Neuronal migration disorders: Heterotopic neocortical neurons in CA1 form a bridge between the hippocampus and the neocortex. *Proc. Natl. Acad. Sci. USA* **95**, 10263–10268.

Chevassus-au-Louis, N., Rafiki, A., Jorquera, I., Ben-Ari, Y. & Represa, A. (1998c): Neocortex in the hippocampus: morpho-functional analysis of CA1 heterotopias after prenatal treatment with methylazoxymethanol in rats. *J. Comp. Neurol.* **394**, 520–536.

Colacitti, C., Sancini, G., Franceschetti, S. *et al.* (1998): Altered connections between neocortical and heterotopic areas in methylazoxymethanol-treated rats. *Epilepsy Res.* **32**, 49–62.

Dambska, M., Haddad, R., Kozlowski, P.B., Lee, M.H. & Shek, J. (1982): Telencephalic cytoarchitectonics in the brains of rats with graded degrees of micrencephaly. *Acta Neuropath.* **58**, 203–209.

De Feo, M.R., Mecarelli, O. & Ricci, G.F. (1995): Seizure susceptibility in immature rats with micrencephaly induced by prenatal exposure to methylazoxymethanol acetate. *Pharmacol. Res.* **31**, 109–114.

Dubeau, F., Tampieri, D., Lee, N. *et al.* (1995): Periventricular and subcortical nodular heterotopia. A study of 33 patients. *Brain* **118**, 1273–1287.

Eksioglu, Y.Z., Scheffer, I.E., Cardenas, P. *et al.* (1996): Periventricular heterotopia: an X-linked dominant epilepsy locus causing aberrant cerebral cortical development. *Neuron* **16**, 77–87.

Germano, I.M., Zhang, Y.F., Sperber, E.F. & Moshé, S.L. (1996): Neuronal migration disorders increase susceptibility to hyperthermia induced seizures in developing rats. *Epilepsia* **37**, 902–910.

Khalilov, I., Esclapez, M., Khazipov, R. *et al.* (1997): A novel *in vitro* preparation: the intact hippocampal formation. *Neuron* **19**, 743–749.

Leinekugel, X., Medina, I., Khalilov, I., Ben-Ari, Y. & Khazipov, R. (1997): Ca^{2+} oscillations mediated by the synergistic actions of GABAA and NMDA receptors in the neonatal hippocampus. *Neuron* **18**, 243–255.

Li, L.M., Dubeau, F., Andermann, F. *et al.* (1997): Periventricular nodular heterotopia and intractable temporal lobe epilepsy: poor outcome after temporal lobe resection. *Ann. Neurol.* **41**, 662–668.

MacLean, P.D. (1992): The limbic system concept. In: *The temporal lobes and the limbic system*, eds. M.R. Trimble & T.G. Bolwig, pp. 1–15. Petersfield, UK: Wrightson Biomedical Publishing.

Okada, R., Moshé, S.L. & Albala, B.J. (1984): Infantile status epilepticus and future seizure susceptibility in the rat. *Dev Brain Res.* **15**, 177–183.

Popovici, T., Represa, A., Crépel, V., Barbin, G., Beaudoin, M. & Ben-Ari, Y. (1990): Effects of kainic acid-induced seizures and ischemia on c-fos like proteins in rat brain. *Brain Res.* **536**, 183–194.

Raymond, A.A., Fish, D.R., Stevens, J.M., Sisodiya, S.M., Alsanjari, N. & Shorvon, S.D. (1994): Subependymal heterotopia: a distinct neuronal migration disorder associated with epilepsy. *J. Neurol. Neurosurg. Psychiatr.* **57**, 1195–1202.

Smith, A.S., Weinstein, M.A., Quencer, R.M. *et al.* (1988): Association of heterotopic gray matter with epilepsy. *Radiology* **168**, 195–198.

Stafstrom, C.E., Thompson, J.L. & Holmes, G.L. (1992): Kainic acid seizures in the developing brain: status epilepticus and spontaneous recurrent seizures. *Dev. Brain Res.* **65**, 227–236.

Tremblay, E., Nitecka, L., Berger, M.L. & Ben-Ari, Y. (1984): Maturation of kainic acid seizure brain damage in the rat. I: Clinical, electrographic and metabolic observations. *Neuroscience* **13**, 1051–1072.

White, L.E. & Price, J.L. (1993): The functional anatomy of limbic status epilepticus in the rat. I. Patterns of 14C-2-deoxyglucose uptake and fos immunocytochemistry. *J.Neurosci.* **13**, 4787–4809.

Yurkewicz, L., Valentino, K.L., Floeter, M.K., Fleshman, J.W. & Jones, E.G. (1984): Effects of cytotoxic deletions of somatic sensory cortex in fetal rats. *Somatosensory Res.* **1**, 303–327.

Chapter 5

Mesial temporal sclerosis: electroclinical and pathological correlations and applications to limbic epilepsy in childhood

Susan S. Spencer, Edward Novotny[*], Nihal de Lanerolle[†] and Jung Kim[‡]

Departments of Neurology, Pediatrics,[*] Neurosurgery,[†] and Pathology;[‡] Yale University School of Medicine, Department of Neurology, P.O. Box 208018, New Haven, CT 06520–8018, USA

Summary

Mesial temporal sclerosis (MTS) is the penultimate model of nonlesional limbic epilepsy in adults, in whom it has been extensively studied by virtue of its frequent surgical treatment. Its scalp and intracranial EEG characteristics, neuropsychological profile, historical relation to early risk factors, MRI findings and their quantification, and (poor) response to medical treatment have been well documented. Its precise pathological definition varies, and the importance of the components of that definition remain controversial. Whether MTS, defined as neuronal loss of greater than 50 per cent in hippocampal fields CA1 and CA3, with gliosis, and with evidence of synaptic reorganization, is a cause or result of the often uncontrolled complex partial seizures with which it is associated remains a topic of debate, and one to which the study of children might provide considerable insight. Do children of all ages have MTS? Does it have all the pathological and clinical features of adults? Some literature suggests MTS occurs much less commonly in childhood; other reports claim that surgical selection bias is responsible for this conclusion. We find that MTS *true to the adult form pathologically* does *not* occur in children under 12 years, although the electroclinical syndrome it defines does. An anatomical and electroclinical syndrome indistinguishable from that seen in adults occurs later in adolescence. Findings gleaned from the literature as well as an extensive analysis of surgically treated children at our centre with respect to pathology, MRI, EEG, and historical features are presented in support of this view. These investigations lead to the conclusion that at least the synaptic reorganization commonly associated with neuronal loss in the adult variety of MTS and medial temporal lobe epilepsy is a result (or at least not a cause) of the intractable seizure disorder with which it is associated.

Mesial temporal sclerosis (MTS) is also referred to as hippocampal sclerosis (HS) or Ammon's horn sclerosis (AHS). The term describes a distinct pathological substrate that underlies the most common limbic epilepsy in adults and possibly in children, with origin in medial temporal lobe structures. This epilepsy syndrome, characterized by medial temporal lobe onset seizures which are often medically refractory, has allowed intensive patient study because of the frequency of surgical intervention. Preoperative electrographic, structural, functional and clinical investigations have allowed detailed electroclinical description of the syndrome, and surgical resection has allowed intensive pathological evaluation of involved tissue. By virtue of this group of patients, we have a window to the relationship between these various investigations, the living person, the epilepsy, and its structural correlates.

The classical pathology in MTS includes three components: neuronal loss, gliosis, and reorganization (Gloor, 1991; de Lanerolle *et al.*, 1994). Based on both qualitative and quantitative analyses, the neuronal loss is established to be greater than 50 per cent of dentate granular cells and pyramidal cells in most areas of Ammon's horn (Babb *et al.*, 1984a, b; Kim *et al.*, 1990). This amount of cell loss is also obvious on qualitative assessment. Variability, however, occurs in the degree and distribution of neuronal loss, from negligible to profound, although CA2 is relatively spared in most instances (Babb *et al.*, 1984a, b; de Lanerolle *et al.*, 1994: Gloor, 1991; Kim *et al.*, 1990; Margerison & Corsellis, 1966). Somatostatin, substance P, and neuropeptide -Y- containing interneurons in the hilus are selectively lost, even in the absence of detectable pyramidal cell loss in the hilus (de Lanerolle *et al.*, 1989). On the other hand, somatostatin, NPY, and substance P neurons in Ammon's horn survive, even in the face of massive loss of pyramidal neurons (de Lanerolle *et al.*, 1992).

The gliosis in MTS is characterized by a high proportion of fibrous astrocytes. These astrocytes have a high density of sodium channels and can generate neuron-like action potentials (de Lanerolle *et al.*, 1994; O'Connor *et al.*, 1998). They are widely distributed in the areas of neuronal loss, but do not bear a significant inverse relationship to the neuronal counts in the same areas when studied quantitatively.

The reorganization in MTS is characterized by mossy fibre recurrent collateral sprouting into the dentate inner molecular layer (de Lanerolle *et al.*, 1989, 1994; Sutula *et al.*, 1989a; Babb *et al.*, 1991). This phenomenon is also seen in animal models of epilepsy (Cronin & Dudek, 1988; Sloviter, 1991; Sutula *et al.*, 1989b). Sprouting in the dentate molecular layer of fibres immunoreactive for NPY, substance P, and somatostatin is also seen (de Lanerolle *et al.*, 1989, 1994); these findings are not reproduced in animal models. An increase in D2 and VIP receptors in the dentate molecular layer accompanies the reorganization (de Lanerolle *et al.*, 1990; 1994).

While these pathologic findings have been carefully described, quantitated, and analysed, their relationship to the genesis of temporal lobe epilepsy with which they are associated continues to be uncertain. MTS is certainly intimately related to medial temporal lobe epilepsy. This statement is based upon the consistent unique pathology in surgical specimens of temporal lobes resected for uncontrolled medial temporal lobe epilepsy (de Lanerolle *et al.*, 1994; Gloor, 1991; Mathern *et al.*, 1997), as well as (and perhaps more importantly) the EEG evidence of seizure onset within the medial temporal structures in the same patients (Babb *et al.*, 1984b; Spencer *et al.*, 1990), and the cure of seizures in over 90 per cent of patients with medial temporal lobe epilepsy (established by those EEG studies) by resection of this medial temporal lobe tissue (with or without additional temporal neocortex) (Spencer, 1993, 1996). But whether the MTS is a cause or effect of medial temporal lobe epilepsy remains a matter of debate.

Human studies, although somewhat inconsistent, suggest that MTS is a cause of medial temporal lobe epilepsy. First, many patients with chronic, uncontrolled, or even catastrophic epilepsy, do not show features of MTS (Gloor, 1991; Mathern *et al.*, 1997) so seizures themselves do not beget the pathology. Second, there is no reported correlation between seizure frequency, or epilepsy duration, and the degree of cell loss, or of its correlate hippocampal atrophy. Finally, resection limited to the hippocampus often cures the seizures (Spencer, 1993, 1996).

On the other hand, animal data (which is not always consistent) suggests that MTS is an effect of medial temporal lobe epilepsy; the idea that the pathologic findings represent excitotoxic injury has been advanced. In animal models of sustained limbic seizures or intermittent stimulation of limbic pathways, selective neuronal loss in CA1 and CA3 as well as gliosis and axonal sprouting with synaptic reorganization in the dentate gyrus have been seen. These parallel the findings in chronic human medial temporal lobe epilepsy. The changes in the animal models are independent of systemic effects of seizures. The suggestion that this appearance is due to excitotoxic damage comes from several lines of evidence. Glutamate-induced neuronal injury resembles the changes that are seen in humans and animals after seizure occurrence (Meldrum & Corsellis, 1984; Sloviter, 1991; Sutula *et al.*, 1989b). Excitatory amino acids are released in excessive amounts during seizures; this has been documented through microdialysis in humans (During, 1994; During & Spencer, 1993). The most vulnerable hippocampal regions to the findings of MTS have the highest excitatory amino acid receptor densities (Gloor, 1991). Finally, NMDA and nonNMDA antagonists prevent seizure-induced damage in these animal models (Choi, 1988; Croucher *et al.*, 1982).

It is conceivable that study of human pathologic features during development could resolve some of these issues about pathogenesis of MTS and medial temporal lobe epilepsy. The question is, to what extent does MTS appear in childhood, and to what extent does it reproduce the findings of the adult syndrome from which the bulk of the data is generated and from which these questions arise? To address this issue I will describe the syndrome and its clinical, pathological, functional and structural correlates in the adult, investigate the correlations of pathological findings with those features, and then extend the evaluation to reports in children and data from our own centre in children.

The clinical features of medial temporal lobe epilepsy have been well described. An early risk factor or event occurring before the age of four years is highly correlated with development of this type of epilepsy. The risk factor is often febrile convulsions, usually complicated or lengthy ones, but could be infection or trauma (French *et al.*, 1993; Marks *et al.*, 1992, 1995; Wieser *et al.*, 1993). After a variably lengthy latent period, usually lasting years, complex partial seizures begin. They are heralded by an experiential or psychic aura in 80 per cent of patients. The seizures themselves are characterized by arrest of motion, staring, oroalimentary and complex upper extremity automatisms, with contralateral upper extremity dystonia. The seizures develop slowly and recede slowly, are lengthy in duration, and are followed by prolonged postictal confusion. They occur with an average frequency of three to five times per month.

The electrographic findings associated with these seizures have been intensely studied. The scalp interictal EEG shows anterior temporal spikes in approximately 90 per cent of patients; they are bilateral and independent in about half the patients. Ictal scalp EEG recordings including anterior temporal and sphenoidal electrodes classically show rhythmic theta frequency discharge over one temporal region (Williamson *et al.*, 1993). This type of seizure discharge localizes the onset, but onset can occur bilaterally and independently in the temporal lobes in at least 20 per cent of patients.

Intracranial EEG has been performed in this entity more than in any other type of intractable epilepsy (King *et al.*, 1995; Spencer, 1998; Spencer *et al.*, 1993b, 1998). Interictal spikes tend to be medial temporal in location and are almost always bilateral and independent. Ictal onset typically shows a periodic 1–2 Hz spike discharge which recurs for seconds or even minutes and is confined to hippocampal recording electrodes. Upon this periodic discharge is later superimposed a 10–15 Hz low voltage discharge, the appearance of which is associated with propagation and clinical onset. (The seizures may also begin spontaneously with the higher frequency discharge in the absence of the periodic discharge, and both types of onset might occur independently in different seizures of a given patient.) The exact frequency of seizure onset can vary, as can the exact medial temporal location in which these phenomena are recorded, but the periodic discharge appears to be hippocampal in origin. Analysis of tissue resected from patients who had intracranial recording has shown that the presence of more seizures with a periodic spike onset is significantly and directly correlated with glial density in CA2 and CA3 (Spencer *et al.*, 1997). This is one piece of evidence that some of the cellular changes described in association with MTS have a role in modifying the electrical appearance of the seizures, if not in generating them.

Seizures beginning in the hippocampal/medial temporal region also demonstrate a long delay to propagation as recorded by intracranial electrodes (King *et al.*, 1995; Spencer *et al.*, 1998). Propagation of the paroxysmal activity most often occurs to the ipsilateral frontal or temporal neocortex or the contralateral hippocampus. The relationship of propagation time to cellular changes has also been investigated by our group in adult patients and is significantly correlated with neuronal loss in CA4 (Spencer *et al.*, 1992). Our interpretation of this finding is that the loss of neurons in CA4 limits access to the major hippocampal propagation pathway. This finding shows that structural alterations can also affect subsequent seizure evolution. Total electrical seizure duration correlates with glial density in CA2 and CA3, and also with the presence of excitatory post-synaptic potentials in slice experiments performed on this tissue (Spencer *et al.*, 1997). It is noteworthy that there is no correlation of any EEG parameter, ictal or interictal, as measured by intracranial recording in patients with medial temporal lobe epilepsy, with the reorganization or sprouting that has been noted in the subsequently resected tissue, in terms of degree, presence or type.

The structural correlate of MTS recorded by MRI is hippocampal atrophy and increased T2 signal in the hippocampus (Cascino *et al.*, 1991; Kuzniecky *et al.*, 1993a; Lencz *et al.*, 1992; Spencer *et al.*, 1993a). MRI is extraordinarily sensitive to these findings: they are demonstrated in over 90 per cent of patients with MTS. The specificity, however, of the findings of hippocampal atrophy and increased T2 signal to seizure onset in that substrate are less notable. Dual pathology, meaning an additional structural lesion on MRI in addition to the MTS, or bilateral hippocampal atrophy (with or without T2 signal increase) are detected in 15 per cent of patients each (Cendes *et al.*, 1995; King *et al.*, 1995; Raymond *et al.*, 1994). Often the dual pathology is a developmental abnormality such as hamartoma or heterotopia. In those situations, either substrate might be the primary epileptogenic area.

Medial temporal lobe epilepsy has also been studied extensively with functional tests. PET scans with fluorodeoxyglucose show diffuse temporal lobe hypometabolism in well over 90 per cent of patients with this syndrome. The hypometabolism may extend to adjacent lobes. It is thought, based on postoperative PET studies as well as animal data, that the hypometabolism reflects network dysfunction rather than purely structural alterations (Engel *et al.*, 1982; Theodore, 1994). SPECT scanning for cerebral perfusion with HMPAO or other agents is less sensitive in its demonstration of interictal temporal hypoperfusion. Ictal studies, however, are feasible with SPECT and highly localizing with sufficiently expert interpretation. Ictal hyperperfusion is more precisely circumscribed to the area of seizure onset than are interictal studies (either perfusion or metabolism) but can also show perfusion changes in areas of propagated seizure involvement (Spencer et al., 1995; Stefan et al., 1990).

Neuropsychological profiles commonly document hemisphere-specific memory impairment which may be clinically progressive, and presumably reflects hippocampal dysfunction (Loring et al., 1988). Verbal memory impairment correlates significantly with cell loss in the dominant CA3 (Sass et al., 1992).

These studies have played a major role in our ability to localize and therefore treat medial temporal lobe epilepsy surgically. Cure with resection of medial temporal structures is predicted by unilateral hippocampal atrophy; unilateral temporal hypometabolism; CA1 cell loss; asymmetric memory; an early risk factor; and the combination of MTS, a known cause, and absent secondary generalization (Berkovic et al., 1995; Spencer et al., 1994; Manno et al., 1994). After medial temporal lobe resection, over 80 per cent of patients are seizure free for one year, but 15 per cent have longterm relapse (Spencer, 1996). The localization of seizure onset in the relapsed patients has not been systematically documented.

Upon examining these observations for their implications, this author concluded that medial temporal lobe epilepsy has a probable developmental aetiology (Spencer, 1998). The conclusion is supported by the concomitant developmental abnormalities seen in 15 per cent of these patients, by the observation that neuronal heterotopia is increased in the temporal lobe white matter of patients with MTS and medial temporal lobe epilepsy (Jung et al., 1996), and by the presence of well-described familial forms of temporal lobe epilepsy (Berkovic et al., 1996). That longterm relapse occurs after resection suggests that the process is more diffuse than initially thought. Bilaterality of findings in up to 80 per cent of patients by autopsy, EEG, memory testing, spectroscopy, and MRI also support the notion that medial temporal lobe epilepsy is a more diffuse process (Babb & Brown, 1987; King & Spencer, 1995; Margerison & Corsellis, 1966; Mouritzen-Dam, 1982; Spencer, 1998; Spencer et al., 1998; Wieser et al., 1993). In a recent report, Fernandez and co-workers measured hippocampal volume in 23 members of two families each of which included one member with temporal lobe epilepsy, several other members with febrile convulsions, and several family members without any seizure history whatsoever (Fernandez et al., 1998). Left hippocampal atrophy and T2 signal was demonstrated in the family member with medial temporal lobe epilepsy. Left hippocampal atrophy but normal signal was seen in all members without epilepsy but with a history of febrile convulsions, and in many members of the families who were unaffected by seizures at any time. In one family, blurred internal hippocampal architecture on MRI was associated with flattened hippocampal bodies. The other family had smaller hippocampal heads. The pattern of structural alteration in the epilepsy patient in each family showed a correlation with the familial pattern of structural abnormality in the unaffected family members. These observations strongly suggest that hippocampal cell loss and structural hippocampal abnormality may be a pre-existing, genetically determined condition which facilitates febrile convulsions and underlies or contributes to the development of MTS. Whether different insults during development have different critical periods during which they exert their effects, and whether they interact with the same, or related or overlapping genetically determined conditions, are all unknown issues in this scenario. (Why the affected hemisphere was always the left one is also intriguing.)

Can these findings be extended to children and can implications for pathogenesis be derived from those studies? Existing reports on temporal lobe epilepsy and MTS in children are scattered in their detail and information (Adelson *et al.*, 1992; Brockhaus & Elger, 1995; Cross *et al.*, 1996; 1997; 1993; Drake *et al.*, 1987; Duchowny *et al.*, 1992; Fish *et al.*, 1993; Gaillard *et al.*, 1997; Goldstein *et al.*, 1996; Grattan-Smith *et al.*, 1993; Harbord & Manson, 1987; Harvey *et al.*, 1993, 1995, 1997; Holopainen *et al.*, 1997; Hopkins & Klug, 1991; Kuzniecky *et al.*, 1993b; Lawson *et al.*, 1997; Lin *et al.*, 1997; Mathern *et al.*, 1994; 1996; Mizrahi *et al.*, 1990; Murakami *et al.*, 1996; Pelaez *et al.*, 1997; Sinclair *et al.*, 1997; Wang *et al.*, 1997; Wyllie *et al.*, 1993). Still, six reports including 543 patients described MRI evidence of MTS in childhood, while 13 reports including 370 children described temporal lobectomy in children (Adelson *et al.*, 1992; Cross *et al.*, 1993; Duchowny *et al.*, 1992; Fish *et al.*, 1993; Gaillard *et al.*, 1997; Goldstein *et al.*, 1996; Grattan-Smith *et al.*, 1993; Harbord & Manson, 1987; Harvey *et al.*, 1997; Hopkins & Klug, 1991; Kuzniecky *et al.*, 1993b; Lawson *et al.*, 1997; Lin *et al.*, 1997; Mizrahi *et al.*, 1990; Pelaez *et al.*, 1997). PET, SPECT and magnetic resonance spectroscopy are included in at least four reports of childhood medial temporal lobe epilepsy (Cross *et al.*, 1996, 1997; Harvey *et al.*, 1993; Holopainen *et al.*, 1997). Childhood temporal lobe epilepsy was reported in 126 patients with trauma, and temporal lobe masses in children in another report addressing 16 patients (Drake *et al.*, 1987). The bulk of data, combined with analysis of 14 intensively studied children at Yale, allows description of the syndrome in children, its pathologic substrate, and thoughts on its development.

The clinical features of medial temporal lobe epilepsy in children are similar to those described in adults. A febrile seizure or other antecedent is reported in 15–75 per cent of paediatric temporal lobe epilepsy series. The onset of temporal lobe epilepsy in these children is reported at three months to fifteen years of age, with a shorter but definite latent period in the majority. The clinical seizures in children over 6 years are similar to those described in adults except that automatisms are simpler. Under the age of 6, however, more motor and clonic manifestations have been described (Brockhaus & Elger, 1995; Harvey *et al.*, 1997; Wyllie *et al.*, 1993). The reported incidence of secondary generalization is variable at 10–50 per cent.

Interictal scalp EEG in children also usually shows abnormalities but these are more often unilateral. They include temporal sharp waves or spikes as well as slowing in 60–70 per cent, a more unique feature in the childhood group (Brockhaus & Elger, 1995; Cross *et al.*, 1993, 1996, 1997; Gaillard *et al.*, 1997; Goldstein *et al.*, 1996; Grattan-Smith *et al.*, 1993; Harvey *et al.*, 1993, 1995, 1997; Holopainen *et al.*, 1997; Hopkins & Klug, 1991; Lin *et al.*, 1997; Murakami *et al.*, 1996; Pelaez *et al.*, 1997; Sinclair *et al.*, 1997; Wyllie *et al.*, 1993). In the Yale children, all were correctly lateralized on interictal EEG, but only half were *localized* to the anterior temporal region. Ictal scalp recording localizes to a unilateral temporal region in 75–95 per cent of children. The Yale group were all correctly lateralized on ictal scalp EEG recording, and 11 of the 14 were well *localized* to a single temporal region. Thus, bilaterality of EEG findings is less common than in adults, *slow* interictal rhythms were *more* common than in adults, and ictal patterns were more localized. Intracranial EEG studies in childhood temporal lobe epilepsy are sketchy and include only 17 patients in two manuscripts; perhaps this is because localization is better by scalp (Brockhaus & Elger, 1995; Wyllie *et al.*, 1993). The seven Yale patients under 16 who had intracranial EEG included two under the age of 12. They had similar ictal onset patterns to adults, including four of seven with periodic spikes and two of seven with low voltage fast activity as the initial change. Both rhythms were represented across the age spectrum. Although too few children have been analysed with respect to intracranial ictal EEG patterns in temporal lobe epilepsy, the findings in our patients suggest that neuronal loss and gliosis may be of the same qualitative and quantitative degree as in adults, since the intracranial ictal patterns are the same. It bears emphasis that although neuronal loss and gliosis are related to features of the intracranial EEG, sprouting is not; this observation may be important in developing a hypothesis about the aetiology of medial temporal lobe epilepsy, and might even relate to the absence of increased T2 signal in many of these children.

Among reported temporal lobe epilepsy series of children under 17 with MRI, a mean of 45 per cent had MTS while 33 per cent had mass lesions, 22 per cent were normal, 9 per cent had dual pathology, and 1 per cent had developmental abnormalities (Adelson *et al.*, 1992; Brockhaus & Elger, 1995; Cross *et al.*, 1993, 1997; Duchowny *et al.*, 1992; Fish *et al.*, 1993; Gaillard *et al.*, 1997; Goldstein *et al.*, 1996; Grattan-Smith *et al.*, 1993; Harvey *et al.*, 1993, 1995, 1997; Holopainen *et al.*, 1997; Kuzniecky *et al.*, 1993b; Lawson *et al.*, 1997; Lin *et al.*, 1997; Mathern *et al.*, 1994; Murakami *et al.*, 1996; Pelaez *et al.*, 1997; Sinclair *et al.*, 1997; Wang *et al.*, 1997; Wyllie *et al.*, 1993). Among six reported temporal lobe resection series in children under 17, a mean of 34 per cent had mass lesions on pathological exam, while 31 per cent had MTS, 18 per cent were normal, 7 per cent had developmental pathology and 2 per cent had dual pathology. These differ from the adult distribution because mass lesions were more highly represented. However, that may be a result of selection rather than true incidence. Dual pathology is also rarer in the reported childhood series. MTS is still the most common substrate of nonlesional temporal lobe epilepsy. Among three nonlesional temporal lobe resection series totalling 50 children, Yale included, 90–96 per cent had MTS by MRI. The MRI appearance of atrophy is similar to adults but the T2 signal increase is less frequent. MRI evidence is just as highly correlated with the classical pathological features. The frequency of MTS by MRI in childhood suggests that there is considerable underdiagnosis.

Functional studies have been performed on limited numbers of children with MTLE. PET is as sensitive as in adults, showing interictal hypometabolism in the epileptogenic temporal lobe in 90–100 per cent (Adelson *et al.*, 1992; Brockhaus & Elger, 1995; Holopainen *et al.*, 1997; Wyllie *et al.*, 1993). Our data are consistent; five of six patients with PET studies had unilateral temporal hypometabolism, of whom two were under 8 years. SPECT is less sensitive interictally and more sensitive ictally to the temporal lobe epileptogenic region in children, as in adults (Brockhaus & Elger, 1995; Cross *et al.*, 1997). Neuropsychologic testing has not been extensively reported but our data are consistent with findings in the adult population. Of 10 patients, eight had poor epileptic hemisphere-specific memory, but only two of those had reduced memory mediated by the contralateral hemisphere.

In children also, response to surgical resection of medial temporal structures has been good. The seizure-free rate in collected series of mixed temporal lobe resections is 64 per cent in children under 17 and 72 per cent in children under 12 (Brockhaus & Elger, 1995; Duchowny *et al.*, 1992; Fish *et al.*, 1993; Goldstein *et al.*, 1996; Grattan-Smith *et al.*, 1993; Harvey *et al.*, 1995; Hopkins *et al.*, 1991; Lin *et al.*, 1997; Mizrahi *et al.*, 1990; Pelaez *et al.*, 1997; Sinclair *et al.*, 1997; Wyllie *et al.*, 1993). Most of the remaining patients have at least had substantial reductions in seizure frequency. There are few studies of predictive factors or longterm outcome in children. The Yale series shows 57 per cent seizure-free and 86 per cent good response, without a difference across the age spectrum.

Some of this information, gleaned from adult and childhood literature as well as our own experience, can be distilled to make additional observations about childhood temporal lobe epilepsy. In several series, MTS is the most common lesion: thus it is underdiagnosed in childhood (Cross *et al.*, 1993; Grattan-Smith *et al.*, 1993; Kuzniecky *et al.*, 1993b; Pelaez *et al.*,

1997). MTS, as demonstrated by hippocampal atrophy, can be seen as young as age 2 years (Harvey et al., 1995) (Table 1). At least three series have documented that MTS (inferred from the presence of hippocampal atrophy) can be present at the time of a first seizure (Table 1) (Gaillard et al., 1997; Harvey et al., 1997; Lawson et al., 1997). In reports of MTS under the age of 4, T2 signal change is not present (Adelson et al., 1992; Cross et al., 1997; Duchowny et al., 1992; Gaillard et al., 1997; Mathern et al., 1996; Murakami et al., 1996; Wyllie et al., 1993). The structural accompaniment of increased T2 signal may appear at a later time, but at least the initial presence of HA seems to demonstrate MTS is not a secondary lesion. Whether the T2 signal increase reflects gliosis or sprouting is not established by these observations, but it is not tied to cell loss.

Table 1. MTS in children < 5 years

Author	Age (N)			Dual path (N)	Diagnosis made by		
	0–5 yrs	6–10 yrs	> 10 yrs		MR	qual path	quant path
Yale (unpublished)	2	2	9	3			√
Cross et al.	1	←——— 15		11	√		
Duchowny et al.	1	1	0	2	√	√	
Sinclair et al.	←——— 8			0		√	
Kuzniecky et al.	←——— 2		8				
Fish et al.	←——— 13						
Grattan Smith et al.	←——— 30			9	√	√	
Goldstein et al.	←——— 11			6	√		
Harvey et al.	←——— 13*			3	√		
Murakami et al.	1	1	4		√		
Lawson et al.	←——— 44≠				√		
Adelson et al.	3	←——— 2			√		
Gaillard et al.	6[1]	9[1]	19[1]		√		
Wang et al.	←——— 18				√		
Wyllie et al.	1	3	0		√		
Mathern et al.	1	←——— 3					√

*All new onset seizures; ≠ includes 3 with 1st sz; [1]includes 13 with new onset; qual = qualitative, quant = quantitative, path = pathology, Sz = seizure

Tying the observations of the clinical and structural syndrome to the pathology in childhood is more difficult. Published reports of quantatitive cell counts in the hippocampus or immunohistochemistry for assessment of sprouting in resected medial temporal lobe tissue from children unfortunately reflect the experience at only a single centre (Mathern et al., 1994, 1996, 1997). All other published 'verification' of pathology associated with hippocampal atrophy in childhood is based on qualitative impressions of hippocampal neuronal loss in small numbers of specimens. Based on the data published by Mathern & colleagues from UCLA (1994, 1996), children with medial temporal lobe epilepsy undergoing temporal lobe resection had 70 per cent hippocampal and dentate gyrus neuronal loss, which is comparable to that seen in adults. Some mossy fibre sprouting was noted, but the sprouting was more limited than seen in adult specimens. Children with frequent generalized seizures or temporal lobe lesions but without the classic clinical syndrome of medial temporal lobe epilepsy had 30 per cent hippocampal and dentate gyrus neuronal loss and even less mossy fibre sprouting; the quantitative degree of cell loss was unrelated to age or epilepsy duration, suggesting that it is not a progressive or secondary lesion. At Yale, we studied 14 children under the age of 16 who had nonlesional medial temporal lobe epilepsy and medial temporal lobe resection: five of those children were under the age of 10. We quantitated neuronal density and performed immunohistochemistry. The MTS was pathologically similar in all respects to the adult pattern in children over 10. *All* our children under 10, however, had much more restricted cell loss, confined to CA1 and the hilus, and *no* evidence of reorganization or sprouting. We found highly significant correlations between the presence of sprouting and the age at surgery (ANOVA, $P = 0.005$) or duration of epilepsy ($P < 0.005$) suggesting that this reorganization is a secondary, progressive lesion. But we found no significant relationship between the degree of cell loss, the clinical seizure features, MRI, functional studies, or surgical outcome and the age at surgery or the duration of epilepsy (Table 2), suggesting that, different from the sprouting, the cell loss is not progressive.

Table 2. Cell loss does not increase significantly with age at surgery in MTS

Region	Mean cell counts		
	under 10 ($n = 5$)	10–16 ($n = 9$)	adults ($n = 53$)
CA1	5868	5110	5642
CA2	9238	13459	12655
CA3	9697	9043	9376
CA4	4898	3741	4352
Gran.	199945	187901	173777

All but one of our MTS specimens in children under 16 who had febrile convulsions involved the left hippocampus. Right medial temporal epilepsy occurred in only three of our 14 children, all with additional MRI documented developmental abnormalities or very early seizure onset (under the age of 6 months). These observations, along with those of Fernandez *et al.* (1998), again suggest that the pathologic findings may reflect genetic determinants of certain temporal lobe epilepsy syndromes. Several other reports show a preponderance of *left* MTS in patients with temporal lobe epilepsy and a febrile convulsion history.

These observations can be unified into a single hypothesis. Classical MTS, with hippocampal cell loss greater than 50 per cent, gliosis, and sprouting is likely to be partly essential to, and partly a result of, medial temporal lobe epilepsy. This conclusion comes from comparison of the findings in adults and children, and from the correlations of clinical and electrical variables with pathologic features. Equivalent degrees of at least 50 per cent cell loss in CA1 and the hilus with or without dentate gyrus, and gliosis, appear to be the essential common substrate underlying medial temporal lobe epilepsy at all ages. It is possible that one or more syndromes account for the variable distribution of cell loss in adults, but it is more confined to CA1 and the hilus in children. It is the cell loss and gliosis that are related to the electrical pattern of intracranially recorded temporal lobe seizures (that is common across all age groups) and by extension to the clinical semiology of the syndrome. Hippocampal atrophy is a measurable correlate of this cell loss. On the other hand, sprouting of mossy fibres and fibres immunoreactive for substance P and somastostatin into the inner molecular layer of the dentate is progressive (i.e. related to duration of epilepsy). Hippocampal increased T2 signal may be a measurable correlate of the sprouting since it seems also to be progressive and not essential to the MTLE syndrome: no child under four years has ever been reported with more than minimal sprouting of the mossy fibres, with sprouting of substance P or somatostatin fibres, or with increased T2 signal. The presence and degree of sprouting is, in our patients, directly and significantly related to the age at tissue examination and/or the duration of epilepsy (hard to distinguish from one another). The functional role of this sprouting remains unknown.

This glance into the clinical, electrical, structural and pathologic features of childhood and adult limbic epilepsy of the medial temporal variety provides insight into pathogenesis that has not previously been obtained by study of animal models or adults with this syndrome. This assessment allows approaches to children with temporal lobe epilepsy to utilize experience obtained with adults, as well as provides reasons to investigate developmental determinants of these epileptic syndromes that could open new therapeutic avenues.

References

Adelson, P.D., Peacock, W.J., Chugani, H.T., Comair, Y.G., Vinters, H.V., Shields, W.D. & Shewmon, D.A. (1992): Temporal and extended temporal resections for the treatment of intractable seizures in early childhood. *Pediatr. Neurosurg.* **18**, 169–178.

Babb, T.L. & Brown, W.J. (1987): Pathological findings in epilepsy. In: *Surgical treatment of the epilepsies*, ed. J. Engel, Jr., pp. 511–540. New York: Raven Press.

Babb, T.L., Brown, W.J., Pretorius, J., Davenport, C., Lieb, J.P. & Crandall, P.H. (1984a): Temporal lobe volumetric cell densities in temporal lobe epilepsy. *Epilepsia* **25**, 729–740.

Babb, T.L., Lieb, J.P., Brown, W.J., Pretorius, J. & Crandall, P.H. (1984b): Distribution of cell density and hyperexcitability in the epileptic human hippocampal formation. *Epilepsia* **25**, 721–728.

Babb, T.L., Kupfer, W.R., Pretorius, J.K., Crandall, P.H. & Levesque, M.F. (1991): Synaptic reorganization by mossy fibers in human epileptic *fascia dentata*. *Neuroscience* **42**, 351–363.

Berkovic, S.F., McIntosh, A.M., Kalnins, R.M., Jackson, G.D., Fabinyi, G.C., Brazenor, G.A., Bladin, P.F. & Hopper, J.L. (1995): Preoperative MRI predicts outcome of temporal lobectomy: an actuarial analysis. *Neurology* **45**, 1358–1363.

Berkovic, S.F., McIntosh, A., Howell, R.A., Mitchell, A., Sheffield, L.J. & Hopper, J.L. (1996): Familial temporal lobe epilepsy: a common disorder identified in twins. *Ann. Neurol.* **40**, 227–235.

Brockhaus, A. & Elger, C.E. (1995): Complex partial seizures of temporal lobe origin in children of different age groups. *Epilepsia* **36**, 1173–1181.

Cascino, G.D., Jack, C.R. Jr. & Parisi, J.E. (1991): Magnetic resonance imaging-based volume studies in temporal lobe epilepsy: pathological correlations. *Ann. Neurol.* **30**, 31–36.

Cendes, F., Cook, M.J., Watson, C., Andermann, F., Fish, D.R., Shorvon, S.D., Bergin, P., Free, S., Dubeau, F. & Arnold, D.V. (1995): Frequency and characteristics of dual pathology in patients with lesional epilepsy. *Neurology* **45**, 2058–2064.

Choi, D.W. (1988): Glutamate neurotoxicity and diseases of the nervous system. *Neuron* **1**, 623–634.

Cronin, J. & Dudek, F.E. (1988): Chronic seizures and collateral sprouting of dentate mossy fibers after kainic acid treatment in rats. *Brain Res.* **474**, 181–184.

Cross, J.H., Jackson, G.D., Connelly, A., Kirkham, F.J., Boyd, S.G., Pitt, M.C. & Gadian, D.G. (1993): Early detection of abnormalities in partial epilepsy using magnetic resonance. *Arch. Dis. Child.* **69**, 104–109.

Cross, J.H., Connelly, A., Jackson, G.D., Johnson, C.L., Neville, B.G.R. & Gadian, D.G. (1996): Proton magnetic resonance spectroscopy in children with temporal lobe epilepsy. *Ann. Neurol.* **39**, 107–113.

Cross, J.H., Gordon, I., Connelly, A., Jackson, G.D., Johnson, C.L., Neville, B.G. & Gadian, D.G. (1997): Interictal 99Tcm HMPAO SPECT and HMRS in children with temporal lobe epilepsy. *Epilepsia* **38**, 338–345.

Croucher, M.J., Collins, J.F. & Meldrum, B.S. (1982): Anticonvulsant actions of excitatory amino acid antagonists. *Science* **216**, 899–901.

de Lanerolle, N.C., Kim, J.H., Robbins, R.J. & Spencer, D.D. (1989): Hippocampal interneuron loss and plasticity in human temporal lobe epilepsy. *Brain Res.* **495**, 387–395.

de Lanerolle, N.C., Tompkins, J.R. & Spencer, D.D. (1990): Hippocampal dopamine receptor changes in human temporal lobe epilepsy. *Soc. Neurosci. Abstr.* **16**, 308.

de Lanerolle, N.C., Brines, M.L., Kim, J.H., Williamson, A., Philips, M. & Spencer, D.D. (1992): Neurochemical remodelling of the hippocampus in human temporal lobe epilepsy. In: *Molecular neurobiology of epilepsy*, eds. J. Engel, C. Wasterlain, E.A. Cavalheiro, U. Heinemann & G. Avanzini. *Epilepsy Res.* (Suppl. 9), pp. 205–220. Amsterdam: Elsevier.

de Lanerolle, N.C., Kim, J.H. & Brines, M.L. (1994): Cellular and molecular alterations in partial epilepsy. *Clin. Neurosci.* **2**, 64–81.

Drake, J., Hoffman, H.H., Kobayashi, J., Havarig, P. & Becker, L.F. (1987): Surgical management of children with temporal lobe epilepsy and mass lesions. *Neurosurgery* **21**, 792–797.

Duchowny, M., Levin, B., Jayakar, P., Resnick, T., Alvarez, L., Morrison, G. & Dean, P. (1992): Temporal lobectomy in early childhood. *Epilepsia* **33**, 298–303.

During, M.J. (1994): Dynamic neurochemical alterations in human temporal lobe epilepsy. *Clin. Neurosci.* **2**, 53–63.

During, M.J. & Spencer, D.D. (1993): Extracellular hippocampal glutamate and spontaneous seizure in the conscious human brain. *Lancet* **340**, 1607–1610.

Engel, J. Jr., Brown, W.J., Kuhl, D.E., Phelps, M.E., Mazziotta, J.C. & Crandall, P.H. (1982): Pathological findings underlying focal temporal lobe hypometabolism in partial epilepsy. *Ann. Neurol.* **12**, 518–529.

Fernandez, G., Effenberger, O., Vinz, B., Steinlein, O., Elger, C.E., Dohring, W. & Hemze, H.J. (1998): Hippocampal malformation as a cause of familial febrile convulsions and subsequent hippocampal sclerosis. *Neurology* **50**, 909–917.

Fish, D.R., Smith, S.J., Quesney, L.F., Andermann, F. & Rasmussen, T. (1993): Surgical treatment of children with medically intractable frontal or temporal lobe epilepsy: results and highlights of 40 years' experience. *Epilepsia* **34**, 244–247.

French, J.A., Williamson, P.D., Thadani, V.M., Darcey, T.M., Mattson, R.H., Spencer, S.S. & Spencer, D.D. (1993): Characteristics of medial temporal lobe epilepsy: I. Results of history and physical examination. *Ann. Neurol.* **34**, 774–780.

Gaillard, W.D., Phulwani, P., Dubovsky, E.C., Conry, J., Weinstein, S. & Vezina, L.G. (1997): Mesial temporal sclerosis in children and adolescents. *Epilepsia* **38** (Suppl. 8), 137.

Gloor, P. (1991): Mesial temporal sclerosis: historical background and an overview from a modern perspective. In: *Epilepsy surgery*, ed. H. Lüders, pp. 689–703. New York: Raven Press.

Goldstein, R., Harvey, A.H., Duchowny, M., Jayakar, P., Altman, N., Resnick, T., Levin, B., Dean, P. & Alvarez, L. (1996): Preoperative clinical, EEG, and imaging findings do not predict seizure outcome following temporal lobectomy in childhood. *J. Child. Neurol.* **11**, 445–450.

Grattan-Smith, J.D., Harvey, A.S., Desmond, P.M. & Chow, C.W. (1993): Hippocampal sclerosis in children with intractable temporal lobe epilepsy: detection with MR imaging. *AJR* **161**, 1045–1048.

Harbord, M.G. & Manson, J.I. (1987): Temporal lobe epilepsy in childhood: reappraisal of etiology and outcome. *Pediatr. Neurol.* **3**, 263–268

Harvey, A.S., Bowe, J.M., Hopkins, I.J, Shield, L.K., Cook, D.J. & Berkovic, S.F. (1993): Ictal 99m Tc HMPAO single photon emission computed tomography in children with temporal lobe epilepsy. *Epilepsia* **34**, 869–877.

Harvey, A.S., Grattan-Smith, J.D., Desmond, P.M., Chow, C.W. & Berkovic, S.F. (1995): Febrile seizures and hippocampal sclerosis: frequent and related findings in intractable temporal lobe epilepsy in childhood. *Pediatr. Neurol.* **12**, 201–206.

Harvey, A.S., Berkovic, S.F., Wrennall, J.A. & Hopkins, I.J. (1997): Temporal lobe epilepsy in childhood: clinical, EEG, and neuroimaging findings and syndrome classification in a cohort with new-onset seizures. *Neurology* **49**, 960–968.

Holopainen, I.E., Lundbom, N.M., Metsahonkala, E., Komu, M.E., Sonninen, P.H., Haaparanta, M.T., Bergmann, J.R. & Sillanpaa, M.L. (1997): Temporal lobe pathology in epilepsy: proton magnetic resonance spectroscopy and positron emission tomography study. *Pediatr. Neurol.* **16**, 98–104.

Hopkins, I.J. & Klug, G.L. (1991): Temporal lobectomy for the treatment of intractable complex partial seizures of temporal lobe origin in early childhood. *Dev. Med. Child. Neurol.* **33**, 26–31.

Jung, Y.T., Kim, J.H., de Lanerolle, N., Spencer, S.S. & Spencer, D. (1996): Quantitative study of neuronal heterotopia in temporal lobe epilepsy [Abstract]. *Epilepsia* **37**, 142.

Kim, J., Guimares, P., Shen, M., Masukawa, L. & Spencer, D. (1990): Hippocampal neuronal density in temporal lobe epilepsy with and without gliomas. *Acta Neuropathol.* **80**, 41–45.

King, D. & Spencer, S.S. (1995): Invasive EEG in mesial temporal lobe epilepsy. *J. Clin. Neurophysiol.* **12**, 32–45.

King, D., Spencer, S.S., McCarthy, G., Luby, M. & Spencer, D.D. (1995): Bilateral hippocampal atrophy in medial temporal lobe epilepsy. *Epilepsia* **36**, 905–910.

Kuzniecky, R., Burgard, S., Faught, E., Morawetz, R. & Bartolucci, A. (1993a): Predictive value of magnetic resonance imaging in temporal lobe epilepsy surgery. *Arch. Neurol.* **50**, 65–69.

Kuzniecky, R., Murro, A., King, D., Morawetz R., Smith, J., Powers, R., Yaghmai, F., Faught, E., Gallagher, B. & Snead, O.C. (1993b): Magnetic resonance imaging in childhood intractable partial epilepsies: pathologic correlations. *Neurology* **43**, 681–687.

Lawson, J.A., Cook, M.J., Bleasel, A.F., Nayanar, V., Morris, K.F. & Bye, A.M.E. (1997): Quantitative MRI in outpatient childhood epilepsy. *Epilepsia* **38**, 289–293.

Lencz, T., McCarthy, G. & Bronen, R.A. (1992): Quantitative magnetic resonance imaging in temporal lobe epilepsy: relationship to neuropathology and neuropsychological function. *Ann. Neurol.* **31**, 629–637.

Lin, E., So, G.M., Schmid, R. et al. (1997): Outcome of temporal lobectomy in children with bitemporal EEG abnormalities. *Epilepsia* **38** (Suppl. 8), 51.

Loring, D.W., Lee, G.P., Martin, R.C. & Meador, K.J. (1988): Material-specific learning in patients with partial complex seizures of temporal lobe origin: convergent validation of memory constructs. *J. Epilepsy* **1**, 53–59.

Manno, E.M., Sperling, M.R., Ding, X., Jaggi, J. Alavi, A., O'Connor, M.J. & Reivich, M. (1994): Predictors of outcome after anterior temporal lobectomy: positron emission tomography. *Neurology* **44**, 2331–2336.

Margerison, J.H. & Corsellis, J.A.N. (1966): Epilepsy and the temporal lobes: a clinical, electroencephalographic and neuropathologic study of the brain in epilepsy with particular reference to the temporal lobes. *Brain* **89**, 499–563.

Marks, D.A., Kim, J., Spencer, D.D. & Spencer, S.S. (1992): Characteristics of intractable seizures following meningitis and encephalitis. *Neurology* **42**, 1513–1519.

Marks, D.A., Kim, J., Spencer, D.D. & Spencer, S.S. (1995): Seizure localization and pathology following head injury in patients with uncontrolled epilepsy. *Neurology* **45**, 2051–2058.

Mathern, G.W., Lete, J.P., Pretorius, J.K., Quinn, B., Peacock, W.J. & Babb, T.L. (1994): Children with severe epilepsy: evidence of hippocampal neuron losses and aberrant mossy fiber sprouting during postnatal granule cell migration and differentiation. *Dev. Brain Res.* **78**, 70–80.

Mathern, G.W., Babb, T.L., Mischel, P.S., Vinters, H.V., Pretorius, J.K., Leite, J.P. & Peacock, W.J. (1996): Childhood generalized and mesial temporal epilepsies demonstrate different amounts and patterns of hippocampal neuron loss and mossy fiber synaptic reorganization. *Brain* **119,** 965–987.

Mathern, G.W., Kuhlman, P.A., Mendoza, D. & Pretorius, J.K. (1997): Human *fascia dentata* anatomy and hippocampal neuron densities differ depending on the epileptic syndrome and age at first seizure. *J. Neuropath. Exp. Neurol.* **56,** 199–212.

Meldrum, B.S. & Corsellis, J.A.N. (1984): In: *Greenfield's neuropathology,* eds. J.H. Adams, J.A.N. Corsellis & L.W. Duchen, pp. 921–95. New York: Wiley.

Mizrahi, E.M., Kellaway, P., Grossman, R.G., Rutecki, P.A., Armstrong, D., Rettig, G. & Loewen, S. (1990): Anterior temporal lobectomy and medically refractory temporal lobe epilepsy of childhood. *Epilepsia* **31,** 302–312.

Mouritzen-Dam, A. (1982): Hippocampal neuron loss in epilepsy and after experimental seizures. *Acta Neurol. Scand.* **66,** 601–642.

Murakami, N., Ohno, S., Oka, E. & Tanaka, A. (1996): Mesial temporal lobe epilepsy in childhood. *Epilepsia* **37** (Suppl. 3), 52–56.

O'Connor, E.R., Sontheimer, H., Spencer, D.D. & de Lanerolle, N.C. (1998): Astrocytes from human hippocampal epileptogenic foci exhibit action potential-like responses. *Epilepsia* **39**.

Pelaez, J., Wyllie, E. & Bulacio, J. (1997): Epilepsy surgery for hippocampal sclerosis in preadolescent children. *Epilepsia* **38** (Suppl. 8), 72.

Raymond, A.A., Fish, D.R., Stevens, J.M., Cook, M.J., Sisodiya, S.M. & Shorvon, S.D. (1994): Association of hippocampal sclerosis with cortical dysgenesis in patients with epilepsy. *Neurology* **44,** 1841–1845.

Sass, K.J., Sass, A., Westerveld, M., Lencz, T., Novelly, R.A. Kim, J.H. & Spencer, D.D. (1992): Specificity in the correlation of verbal memory and hippocampal neuron loss: dissociation of memory, language, and verbal intellectual ability. *J. Clin. Exp. Neuropsychol.* **14,** 662–672.

Sinclair, D.B., Aronyk, K., Bhargava, R. *et al.* (1997): 'Pure mesial temporal sclerosis' in paediatric temporal lobectomy. *Epilepsia* **38** (Suppl. 8), 221.

Sloviter, R.S. (1991): Permanently altered hippocampal structure, excitability, and inhibition after experimental status epilepticus in the rat: the 'dormant basket cell' hypothesis and its possible relevance to temporal lobe epilepsy. *Hippocampus* **1,** 41–66.

Spencer, S.S. (1993): Temporal lobectomy: selection of candidates. In: *The treatment of epilepsy: principles and practice*, ed. E. Wyllie, pp. 1062–1074. Malvern, PA: Lea and Febiger.

Spencer, S.S. (1996): Longterm outcome after epilepsy surgery. *Epilepsia* **37,** 807–813.

Spencer, S.S. (1998): Substrates of localization-related epilepsies: biologic implications of localizing findings in humans. *Epilepsia* **39,** 114–123.

Spencer, S.S., Williamson, P.D., Spencer, D.D. & Mattson, R.H. (1990): Combined depth and subdural electrode investigations of uncontrolled epilepsy. *Neurology* **40,** 74–79.

Spencer, S.S., Marks, D., Katz, A., Kim, J. & Spencer, D.D. (1992): Anatomical correlates of interhippocampal seizure propagation time. *Epilepsia* **33,** 862–873.

Spencer, S.S., McCarthy, G. & Spencer, D.D. (1993a): Diagnosis of medial temporal lobe seizure onset: relative specificity and sensitivity of quantitative MRI. *Neurology* **43,** 2117–2125.

Spencer, S.S., So, N.K., Engel, J., Williamson, P.D., Levesque, M.F. & Spencer, D.D. (1993b): Depth electrodes. In: *Surgical treatment of the epilepsies,* 2nd edn., ed. J. Engel, Jr., pp. 359–376. New York: Raven Press.

Spencer, S.S., Berg, A.T. & Spencer, D.D. (1994): Predictors of remission one year after resective epilepsy surgery. *Epilepsia* **34** (Suppl. 6), 27.

Spencer, S.S., Berkovic, S. & Theodore, W. (1995): Clinical applications: MRI, SPECT and PET. *Magn. Reson. Imaging* **13,** 1119–1124.

Spencer, S., Kim, J., de Lanerolle, N. & Spencer, D. (1997): Intracranial EEG seizure patterns and pathology in temporal lobe epilepsy [Abstract]. *Epilepsia* **38** (Suppl. 8), 212.

Spencer, S.S., Sperling, M. & Shewman, A. (1998): Intracranial electrodes. In: *Epilepsy, a comprehensive textbook*, eds. J. Engel, Jr. & T.A. Pedley, pp. 1719–1748. New York: Lippincott-Raven.

Stefan, H., Bauer, J., Feistel, H., Schulemann, H., Neubauer, U., Wenzel, B., Wolf, F., Neundorfer, B. & Huk, W.J. (1990): Regional cerebral blood flow during focal seizures of temporal and frontocentral onset. *Ann. Neurol.* **27**, 162–166.

Sutula, T., Cascino, G., Cavazos, J., Pavada, I. & Ramirez, L. (1989a): Mossy fiber synaptic reorganization in the epileptic human temporal lobe. *Ann. Neurol.* **26**, 321–330.

Sutula, T., Xiao-Xian, H., Cavazos, J. & Scott, G. (1989b): Synaptic reorganization in the hippocampus induced by abnormal functional activity. *Science* **239**, 1147–1150.

Theodore, W.H. (1994): Insights from functional neuroimaging in the localization and definition of focal epilepsy. *Clin. Neurosci.* **2**, 89–95.

Wang, P., Lin, H., Fan, P. *et al.* (1997): Magnetic resonance imaging in symptomatic/cryptogenic partial epilepsies of infants and children. *Acta Paed. Sing.* **38**, 127–136.

Wieser, H.G., Engel, J. Jr., Williamson, P.D., Babb, T.L. & Gloor, P. (1993): Surgically remediable temporal lobe syndromes. In: *Surgical treatment of the epilepsies*, ed. J. Engel, Jr., pp. 49–63. New York: Raven Press.

Williamson, P.D., French, J.A., Thadani, V.M., Kim, J.H., Novelly, R.A., Spencer, S.S., Spencer, D.D. & Mattson, R.H. (1993): Characteristics of medial temporal lobe epilepsy: II. Interictal and ictal scalp electroencephalography, neuropsychological testing, neuroimaging, surgical results, and pathology. *Ann. Neurol.* **34**, 781–787.

Wyllie, E., Chee, M., Granstrom, M., del Guidice, E., Estes, M., Conair, V., Pizzi, M., Kotagal, P., Bourgeovis, B. & Lüders, H. (1993): Temporal lobe epilepsy in early childhood. *Epilepsia* **34**, 859–868.

Chapter 6

Loss of contact and impairment of consciousness

Roberto Mai, Stefano Francione, Francesco Cardinale, Giorgio Lo Russo and Claudio Munari

Centro Regionale per la Chirurgia dell'Epilessia, Ospedale Niguarda Ca' Granda, Piazza Ospedale Maggiore 3, 20162 Milan, Italy

Summary

Despite the ILAE International Classification guidelines, the definition of consciousness remains somewhat difficult for the neurologist, mostly in terms of basic neuronal mechanisms. The aim of the present study is to examine a group of children with symptomatic partial epilepsy in order to investigate whether loss of contact is related to the involvement of limbic structures by seizure activity. The role of these structures is assessed as to the production of the symptom 'loss of contact' by analysing electroclinical correlations.

Our investigation in a limited number of children shows that limbic structures can be involved in seizures with or without loss of contact. These results are preliminary because of the heterogeneity and the small number of the population. In any case, loss of contact does not seem to present a localizing value, especially as far as the limbic structures are concerned. These data are in agreement with other authors who found that ictal loss of contact may occur during seizures that arise in the temporal neocortex and never involve mesial temporal limbic structures. Therefore, the impairment of contact appears to be related more to the extent, duration and/or modalities of the discharge rather than to the involvement of a precise anatomical structure.

Introduction

The fundamental distinction between simple partial and complex partial seizures is the presence or the impairment of the fully conscious state (Commission on Classification, 1981). In fact 'a partial seizure is classified primarily on the basis of whether or not consciousness is impaired during the attack' (Commission on Classification, 1981). Moreover the same classification states that 'in patients with impaired consciousness aberrations of behaviour (automatisms) may occur'. Finally we got a definition of impaired consciousness 'as the inability to respond normally to exogenous stimuli by virtue of altered awareness and/or responsiveness'.

Despite the guidelines of the International Classification, the definition of consciousness remains somewhat difficult for the neurologist (and the philosopher, too) especially in terms of the basic neuronal mechanisms. Gloor in 1986 wondered whether 'consciousness really represents a workable neurological concept in epileptology and in neurology in general'; after several thoughtful pages he concluded that in epileptology the terms 'loss' or 'impairment of consciousness' were inadequate. For these reasons we prefer to speak of 'loss of contact'.

In clinical practice the common way to ascertain loss of contact is to ask relevant questions and to do relevant manoeuvres, but this requires the observer to:

- Be there at the very beginning of the seizure;
- Be prepared to the particular seizure of the patient;
- Be prepared to test those functions that could be impaired in the individual seizure (motor, verbal, visual, etc).

However testing the contact of the patient during the seizures remains a difficult task for several reasons, such as:

- Lack of motor response;
- Lack of verbal output (anarthria);
- Aphasia;
- Diversion of attention (i.e. hallucinations).

The aim of the present study is to examine a group of children with symptomatic partial epilepsy to investigate whether loss of contact is related to involvement of limbic structures by seizures activity, assessing the role of these structures in producing the symptom 'loss of contact' by analysing electroclinical correlations.

Material and methods

From May 1996 to February 1998, 13 children (i.e. age under 16 years) with drug-resistant partial epilepsy were investigated at the Regional Centre for Epilepsy Surgery of the Niguarda Hospital in Milan by mean of stereoelectroencephalography (SEEG) exploration (Bancaud et al., 1965) in view of surgical intervention (Talairach et al., 1974). Among them nine children had at least one electrode exploring an anatomical component of the limbic system.

The children were seven males and two females. The mean age at the time of SEEG investigation was 7.6 years (range 5–15 years). The mean age of onset of epilepsy was 2.7 years (range 1 month–12 years). The mean duration of epilepsy was 5.2 years (range 1–10 years). The seizure frequency was daily in all patients.

Three patients were investigated bilaterally, although only one had a bilateral symmetric implantation, while five patients were investigated in the right hemisphere and one patient in the left hemisphere only. The investigations were performed with 114 multilead (5–15 contacts) electrodes implanted on the basis of previously gathered individual anatomical and electroclinical data. There were 34 in the left hemisphere and 80 in the right hemisphere (Fig. 1). Among these, 42 electrodes investigated an anatomical structure of the limbic structures (13 in left hemisphere and 29 in right hemisphere) (Fig. 2). We recorded a total of 63 seizures that were analysed on the basis of both direct observation and videotape recording.

For each seizure we ascertained the onset of loss of contact and in the corresponding EEG

Results

Out of the total 63 recorded seizures, 25 in five patients were not suitable for assessment (i.e. seizure too short, patient sleeping, outside of the camera, etc.), and seven in four patients were not assessed or assessment was inadequate. Twelve seizures in four patients did not include loss of contact; 19 seizures in seven patients presented with loss of contact.

Table 1 illustrates recorded seizures for each patient in detail, specifying, for each reliably assessed seizure, discharge localization with reference to presence or absence of loss of contact. In one patient all seizures were too short to assess (despite the high number recorded); in four patients all seizures were with loss of contact; three patients had seizures both with and without loss of contact and only one had seizures without loss of contact.

Table 1.

Pt	Recorded seizures	With loss of contact	EEG activity	Without loss of contact	EEG activity	Epileptogenic zone
F.A.	8	7	2 theta rhythmic discharge in A; 1 LVFA in A, H and TN; 1 SW in A, H and TN; 3 theta rhythmic discharge in A, H and TN	0	–	Right and left temporal
Z.D.	8	3	3 LVFA in mesial preR and R region	1	1 LVFA in mesial R region	Left parieto-central
Br. M.	5	2	2 SW and LVFA in mesial rolandic region	1	1 flattening in mesial rolandic region	Right parieto-centro-temporal
L.A.	7	1	1 LVFA in F3 (inferior frontal gyrus)	2	1 flattening in A and H associated with SW in F3	Right fronto-central
R.F.	2	1	1 SW in FC region	0	–	Right fronto-precentral
N.S.	4	3	3 SW in fronto-basal (orbital cortex) and TN	0	–	Right frontal
B.M.	8	0	–	8	8 flattening in F2 (middle frontal gyrus)	Right frontal
C.V.	3	2	2 LVFA in FC region and anterior GC	0	–	Right centrral

A = amygdala; H = hippocampus; TN = temporal neocortex; preR = prerolandic; R = rolandic; FC = fronto-central; GC = gyrus cinguli; LVFA = low voltage fast activity; SW = spike-wave.

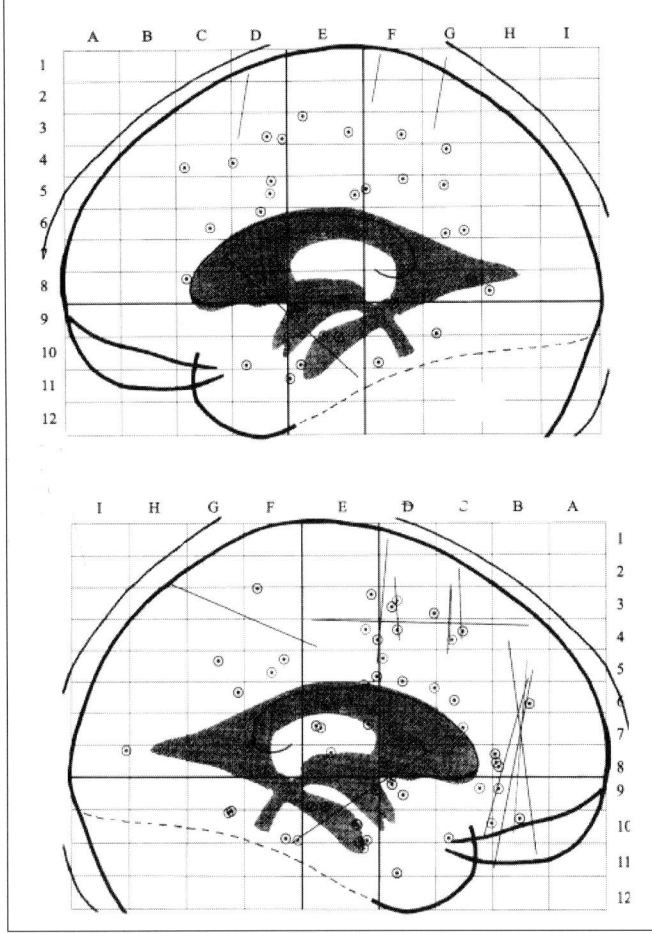

Fig. 1.

Out of 12 seizures without loss of contact (Table 2) none involved exclusively the limbic structure, 11 seizures started outside the limbic lobe and only one seizure involved both limbic structures (amygdala and hippocampus) and the inferior frontal gyrus.

Among 19 seizures with loss of contact (Table 3) two involved only the amygdala, seven seizures involved both limbic and extralimbic structures, and 10 involved only structures outside the limbic system.

Discussion

The study of epileptic patients in a surgical perspective requires a correct assessment of the localizing value of clinical symptoms, especially at the onset of the epileptic seizures. First and foremost, we must point out that 32 seizures (more than 50 per cent) could not be assessed for technical or clinical reasons. This appears even more relevant given that these data come from a Centre where direct surveillance of patients by skilled examiners is given primary importance, rather than letting the camera document the seizures. This observation emphasizes the difficulty to assess such an elusive clinical sign as loss of contact.

Table 2. Twelve seizures without 'loss of contact' (SEEG analysis)

B	1 flattenining in amygdala and hippocampus associated with SW in F3
E	8 flattening in F2 (middle frontal gyrus)
E	1 flattening in F3 (inferior frontal gyrus)
E	1 flattening in mesial rolandic region
E	1 LVFA in mesial rolandic region

L = limbic structures; B = both limbic and extralimbic structures; E = extralimbic structures.

As far as patients are concerned:

— The only one who presents exclusively seizures without loss of contact has a right frontal epileptogenic zone with discharges limited to F2;

— Four patients present only seizures with loss of contact;

— Three patients present both seizures with and without loss of contact.

Although seizures without loss of contact seem to be more often related to discharges involving extralimbic structures (11/12 – see Table 1), in some cases discharges extending to limbic structures do not produce loss of contact. By the same token, loss of contact may follow an 'isolated' discharge in one or more limbic structure(s), but it is by no means rare that this symptom be brought about by discharges involving extralimbic structures (10/19 – see Table 1).

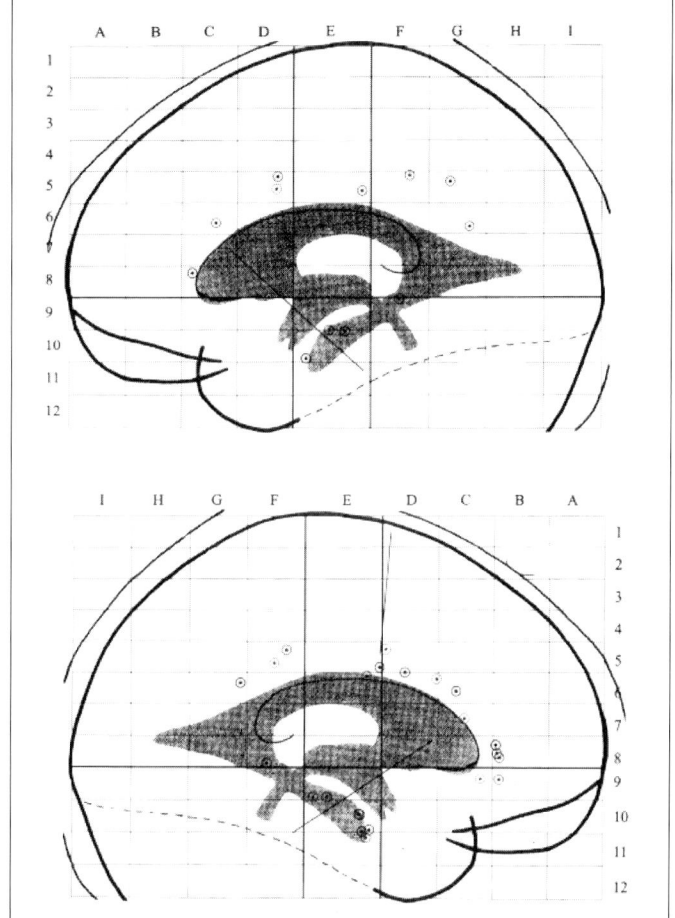

Fig. 2.

Table 3. Nineteen seizures with 'loss of contact' (SEEG analysis)

L	2 theta rhythmic discharge in amygdala
B	2 LVFA in fronto-central region and anterior gyrus cinguli
B	1 LVFA in amygdala, hippocampus and temporal neocortex
B	3 theta rhythmic discharge in amygdala, hippocampus and temporal neocortex
B	1 SW in amygdala, hippocampus and temporal neocortex
E	2 SW and LVFA in mesial rolandic region
E	3 LVFA in mesial prerolandic and rolandic region
E	1 SW in fronto-central region
E	3 SW in fronto-basal (orbital cortex) and temporal neocortex
E	1 LVFA in F3 (inferior frontal gyrus)

L = limbic structures; B = both limbic and extralimbic structures; E = extralimbic structures.

Our investigation in a limited number of children shows that limbic structures can be involved in seizures with or without loss of contact. These results are preliminary because of the heterogeneity and the small number of the population. In any case loss of contact does not seem to have a localizing value, especially as far as the limbic structures are concerned. Our data are in agreement with other authors who found that ictal loss of contact may occur during seizures that arise in the temporal neocortex and never involve mesial temporal limbic structures (Williamson, *et al.*, 1985). Therefore, the impairment of contact appears to be related more to the extent, duration and/or modalities of the discharge rather than to the involvement of a precise anatomical structure (Munari *et al.*, 1980; Munari *et al.*, 1982).

References

Bancaud, J., Talairach, J., Bonis, A., Schaub, C., Szikla, G., Morel, P. & Bordas-Ferrer, M. (1965): *La stéréo-électro-encéphalographie dans l'épilepsie*. Paris: Masson.

Commission on Classification and Terminology of the International League Against Epilepsy (1981): Proposal for revised clinical and electroencephalographic classification of epileptic seizures. *Epilepsia* **22**, 489–501.

Gloor, P. (1986): Consciousness as a neurological concept in epileptology: a critical review. *Epilepsia* **27**(2), S14–S26.

Munari, C., Bancaud, J., Bonis, A., Stoffels, C., Szikla, G. & Talairach, J. (1980): Impairment of consciousness in temporal lobe seizure: a stereoelectroencephalographic study. In: *Advances in epileptology: XIth Epilepsy International Symposium,* eds. R. Canger, F. Angeleri, K. Penry, pp. 111–114. New York: Raven Press.

Munari, C., Stoffels, C., Bossi, L., Brunet, P., Bonis, A., Bancaud, J. & Talairach, J. (1982): Partial seizures with elementary or complex symptomatology: a valid classification for temporal lobe seizures? In: *Advances in epileptology: XIIIth Epilepsy International Symposium*, eds. H. Akimoto, H. Kazamatsuri, M. Seino & A. Ward, pp. 25–27. New York: Raven Press.

Talairach, J., Bancaud, J., Szikla, G., Bonis, A., Geier, S. & Vedrenne, C. (1974): Approche nouvelle de la neurochirurgie de l'épilepsie. Méthodologie stéréotaxique et résultats thérapeutiques. *Neurochirurgie* **20**(1), 1–240.

Williamson, P.D., Spencer, D.D., Spencer, S.S., Novelly, R.A. & Mattson, R.H. (1985): Complex partial seizures of frontal lobe origin. *Ann. Neurol.* **18**, 497–504.

Chapter 7

Neuro-vegetative manifestations in temporo-limbic seizures

Dominique Broglin

Centre Saint Paul, Hôpital Henri Gastaut, 300 Boulevard Sainte-Marguerite, 13009 Marseille, France

Summary

Observed in virtually all types of seizures, autonomic manifestations (AM) have undoubtedly their most prominent basis in partial seizures, especially those originating from, or involving, the mesio-temporal and limbic structures. In these seizures, sensorial and motor, polymodal AM are very common, especially as aura or early signs. Their main characteristics and meaning, summarized below, are well known in adults and adolescents. Conversely, in children and even more in infants, until now only few data are available; however, from literature studies and personal results, in proven temporal lobe seizures, some age-specific features appear. In young patients, AM are globally the same as, and when specially studied, about as frequent as in older ones, with most commonly cardio-vascular, ocular, digestive and respiratory AM. Of course, before the age of speech, viscero-motor signs, particularly vasomotor, respiratory and digestive, are predominant. But very young children prove they are able to correctly describe many subjective AM, especially epigastric feelings or 'aura' which appear, like in adults, as the most significant vegetative symptom among very numerous AM. So, even from this very young age, thorough questioning is paramount. As in adults, AM have no localizing value if taken in isolation, but only an indicative value in the global ictal pattern. Epigastric aura followed by early chewing automatisms are highly suggestive of an involvement of the amygdala by the discharge; AM associated with negative affective symptoms, such as fear, suggest strongly a temporo-limbic or even more fronto-cingulate discharge. Otherwise, the global pattern of temporal lobe seizures appears similar to adults in children over 6 years; under this age, the younger the children are, the more crude and predominantly motor the ictal pattern is.

For many centuries, in fact as early as the Hippocratic era, neuro-vegetative symptoms and signs had been described as occurring in different fits affecting the humans (Temkin, 1945). Retrospectively, in a few exemplary descriptions the epileptic nature of the attacks may appear to us probable or even almost sure. However it is only much more recently, during the 19th century, that the clinical phenomenology of such fits, including epileptic seizures, has been rationally studied. Several famous doctors provided very accurate descriptions and sharp interpretations (Gowers, 1885; Herpin, 1867; Trousseau, 1868; Jackson (see Taylor, 1931)). Especially they presumed or maintained: firstly the epileptic origin of numerous neuro-vegetative paroxysmal manifestations observed in their practice; secondly the high frequency of neuro-vegetative manifestations in epileptic seizures; and thirdly their often inaugural or early occurence in the course of a seizure. Later descriptions, many of them no longer based only on the clinical signs but on the correlation between the clinical seizure and the EEG, confirmed that neuro-vegetative – or autonomic – manifestations are very common in epileptic seizures (Lennox & Cobb, 1933; Marchand & de Ajuriaguerra, 1948; Penfield & Kristiansen, 1951; Mulder *et al.*, 1954; Penfield & Jasper 1954).

Autonomic manifestations in epileptic seizures

Autonomic manifestations (AM) occur in virtually all types of seizures (Gastaut & Broughton, 1972). For instance, AM are constant and massive in generalized tonic–clonic seizures, either spontaneous or induced (Wannamaker, 1985), and usual in tonic seizures (Beaumanoir & Dravet, 1992); but careful observations show that AM are also quite common in the non-convulsive generalized absence seizures (Penry *et al.*, 1975; Loiseau, 1992).

However, AM undoubtedly present a particular interest in partial seizures due to their frequency, diversity and richness and finally because they raise the question of their potential localizing value. Modern tools and methods – recordings of spontaneous seizures, results of cortical electrical stimulations, and more recently long-term video-EEG monitoring ideally coupled with an active perictal examination – have all greatly improved our knowledge of the semiology of partial seizures. In this respect, some points are crucial: first, the initial manifestations which may be subjective symptoms – the aura – and/or objective signs; second, the spatio-temporal occurrence of ictal symptoms and signs and the relationship between them; and finally the global pattern (the 'Gestalt') of the seizure taken as a dynamic entity whose components do not occur randomly but are meaningfully interrelated according to the brain structures the ictal discharge involves.

On these conceptual grounds, several authors have confirmed, in adolescents and adults, the high frequency of AM in partial seizures as well as their very common early occurrence (Penfield & Kristiansen, 1951; Penfield & Jasper 1954; Daly, 1975; Bancaud, 1976; Wieser & Williamson 1993) especially, but not only, in seizures of temporal lobe origin (Gastaut, 1980; Bancaud, 1987; Wieser, 1983, 1986, 1987; Broglin & Bancaud, 1991; French *et al.*, 1993; Wieser *et al.*, 1993) and frontal (Swartz & Delgado-Escueta, 1987; Bancaud & Talairach, 1992; Broglin *et al.*, 1992; Chauvel *et al.*, 1992).

Conversely, the data remain rather scarce in children, notably the youngest ones. This appears due to two main reasons: first of all, the difficulty of studying ictal semiology in young children, especially before the age of fluent speech; and also the relatively recent development of surgical treatment in children with partial epilepsy, since an important part of our knowledge of the semiology of partial seizures remains indeed derived from ictal video-EEG recordings performed during pre-surgical evaluations (Wyllie *et al.*, 1993, Wyllie, 1995). We summarize some of the most significant published data on proven temporal lobe seizures in children and infants, and then add personal data, some of them concerning pre-adolescents and children.

Autonomic manifestations in temporal lobe seizures in children: the literature

Numerous papers (Glaser, 1967; Holmes, 1986; Duchowny, 1987; Yamamoto *et al.*, 1987; Blume, 1989; Dravet *et al.*, 1989; Luna *et al.*, 1989; Jayakar & Duchowny, 1990; Wyllie *et al.*, 1993; Aicardi, 1994; Bye & Foo, 1994; Brockhaus & Elger, 1995; Harvey *et al.*, 1997; Rathgeb *et al.*, 1998) have dealt with the semiology of partial seizures, especially complex partial, in young adolescents, children and infants. However, in many of these studies the modes of selection of patients differ, as well as the methods used to investigate both the semiology of the seizures and the underlying epileptic syndrome. Therefore: firstly, the results are unavoidably heterogenous and difficult to compare; secondly, these studies undoubtedly include partial seizures of different localization, mainly temporal and frontal, but also originating from other brain regions; and finally the exact seizure origin or localization may remain doubtful, particularly because EEG data are only based upon scalp-ictal, or even in some cases scalp-inter-ictal, recordings. In addition, none of these studies was especially dedicated to the analysis of AM; and in some of them AM are not at all mentioned. Actually only a small number of studies include either a confident or a sound determination of the seizure localization, and even fewer published studies dealing only with partial seizures of temporal lobe origin or in which the temporal lobe origin was definitely proven by depth-EEG recordings and/or long-term disappearance of seizures after temporal lobe surgery.

Bye & Foo (1994) analysed 87 complex partial seizures recorded in 17 patients, aged 7 months to 10 years (mean 6.5 years), 15/17 suffering from a medically intractable partial epilepsy. All patients underwent a video-scalp-EEG monitoring and three had an intra-cranial ictal recording. Nine patients showed a brain lesion on the MRI. Seizure localization was temporal in five patients, frontal in five patients and remained unknown in the others, except two. The authors found an aura in nine children (53%). There was a clear predominance of digestive manifestations: six/nine children, five with an 'abdominal discomfort' and one with nausea. Four of these six patients had a temporal lobe origin of seizures. Autonomic objective signs occured in six patients, mainly vasomotor and ocular manifestations (five/six).

Harvey *et al.* (1997) studied 63 children aged 3 months to 16 years (mean 7.5 years) with a diagnosis of a new- or recent-onset temporal lobe epilepsy, founded on clinical, EEG and MRI investigations. Temporal lobe epilepsy diagnosis was made 'when there was agreement that the child's episodes were typical or, at least consistent with, partial seizures of temporal lobe origin and that no alternate diagnosis was likely'. Clinical seizures were directly observed in all children but recorded by video-scalp-EEG in only 18. The authors state that 'autonomic features were prominent in most children', mainly of visceromotor types: various vaso-motor changes (71 times in the 63 children); tachycardia (nine times); retching or vomiting (12 times); pupillary changes (nine times) and lacrimation (three times); apnoea (six times) and micturition (14 times). An aura was present (23 children) or likely (19 children) without an available description of the content.

Jayakar and Duchowny (1990) studied retrospectively 126 complex partial seizures, only of temporal lobe origin, in 26 young patients. A majority of subjects under 6 years with a significant number of infants was enrolled in this study. Patients were divided into three categories by age: infants (2 years, 11 patients), pre-school children (2–6 years, seven patients) and pre-adolescents (6–12 years, eight patients). The unilateral temporal lobe origin of partial seizures was documented by ictal video-EEG recordings and the onset of the discharge was always on the same side in 24/26 patients. In the whole population, the authors reported very few AM, either as initial clinical ictal manifestations or later during the seizures. Seemingly, no AM was observed or reported in the 18 patients under 6 years; however, the authors recorded 22 seizures in eight patients in the two subgroups of age 6 with 'uncertain' initial clinical manifestations. Indeed only two children, in the oldest subgroup, had ictal autonomic manifestations, which were objective viscero-motor signs in both cases, vomiting and salivation respectively. Three patients between 6 and 12 years showed a facial expression change (smile in two patients, appearance of fear in the third) without further description of a possible associated subjective content. And finally no patient was reported as presenting with an aura and/or initial ictal signs comprising one or several AM. Several explanations of low occurrence of AM may be conceivable. First, the young age of patients with a high proportion of infants; then, initial manifestations of seizures were often missed by parents or nurses, especially in infants, therefore slight or purely subjective AM may have been unrecognized, and the authors did not expressly study the AM or report especially on subjective symptoms, even in the oldest children.

Wyllie et al. (1993) reported on 14 children who were seizure-free after anterior temporal lobectomy, with a post-operative follow-up from 6 months to 3 years (mean 16 months). At the time of video-EEG, patients were aged 16 months to 12 years (mean 8 years); actually, all children but one were 5 years or more and 11/14 between 8 and 12 years. In all patients a detailed pre-surgical evaluation was performed, including video-EEG ictal recordings for all subjects included in the study. Overall, 151 videotaped complex partial seizures were reviewed (one to 29 seizures per patient, mean 11). The dominant aetiology was low grade brain tumor in nine patients and otherwise one case of cortical dysplasia and four cases with MRI suggestive of unilateral Ammon's horn sclerosis (without available pathological confirmation). Globally, AM are rather uncommon but this study was not at all specially focused on AM. Four children (between 5 and 9 years) had an abdominal ('stomach ache', two/four patients) or a gustatory ('bad or funny taste') aura, all of them presenting with a presumed Ammon's horn sclerosis on the MRI and a seizure-free post-operative outcome. According to the authors, these auras 'were typical of those described by adolescents and adults with mesiotemporal lobe epilepsy'. Otherwise, the authors consider implicitly the gustatory feelings they observed as suggestive of a mesiotemporal origin of the discharge; this may remain a matter of debate since, according to others, gustatory hallucinations depend on discharges involving the supra-sylvian opercular neo-cortex (Bancaud, 1987; Hausser-Hauw & Bancaud, 1987). Otherwise, two children reported an aura with possible some autonomic features, namely unpleasant head feeling, without further available details. Finally, an 8-year-old child with a ganglioglioma had gagging, retching or vomiting during his seizures.

Brockhaus and Elger (1995) studied 83 complex partial seizures of temporal lobe origin (1–10 seizures per patient, mean three) in a selected population of 29 children who underwent a resective temporal lobe neurosurgery for a medically intractable partial epilepsy. As part of the pre-surgical evaluation, a continuous video-EEG (all patients) or ECoG (13 patients) monitoring was performed. On the whole, patients were 18 months to 16 years old (mean 11 years), with a majority (23/29) after the age of 6. They were divided into three subgroups by age: pre-school (18 months–6 years, 6 patients), school age (7–12 years, 10 patients) and adolescents (13–16 years, 13 patients). MRI was negative in five patients and showed a unilateral temporal lesion in the 24 others, a low grade tumour in 18/24 cases. Surgical resections were as follows: anterior two-thirds temporal lobe resection (17 patients) with hippocampectomy in 13; lesionectomy with or without hippocampectomy (10 patients); and selective amygdalohippocampectomy in two patients. The unilateral temporal lobe origin of seizures was confirmed on the basis of all pre-surgical data – especially the electroclinical pattern of the seizures – as well as of the post-operative outcome. From this point of view, with a mean post-operative follow-up of 21.5 months, 24/29 patients were seizure-free, one patient had isolated auras and four had at least a 75 per cent reduction of pre-surgery seizure frequency. As in several other studies considered above, ictal AM appeared rather uncommon in this population. Indeed, the authors found only five children over 6 years, who reported an epigastric sensation as the aura of their seizures. Otherwise, six children had a fearful expression at the start of their seizures; but there seemed to be no eventual concomitant AM. Again, several explanations of these facts can be hypothesized. Firstly, as in the study by Wyllie *et al.* (1993), AM were not particularly studied. Secondly, auras were noted only according to visible signs on the videotape or to spontaneous verbal announcement of subjective symptoms by children. And so, rather unsurprisingly an aura was reported by almost half of the children aged over 6 years, but only by one of the six patients under 6.

Michel (1999) studied a small series of five children, aged 10 to 14 years (mean 12 years). Twenty-three seizures were recorded (three to eight seizures per patient), 13 of them during a stereo-electroencephalography (SEEG). All children became seizure-free after an individually tailored temporal cortectomy, with a post-surgery follow-up of at least 2 years. In contrast to some of the above mentioned results, AM appeared more frequent in this very small sample: four children reported an epigastric aura, and the last had an impossible-to-describe feeling then a sensation in her mouth; fear was associated in three patients; finally vaso-motor changes in the face were very common.

Autonomic manifestations in temporal lobe seizures: personal data

We previously studied a population of 233 patients, mainly young adults, hospitalized at the neurosurgical department of the Sainte Anne Hospital, Paris, because of intractable partial epilepsy and who were eligible for a pre-surgical evaluation (Broglin & Bancaud, 1991). Out of all patients, 26 were preadolescents or children and aged 4 to 15 years (mean 11 years) with the majority of them aged 8 or more (21 patients). During the pre-surgical evaluation, 1707 partial seizures were recorded in these 233 patients (one to 13 seizures per patient), and 103 seizures in the paediatric sugbgroup (one to nine seizures per patient). In all seizures, a direct observation and an interactive examination were performed by a neurologist or by a well-trained observer; and in most of them a videotape recording was available.

The temporal lobe origin of these seizures was proven by SEEG, performed in all patients, according to the methodology described by Bancaud & Talairach (Bancaud *et al.*, 1965). In the vast majority of these seizures, the epileptic discharge involved, from the start or during the first twenty seconds, mesiotemporal limbic structures (amygdala, hippocampus and para-hippocampal gyrus) and some limbic cortical areas, such as temporo-polar cortex, cingulate gyrus or orbito-frontal cortex. On this sample, representative of temporo-limbic seizures, we specially analysed ictal AM, with a particular attention paid to those occuring initially and/or early in the course of the seizure.

Analytical semiology

Autonomic manifestations reported in the literature and actually observed in our temporo-limbic seizures are very numerous and varied, resulting frequently in compound symptoms and signs with spatio-temporally complicated course and patterns, highly variable from one patient to another. Therefore, it is useful to attempt to classify these AM, but we keep in mind that such a classification unavoidably results in an oversimplification and is unable to encompass all the possible semiological pictures.

First, it is certainly useful to differentiate subjective or viscero-sensitive symptoms and objective or viscero-motor signs (Wieser, 1987). Both may be associated, or not, within a same autonomic phenomenon; for instances, a sensation of nausea may be associated with retching or vomiting, a shiver or more rarely a 'gooseflesh' phenomenon may accompany a feeling of cold.

A second categorization concerns the visceral organ or system which is involved, though even such a distinction may be very difficult in some cases, or irrelevant in others. However, we can distinguish: digestive, cardio-vascular, ocular, respiratory, uro-genital, and thermo-regulatory AM. The qualitative features of AM in our patients, for these different organs or functions, are summarized in Table 1. Short-term hormonal changes induced by partial seizures, like a rise of prolactine serum level, must also be included in autonomic manifestations (Wannamaker, 1985; Wieser, 1987); but we will not consider them here.

Table 1. Principal autonomic manifestations in temporo-limbic seizures

	Viscero-sensitive symptoms	Viscero-motor signs
Digestive tract	Epigastric aura Nausea Abdominal, pelvic sensations Hunger, thirst	Belches, retching, vomiting Rumblings, winds Defecation urge, faecal incontinence
Cardio-vascular system	Tachycardia, palpitations Precordial constriction	Heart rhythm changes Blood pressure changes Pallor, flush
Eyes and annexes		Mydriasis, myosis Gaze brightness, watering
Respiratory tract	Dyspnea, stifling feeling Chest or laryngeal constriction	Tachypnea, bradypnea, apnea Cough, sneeze, hiccups
Urogenital tract	Bladder discomfort Urge to urinate Vague perineal/genital feelings	Loss of urine Erection, ejaculation
Body temperature regulation	Cold or warm feelings, shivering	Shivers, horripilation Sweating Body temperature changes

Digestive autonomic manifestations are not the most frequent of AM (Table 2). Nevertheless, we will describe them in the first place because they have certainly the most important semiological meaning (Bancaud *et al.*, 1965; Gupta *et al.*, 1983; Wieser, 1983; Bancaud, 1987). Digestive AM are viscero-sensitive in more than two thirds of cases. Undoubtedly, the most significant are the various epigastric feelings which are also the most frequent digestive phenomena, since they account for 55 per cent of digestive AM in our series. These sensations are usually median and typically located in the supra-umbilical and xiphoid process regions. With very few exceptions, these feelings are very unpleasant or even, more seldom, really painful like a stomach cramp. To describe these often difficult-to-characterize feelings, adult patients use numerous and varied words or expressions (such as 'butterflies in the stomach', 'sinking', 'vacuum' ...), so attempting to express the idea of constriction, pressure, blocking, warmness, heaviness or emptiness; often it is simply an impossible-to-describe 'malaise' or discomfort (Penfield & Kristiansen, 1951). In two thirds of cases, the epigastric sensation is moving, typically upwards in the chest, to the retro-sternal and then the pharyngo-laryngeal region where it results in a feeling of constriction (Penfield & Kristiansen, 1951; Van Buren, 1963; Bancaud, 1987). Interestingly, we noted that in complex partial seizures the loss of consciousness, or more accurately for the majority of cases disturbances of the normal perception and contact with people and environment, occurs commonly at this moment in the course of the seizure. A true nausea or a nauseous quality of the epigastric sensation are also common. In some cases, simultaneous changes in the gastric motility accompany epigastric feeelings; conversely, it is not the case in other instances, so that these latter may represent genuine visceral hallucinations (Penfield & Faulk, 1955; Penfield, 1958; Van Buren, 1963).

In the nineteenth century, Herpin (1867) and Gowers (1885) gave very thorough descriptions of these digestive visceral symptoms. In addition, Gowers named them 'epigastric aura', because he observed that these sensations very often represent the starting symptoms of a partial seizure. Similarly, in our mono- or pauci-symptomatic population, brief, simple partial seizures may be rather commonly limited or almost limited to these epigastric feelings. Obviously, these purely subjective symptoms are true simple partial seizures and, as such, have a high semiological value. But, so isolated, they are frequently very brief and/or subtle; in other cases patients do not even suspect the ictal nature of these symtoms, or they have become used to these symptoms over a long period, or even consider them normal. Whatever the reason, patients may have a tendency to neglect these symptoms and not to mention them. Keeping this fact in mind, it is especially important to search for such isolated epigastric symptoms by repeated and thorough interviews, especially in children. In other cases the simple partial seizure evolves to a complex partial one. Otherwise localized abdominal sensations, such as hypogastric, suprapubian, perineal or ano-rectal discomfort or pain are much more rare and we did not observe them in our children subgroup, except as a vague and ill-localized feeling of abdominal discomfort in two children.

Digestive motor signs are much less frequent than the sensitive symptoms. These digestive motor AM are rarely isolated and conversely in almost all cases they are associated with, and follow, viscero-sensitive symptoms. In a few cases, we observed belches, hiccups, rumblings, and exceptionally intestinal winds or even defecation urge. But the most common motor digestive sign is retching accompanying nausea and sometimes resulting in vomiting. Some authors reported ictal vomiting to be rather common, either in surgically-treated temporal lobe epilepsy (Kotagal *et al.*, 1995) or in pre-puberty children presenting with partial seizures, mainly partial idiopathic epilepsies, especially the 'benign childhood epilepsy with occipital paroxysms' (Panayiotopoulos, 1988). However, in our present series of non-idiopathic partial epilepsies, ictal vomiting remains rather rare, even in the paediatric age group.

Hypersalivation with occasional slobbering is also rare and usually associated with other AM, as well as with somato-motor and/or somesthetic oro-facial signs, suggesting that ictal discharge has involved or reached extra-limbic structures, namely the supra-sylvian opercular area (Bancaud, 1987). Indeed, we did not observe hypersalivation in the cases of ictal discharges remaining limited to limbic structures.

Feelings of hunger and/or thirst, or more complex eating or drinking ictal conducts, are exceptional in our population as in the literature. These signs must be considered more as instinctivo-affective and behavioural than properly viscero-sensitive. We did not observe them in our children subgroup.

Cardio-vascular autonomic manifestations (Jallon, 1997) appear among the most frequent of AM and we observed them in 15.6 per cent of the temporo-limbic seizures we studied (Table 2); they are associated with other AM in more than two thirds of cases. Viscero-motor signs are undeniably more frequent than isolated subjective symptoms. Vaso-motor changes are the most common objective phenomena: flush or rubefaction – sometimes accompanied by a feeling of warmth – pallor or cyanosis, which may follow each other in the same seizure. Most often they are localized to the face or to the upper part of the body. Interestingly, these vaso-motor changes represent a warning sign readily reported by the witnesses of the seizure.

Cardiac rhythm modifications are also very frequent and consist mainly of tachycardia (and blood pressure elevation when monitored) and, much less frequently, bradycardia or irregular heart beats. Heart rhythm changes may be conscious with concomitant tachycardia, palpitations or irregular beating feeling. Marked and lasting bradycardia was rare in our series and we observed only one case of per-ictal brief cardiac arrest in an adult patient. Cases of cardiac arrest occuring in partial seizures are reported, which probably explain a significant part of unexpected sudden deaths which happen in patients with partial epilepsy (Nashef et al., 1996; Jallon, 1997). Other cardio-thoracic symptoms include distressing or even painful sensations of discomfort, heaviness or constriction, localized in the precordial region or more diffuse in the chest.

Various symptoms localized in the head are classically reported in partial seizures. Often these symptoms are very difficult to describe for the patient, and their accurate categorization may remain uncertain – thus, they are described sometimes as viscero-sensitive phenomena (Wieser, 1983), sometimes as somato-sensitive (Gastaut & Broughton, 1972), or even discussed under both these headings (Penfield & Jasper, 1954) – as well as their definite interpretation: are these symptoms directly resulting from an epileptic discharge? or only indirectly, via vaso-motor or haemodynamic ictal changes in the facial, meningeal or brain loco-regional blood circulation and vessels? Again, adult patients use several words to depict these often unlocalized, ill-defined and difficult-to-describe head sensations: constriction, pressure, heaviness or emptiness, beating, swelling, warmth, etc. but also often simply 'something in the head'. These cephalic feelings appear common in our patients when they are associated with other AM, notably digestive – especially a rising epigastric discomfort – and cardio-vascular/thoracic. Conversely, rare (1.2 per cent of seizures, Table 2) are the cases with cephalic symptoms really at the forefront of the early ictal semiology and resulting then in a true 'cephalic aura', which may be, however, isolated or almost. No child in our series reported such a true isolated cephalic aura.

Ocular and pupillary autonomic manifestations are also frequent since they are observed in more than 15 per cent of temporo-limbic seizures (Table 2). In a vast majority of cases (about 90 per cent), they consist of pupillary changes, namely bilateral mydriasis. Usually it is accompanied by a modification of the expression of gaze comprising brightness with more or less typical staring and rather commonly by a fearful facial expression. A small increase of lacrymal secretion with a moist appearance of the eyes is commonly associated. On the contrary, a true watering or *a fortiori* tears without emotional content are exceptional and we did not observe them in our children patients. Myosis may also occur but much more rarely.

Respiratory autonomic manifestations occurred in about 5 per cent of our temporo-limbic seizures (Table 2). They are associated in the majority of cases with other AM. Viscero-sensitive respiratory symptoms consists of dyspnoeic feelings such as breathlessness or sensation of suffocation, usually retro-sternal and medio-thoracic, sometimes difficult to clearly differentiate from an epigastric sensation. Frequently, these respiratory symptoms are rising and result in a sensation of laryngeal constriction.

In our population, motor respiratory signs consist mainly of polypnea or increased amplitude of respiratory movements or more rarely bradypnea; these signs may be conscious but irrepressible. They occur usually in combination with respiratory subjective symptoms and sometimes they appear as a more or less voluntary and well-adapted reaction of the patient to respiratory unpleasant feelings. Cough, sneeze and hiccups are much more rare. A lasting apnoea may occur during a partial seizure, notably in infants or children. Nashef et al. (1996) addressed specifically this question in 17 adult patients and reported a quite common occcurence of ictal apnoea (10/17 patients and 20/47 clinical seizures). We observed merely a few cases in our population and only one child with an ictal apnoea, perhaps because we did not perform such detailed respiratory investigations.

Urinary and genital autonomic manifestations are globally infrequent (<2 per cent of seizures, Table 2) and they appear even more uncommon in children. They are much more frequent in men than in women. Both types of symptoms – urinary and genital – may be associated, especially in men; however such a combination is rare. Urinary manifestations consist of feelings such as hypogastric pressure or tension, or sensation of repletion of the bladder sometimes accompanied by an urge to urinate. A loss of urine, usually unconscious, may also occur, with or without this warning; such a loss remains rare in our patients except in partial seizures evolving to a secondary tonic–clonic generalization. Imprecise and difficult-to-describe feelings in the genitalia, also much more frequent in men, consist of shivers, warm or cold feeling, tension or swelling sensations. Exceptionally these feelings have sexual and erotic features, such as pleasure or even orgasmic sensations, which occured only in very few cases of our adult patients. In fact, we did not observe uro-genital AM in our young patients, except two children with hypogastric discomfort or urge to urinate.

Thermo-regulatory autonomic manifestations are observed in 3.5 per cent of seizures (Table 2). They mainly have difficult to describe feelings of warm or cold, ill-localized or more or less diffuse. Other manifestations may be associated: vaso-motor changes; sweating with warmth feeling; shivers or horripilation and 'goose flesh' phenomenon with cold sensation. Such a horripilation may happen as the first-rank sign or among the first-rank signs in the so-called pilo-motor seizures recently reviewed by Roze *et al.* (2000), but this occurrence is rare in our series (12/1707 seizures), with no case in the paediatric sub-group.

Table 2. Frequency of different types of autonomic manifestations in temporo-limbic seizures

Autonomic manifestations	% of seizures ($n = 1707$)
Viscero-motor	38%
Viscero-sensitive	27%
Cardio-vascular	15.6%
Eyes and annexes	15.6%
Digestive	10.6%
Respiratory	5.1%
Thermo-regulation	3.5%
Uro-genital	1.8%
'Cephalic aura'	1.2%

Overall semiological features

These data confirm the high frequency of AM in partial seizures of temporo-limbic origin as well as they commonly represent all or part of the early ictal phenomena. So, on the whole early AM – i.e. in the first 20 s – occur in 65 per cent of seizures (Table 2). As reported before by Wieser (1983), viscero-motor signs are more frequent in our population (38 per cent of of seizures) than viscero-sensitive symptoms (27 per cent of seizures). This fact results mainly from the high frequency of vaso-motor and pupillary manifestations, respectively.

Autonomic manifestations, especially subjective symptoms, either in isolation or associated with other ictal phenomena, often represent a significant part of a simple partial seizure or the so-called aura of a complex partial seizure (Gupta et al., 1983; Taylor & Lochery, 1987). However, a more complex pattern of AM is quite common, with occurrence of AM later in, or all through, the seizure. These later manifestations are generally in relation with the cortical and sub-cortical spread of the discharge; and therefore they have less or no localizing value.

If autonomic manifestations show a large inter-individual variability, conversely they appear very similar from one seizure to another in a given subject. Usually, they are distressing and even, although rarely, quite painful. Subjective AM may be very hard to describe for the patient. Therefore, careful and repeated interviews with the patient and relatives, and ictal and post-ictal examinations are essential; the video-camera alone cannot replace them. Subjective AM sometimes correspond to the perception of a viscero-motor phenomenon, sometimes not, then appearing as visceral hallucinations. Objective AM may be slight or quite subtle. In some cases, they may be perceived by the patient himself; in some others they are not, either due to a simultaneous disturbance or loss of consciousness or because the fact that some neuro-vegetative phenomena (e.g. a change in the size of the pupil) do not normally reach consciousness.

Most often, AM mean *per se* the involvement by the ictal discharge of brain anatomo-functional structures controlling the autonomic functions, directly or by their efferent projections. In some other instances, AM may seem to be reactive to other ictal phenomena such as a deep emotion, a strong fright or an intense motor activity (Wieser, 1987).

Very often, several AM combine in a same seizure, involving different anatomo-functional subdivisions of the autonomic nervous system and several territories of the body. The most frequently associated are digestive, cardio-vascular and respiratory AM. Ocular manifestations occur almost always associated with other AM. Likewise, uro-genital and thermo-regulatory AM as well as cephalic feelings combine usually with digestive or cardiac symptoms or signs.

Even though seizures with very prominent or even isolated, or almost, autonomic phenomena may occur, notably in infants or children (Drake, 1984; Aicardi, 1994), AM almost always are actually associated with other ictal phenomena, resulting finally in a countless number of possible ictal patterns. However several evocative associations and clusters of ictal phenomena stand out (see below).

Do autonomic manifestations have a localizing value?

In the seizures we studied, the temporo-limbic localization of the discharges was founded on depth electrode-SEEG recordings. Despite some possible and essentially unavoidable sampling limitations, SEEG undoubtedly gives us very valuable clues or proofs of the localization of the discharge. On the other hand, it is advisable to remember that 'many, and often all, of the clinical manifestations of seizures reflect spread from the region of origin' (Wieser & Williamson, 1993). Accepting these intrinsic limitations, some comments can be made.

It is known that a single ictal symptom or sign may have a definite localizing value, only when it depends on a discharge involving a primary cortex. Firstly, this is rather rare in temporal lobe seizures. Secondly, it is not the case for AM. Like most ictal phenomena, AM are devoid of a clear-cut localizing value if taken in isolation. However, they may contribute to the hypothesis of localization provided they are always considered together with the other ictal manifestations, in the global dynamic pattern of the seizure. Viscero-sensitive symptoms, although less frequent, appear endowed with a more significant localizing value than viscero-motor signs. Autonomic manifestations are exceptionnally lateralized in the body and they do not have any reliable lateralizing value.

As mentioned above, some semiological clusters comprising important or prominent AM are very suggestive. A first salient association of ictal phenomena consists of initial digestive AM, above all a rising epigastric aura, and early oro-alimentary automatisms of chewing, this association being especially suggestive of a discharge involving the amygdala and its efferences (Bancaud et al., 1965, 1986; Wieser, 1983; Maldonado et al., 1988). We observed other automatic activities, classically suggestive of temporo-limbic seizures such as repetitive gestures of one arm or both; most often these gestures appear purposeless but in other instances they seem reactive to viscero-sensitive symptoms such as rubbing movements of the epigastric region, the chest or the genitalia.

Secondly, affective ictal manifestations are strikingly associated with AM – particularly of digestive, ocular, cardio-vascular and respiratory types – especially at the early phase of the seizures, as already reported by several authors mainly in adults (McRae, 1954; Penfield & Jasper, 1954; Williams, 1956; Daly, 1958; Gastaut, 1980; Gloor, 1986) but also in children (Dalla Bernardina et al., 1992). With very few exceptions, these emotional symptoms are distressing: anxiety, fright or terror, sadness; or very seldom feeling of well-being, joviality or pleasure. As a rule, facial expression changes in accordance with the content of the affective experience occurring, especially a fearful expression accompanying painful emotions. Such a pattern strongly suggests a discharge involving either mesiotemporo limbic structures, or even more the frontocingular cortex, or both.

The insular cortex, closely related to mesiotemporal limbic structures, appears involved in cardio-vascular (Oppenheimer et al., 1992) respiratory or uro-genital AM. But above all, it surely plays an essential role at the origin of the epigastric aura. Stimulation studies suggests such a role as well as the probable existence of a somatotopic representation of the digestive tract at this level (Penfield & Faulk, 1955; Van Buren, 1961, 1963; Bancaud, 1987). More recently this issue was addressed in adult epileptic patients undergoing a chronic SEEG exploration (Isnard et al., 1998; Ostrowski et al., 2000). One or several of the depth electrodes was implanted directly in the insular cortex. Isnard et al. (1998) observed ictal viscero-sensitive symptoms occurring simultaneously with polyspike discharges in both insular cortex and hippocampus. Moreover, stimulating the insular cortex, Ostrowski et al. (2000) reported mainly viscero-sensitive symptoms, as well as chewing and lipsmacking (which they classified as viscero-sensitive signs). Most of these symptoms and signs were elicited by anterior insular cortex stimulations. These elicited AM appeared similar to those evoked by temporo-mesial structure stimulations; nevertheless most patients were able to perceive subtle differences between the symptoms triggered by insular or by tempor-mesial stimulation respectively.

Autonomic manifestations are certainly very common and of a special value in temporal lobe seizures. However, they occur not only in seizures originating from temporo-limbic structures but also from other areas of the temporal cortex such as the temporal neo-cortex; furthermore they are by no means specific to a temporal lobe localization. Indeed, AM occur also in many partial seizures of extra-temporal origin, the most frequent and important being without any doubt frontal lobe seizures, whose AM often constitute a significant phenomenological component (Bancaud & Talairach, 1992; Broglin et al., 1992; Chauvel et al., 1992) although other authors do not reach the same conclusion (Williamson et al., 1985; Veilleux et al., 1992). Various AM may occur in frontal seizures originating from different subdivisions of the frontal lobes. However, as mentioned above, AM at first characterize the seizures involving regions of the frontal lobe which belong to the limbic system: mesial fronto-cingular cortex (Talairach et al., 1973; Bancaud & Tailarach, 1992) and orbito-frontal cortex (Van Buren et al., 1961;

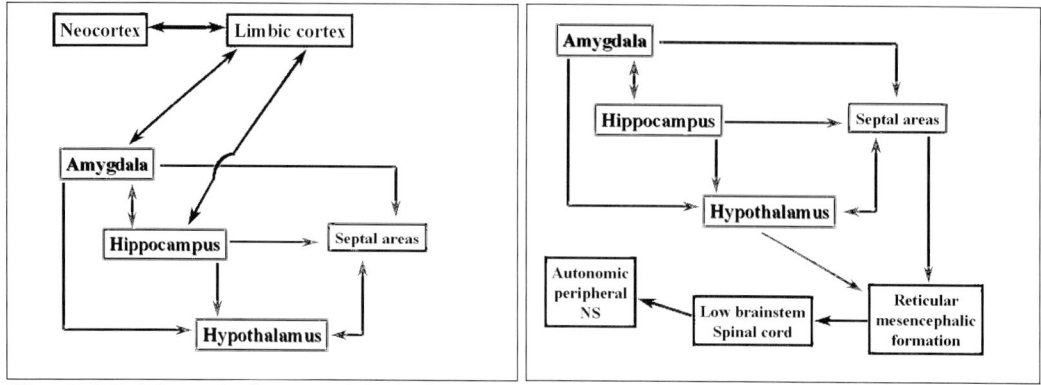

Figs. 1 & 2. Schematic diagram of the limbic system and its main connections.

Munari & Bancaud, 1992). This is not surprising, since frontal and temporal limbic areas are closely interconnected as parts of the same functional unit constituted by the limbic system. Cardio-vascular, ocular, respiratory and urinary AM are usually predominant in these seizures involving limbic frontal areas. In these cases, especially in seizures involving the fronto-cingulate cortex, AM are frequently associated with intense negative affective feelings – fright, terror – and sudden, spectacular behavioural changes – crying, screaming, violent movements and agitation.

Pathophysiological hypotheses

The limbic system is a very complex anatomo-functional entity, comprising numerous brain cortical areas in the temporal and frontal lobes and sub-cortical structures, reciprocally interconnected in a very complex fashion. Briefly, it constitutes a very important anatomic and physiologic relay between the neocortex – its main input – and the hypothalamus and reticular formation – its main output. Actually, many multimodal afferences coming from associative neocortical areas converge, via the so-called 'limbic' neo-cortical frontal and temporal cortex, on the limbic cortex proper and then, principally via the para-hippocampal gyrus, on the hippocampus and the amygdala. The latter have numerous cortical and sub-cortical connections; their main efferent projections are on the septal areas and on the hypothalamus, which themselves are interconnected and send important projections on the limbic mesencephalic area in the brainstem reticular formation. The septal areas, hypothalamus and limbic mesencephalic area form an anatomo-functional complex which is essential in the regulation of visceral functions, by controlling the two-neuron (the first one located in the nevraxis, the second in the autonomic ganglia) centrifugal chain of the autonomic nervous system which project very largely, on all apparatus and tissues of the body, to smooth muscles, heart and various glandular epitheliums (Figs. 1 and 2).

The term 'limbic seizures' was coined by Fulton (1953) fifty years ago in the setting of conceptual and terminological discussions and topographical hypothesis about partial seizures of the 'psychomotor' type according to the denomination in use at that time (Gastaut, 1953). He argued that 'such attacks involve not only the temporal lobe structures but usually also the posterior orbital gyrus, the hippocampus, and the cingulate gyrus'. This term remains rather ill-defined and may be confusing. 'Limbic' seizures may be sometimes more or less confused with the whole of temporal lobes seizures (Wieser, 1987). But all temporal lobe seizures are not limbic seizures and all limbic seizures are not temporal lobe seizures.

It is well-known now that the limbic system, especially through the mesio-temporo-limbic structures, plays a crucial role in many partial seizures in the genesis and/or the propagation of the epileptic discharge and corresponding clinical phenomena, due to its anatomical organization, to the physiological properties of its neuronal networks and to the propensity of these networks to generate excessive and hypersynchronous neuronal discharges.

In other respects numerous studies, in animals but also in humans – observation of seizures (Penfield & Jasper, 1954; Bancaud et al., 1965; Van Buren, 1958, 1963; Van Buren & Ajmone-Marsan, 1960; Wieser, 1983, 1986, 1987; Gloor, 1986; Isnard et al., 1998), results of cortical and deep brain stimulations in patients, epileptic or not (Penfield & Rasmussen, 1950; Penfield & Jasper, 1954; Penfield & Faulk, 1955; Chapman, 1958; Jasper & Rasmussen, 1958; Penfield, 1958; Pampiglione & Falconer, 1960; Van Buren, 1961, 1963; Van Buren et al., 1961; Nelson & Ray, 1968; Talairach et al., 1973; Wieser, 1983; Bancaud et al., 1986; Gloor, 1986; Ostrowski et al., 2000), intra-cellular recordings (Frysinger & Harper, 1990) – have demonstrated that the limbic system plays a leading role in the regulation of visceral organs and functions. It plays also a major role – especially by the amygdaloid complex – in some basic and instinctive behaviour importantly involved in the survival of the individual and the perpetuation of the species such as eating, sexual and safeguard behaviour, and also – especially by the hippocampal formation – in the mnesic processes. So the limbic system, taking into account the past experience and the present stimuli together, notably appears able to govern and modulate emotional and instinctive behaviour, as well as their associated visceral adaptive reactions since, mainly via its hypothalamic connections, it exerts a powerful regulation on the autonomic nervous system.

Taking into consideration the relationships between these physiological functions of the limbic system and the abnormal excessive functioning imposed on it by an epileptic discharge, it is conceivable that an ictal disorganization involving the limbic system activates and releases not only instinctive and/or archaic automatic behaviour but also intense visceral and homeostasis-linked manifestations and emotional reactions, all closely related to these phylogenetically primitive conducts.

Some distinctive features of autonomic manifestations in children

The clinical semiology of partial seizures, notably as to the autonomic manifestations, appears today reasonably well-known in adult and adolescent patients, as well as the meaning of several well-delineated ictal patterns about the origin and propagation of ictal discharges. Conversely, available data are relatively few in pre-adolescents, children and even more so in infants, and hypotheses or interpretations remain controversial. Furthermore, the prevalent pre-surgical mode of recruitment is probably responsible for selection bias and perhaps for skewed observations or conclusions (Wyllie et al., 1993; Brockhaus & Elger, 1995). However, from literature and personal data summarized above, it seems possible to draw some relevant comments or conclusions.

The overall frequency of ictal AM in children differs according to the studies. However this heterogeneity seems to be, possibly or probably, only apparent, depending on whether autonomic manifestations were a specific and deliberate objective of analysis or not. Our explicitly focused study has shown us the frequency of AM in partial seizures of children is rather high, since we observed in fact a significant – and not very much lower than in older patients – proportion of children and pre-adolescent reporting or presenting with one or several AM during at least one of the seizures we analysed (Table 3).

Many features of AM observed in adults appear also in children. However, some distinctive features depend on age. Overall, AM are unsurprisingly more difficult to detect and analyse in children than in older patients and all the more so when the children are younger. Subjective AM certainly exist from the earliest age but they are of course impossible to describe before the age of fluent and meaningful speech. On the other hand, even in pre-school age children, warning viscero-sensitive symptoms appear rather frequently and roughly similarly to older subjects, provided the children succeed in describing them. We agree with Bye & Foo (1994) and others (Landré et al., 1998; Michel, 1999) who emphasized that careful and direct inquiry of such symptoms is essential. This leads us to stress again the prime importance of thorough repeated talks with the children as soon they are able to express themselves, even if imperfectly.

Table 3. Main ictal autonomic manifestations in children with temporo-limbic seizures

Autonomic symptoms or signs	Number of children (Total = 26)
Digestive	
Epigastric aura	12
Pharyngo-laryngeal constriction	7
Other abdominal feelings	2
Nausea [and vomiting]	6 [2]
Cardio-vascular	
Vasomotor changes	15
Sensation of heart rhythm changes	9
Objective heart rhythm change	16
Ill-defined cephalic feeling	4
Ocular	
Mydriasis	14
Respiratory	
Dyspnoea, unpleasant chest feeling	10
Breath rhythm changes [apnoea]	7 [1]
Uro-genital	
Hypogastric discomfort, urge to urinate	2
Thermoregulation	
Cold feeling, shivers	3

Results are expressed as numbers of children presenting with the corresponding autonomic phenomenon, during at least one partial seizure. Commonly several types of autonomic manifestations (AM) are observed in the same child. Slight changes in AM may occur from one seizure to another. Total number of seizures: 103.

Because subjective symptoms may be lacking, subtle, or impossible to describe by the child, objective AM may appear at the first rank of the ictal semiology, all the more if the patient is younger. Ocular and vaso-motor signs appear with a same range of frequency than in older subjects. Probably, some digestive – retching and even vomiting – or respiratory – bradypnoea and even lasting apnoea – signs are more common than in adults, but this has to be confirmed.

Concerning the associated ictal signs, the data from the literature demonstrate an age-related pattern in the temporal lobe seizures in children (Jayakar & Duchowny, 1990; Wyllie et al., 1993; Brockhaus & Elger, 1995). Over 6 years, the ictal patterns are roughly similar to adults. On the contrary, patterns appear different in children aged less than 6 years. In summary, the younger the child, the more crude and less elaborate is the ictal semiology. In infants and youngest children, motor signs, often bilateral and more or less symmetric, and very simple and purposeless automatisms are prominent. Such patterns can be misleading as primarily suggestive of partial frontal lobe or generalized seizures.

To conclude, the clinical expression of an epileptic discharge certainly depends on the stage of the brain maturation. In young patients, probably the incomplete development of the neural connections, notably in the temporal lobe and in the limbic system on the one hand, and possibly the easier and faster propagation of the discharge in an immature brain on the other hand, may explain these peculiar semiological features. Further data and more precise tools to analyse the seizures of children are needed to improve the answers to these questions.

We wish to dedicate the present work to the memory of Jean Bancaud and Claudio Munari.

Acknowledgements: The personal study presented in this paper was carried out at Sainte Anne Hospital, Paris. We are grateful to our colleagues A. Biraben, F. Chassoux, P. Chauvel, J.P. Gagnepain, E. Landré, A. Philippe, D. Toussaint, S. Trottier and J.P. Vignal for their assistance.

References

Aicardi, J. (1994): *Epilepsy in children*, 2nd edn. New York: Raven Press.

Bancaud, J. (1976): Epilepsies. *Encycl. Méd. Chir. Neurologie.* 17045 A10 and A30.

Bancaud, J. (1987): Sémiologie clinique des crises épileptiques d'origine temporale. *Rev. Neurol.* **143,** 392-400.

Bancaud, J. & Talairach, J. (1992): Clinical semiology of frontal lobe seizures. In: *Frontal lobe seizures and epilepsies. Advances in Neurology*, vol. 57, P. Chauvel, A.V. Delgado-Escueta, E. Halgren & J. Bancaud (eds.), pp. 3–58. New York: Raven Press.

Bancaud, J., Talairach, J., Bonis, A., Schaub, C., Szikla, G., Morel, P. & Bordas-Ferrer, M. (1965): *La stéréo-électroencéphalographie dans l'épilepsie*. Paris: Masson.

Bancaud, J., Talairach, J., Morel, P. & Bresson, M. (1986): La corne d'Ammon et le noyau amygdalien: effets cliniques et électriques de leur stimulation chez l'homme. *Rev. Neurol.* **115,** 329–352.

Beaumanoir, A. & Dravet, Ch. (1992): The Lennox–Gastaut syndrome. In: *Epileptic syndromes in infancy, childhood and adolescence,* 2nd edn., eds. J. Roger, M. Bureau, Ch. Dravet, F. E. Dreifuss, A. Perret & P. Wolf, pp. 115–132. London, Paris, Rome: John Libbey.

Blume W.T. (1989): Clinical profile of partial seizures beginning at less than four years of age. *Epilepsia* **30,** 813–819.

Brockhaus, A. & Elger, C.E. (1995): Complex partial seizures of temporal lobe origin in children of different age groups. *Epilepsia* **36,** 1173–1181.

Broglin, D. & Bancaud, J. (1991): Manifestations neuro-végétatives au cours des crises partielles du lobe temporal. In: *Crises épileptiques et épilepsies du lobe temporal, tome I, VIIème Cours de perfectionnement en Epileptologie,* ed. M. Weber, pp. 69–96. Paris: Documentation médicale Labaz.

Broglin, D., Delgado-Escueta, A.V., Walsh, G.O., Bancaud, J. & Chauvel, P. (1992): Clinical approach to the patient with seizures and epilepsies of frontal origin. In: *Frontal lobe seizures and epilepsies, Adv. Neurol.* **57,** eds. P. Chauvel, A.V. Delgado-Escueta, E. Halgren & J. Bancaud, pp. 59–88. New York: Raven Press.

Bye, A.M.E. & Foo, S. (1994): Complex partial seizures in young children. *Epilepsia* **35,** 482–488.

Chapman, W.P. (1958): Studies of the periamygdaloid area in relation to human behavior. In: *The human brain and behaviour. Res. Pub. Ass. Nerv. Ment. Dis.*, pp. 258–277. Baltimore: Williams and Wilkins.

Chauvel, P., Delgado-Escueta, A.V., Halgren, E. & Bancaud, J., eds (1992): *Frontal lobe seizures and epilepsies. Advances in Neurology*, vol. 57. New York: Raven Press.

Dalla Bernardina, B., Colamaria, V., Chiamenti, C., Capovilla, G., Trevisan, E. & Tassinari, C.A. (1992): Benign partial epilepsy with affective symptoms ('benign psychomotor epilepsy') In: *Epileptic syndromes in infancy, childhood and adolescence,* 2nd edn., eds. J. Roger, M. Bureau, Ch. Dravet, F.E. Dreifuss, A. Perret & P. Wolf, pp. 219–223. London, Paris, Rome: John Libbey.

Daly, D.D. (1958): Ictal affect. *Amer. J. Psychiatr.* **115,** 97–108.

Daly, D.D. (1975): Ictal clinical manifestations of complex partial seizures. In: *Complex partial seizures and their treatment, Adv. Neurol.*, **11**, eds. J.K. Penry & D.D. Daly, pp. 57–83. New York: Raven Press.

Drake, M.E. (1984): Isolated autonomic symptoms in complex partial seizures. *J. Neurol. Neurosurg. Psychiatry* **47**, 100–101.

Dravet, C., Catani, C., Bureau, M. & Roger, J. (1989): Partial epilepsies in infancy: a study of 40 cases. *Epilepsia* **30**, 807–812.

Duchowny, M.S. (1987): Complex partial seizures of infancy. *Arch. Neurol.* **44**, 911–914.

French, J.A., Williamson, P.D., Thadani, V.M., Darcey, M., Mattson, R.H., Spencer, S.S. & Spencer, D.D. (1993): Characteristics of medial temporal lobe epilepsy: I. Results of history and physical examination. *Ann. Neurol.* **34**, 774–780.

Frysinger, R.C. & Harper, R.M. (1990): Cardiac and respiratory correlations with unit discharges in epileptic human temporal lobe. *Epilepsia* **31**, 162–171.

Fulton, J.F. (1953): Discussion of Gastaut, H.: So-called 'psychomotor' and 'temporal' epilepsy. *Epilepsia* (Third Series) **2**, 77.

Gastaut, H. (1953): So-called 'psychomotor' and 'temporal' epilepsy. *Epilepsia* (Third Series) **2**, 59–76.

Gastaut, H. (1980): L'épilepsie temporale. *Le Concours Médical* N° 15, Suppl. pp. 3–48.

Gastaut, H. & Broughton, R. (1972): *Epileptic seizures. Clinical and electrographic features, diagnosis and treatment.* Springfield, IL: C.C. Thomas.

Glaser, G.H. (1967): Limbic epilepsy in childhood. *J. Nerv. Ment. Dis.* **144**, 391–397.

Gloor, P. (1986): Role of the human limbic system in perception, memory, and affect: lessons from temporal lobe epilepsy. In: *The limbic system: functional organization and clinical disorders*, eds. B.K. Doane & K.E. Livingston, pp. 159–169. New York: Raven Press.

Gowers, W.R. (1885): *Epilepsy and other chronic convulsive diseases: their causes, symptoms and treatment.* Reprint of the 1st American edn. 1994. Nijmegen: Arts and Boewe.

Gupta, A.K., Jeavons, P.M., Hughes, R.C. & Covanis, A. (1983): Aura in temporal lobe epilepsy: clinical and electroencephalographic correlation. *J. Neurol. Neurosurg. Psychiatry* **46**, 1079–1083.

Harvey, A.S., Berkovic, S.F., Wrennall, J.A. & Hopkins, I.J. (1997): Temporal lobe epilepsy in childhood: clinical, EEG, and neuroimaging findings and syndrome classification in a cohort with new-onset seizures. *Neurology* **49**, 960–968.

Hausser-Hauw, C. & Bancaud, J. (1987): Gustatory hallucinations in epileptic seizures. *Brain* **110**, 339–359.

Herpin, T. (1867): *Des accès incomplets d'épilepsie.* Paris: J. B. Baillière et fils.

Holmes, G.L. (1986): Partial seizures in children. *Pediatrics* **77**, 725–731.

Isnard, J., Ryvlin, P., Guénot, M., Ostrowski, K., Fischer, C., Sindou, M. & Mauguière, F. (1998): Role of the insular cortex in temporo-limbic seizures: a stereo electroencephalographic study. *Epilepsia* **39** (Suppl. 6), 65.

Jallon, P. (1997): Epilepsie et cœur. *Rev. Neurol.* **153**, 173–184.

Jasper, H.J. & Rasmussen, T. (1958): Studies of clinical and electrical responses to deep temporal stimulation in man with some considerations of functional anatomy. In: *The human brain and behaviour. Res. Pub. Ass. Nerv. Ment. Dis.*, pp. 316–334. Baltimore: Williams and Wilkins.

Jayakar, P. & Duchowny, M.S. (1990): Complex partial seizures of temporal lobe origin in early childhood. *J. Epilepsy* **3** (Suppl.), 41–45.

Kotagal, P., Lüders, H.O., Williams, G., Nichols, T.R. & McPherson, J. (1995): Psychomotor seizures of temporal lobe onset: analysis of symptom clusters and sequences. *Epilepsy Res.* **20**, 49–67.

Landré, E., Turak, B., Chassoux, F., Ghossoub, M., Devaux, B., Chagot, D., Gagnepain, J.P. & Chodkiewicz, J.P. (1998): Enregistrements vidéo-EEG. In: *Epilepsies partielles graves pharmaco-résistantes de l'enfant: stratégies diagnostiques et traitements chirurgicaux*, eds. M. Bureau, P. Kahane & C. Munari, pp. 107–112. Paris: John Libbey Eurotext.

Lennox, W.G. & Cobb, S. (1933): Epilepsy, XIII. Aura in epilepsy: a statistical review of 1359 cases. *Arch. Neurol. Psych.* **30**, 374–387.

Loiseau, P. (1992): Childhood absence epilepsy. In: *Epileptic syndromes in infancy, childhood and adolescence,* 2nd edn., eds. J. Roger, M. Bureau, Ch. Dravet, F.E. Dreifuss, A. Perret & P. Wolf, pp. 135–150. London: John Libbey.

Luna, D., Dulac, O. & Plouin, P. (1989): Ictal characteristics of cryptogenic partial epilepsies in infancy. *Epilepsia* **30**, 827–832.

McRae, D. (1954): Isolated fear, a temporal lobe aura. *Neurology* **4**, 497–505.

Maldonado, H.M., Delgado-Escueta, A.V., Walsh, G.O., Swartz, B.E. & Rand, R.W. (1988): Complex partial seizures of hippocampal and amygdalar origin. *Epilepsia* **29**, 420–433.

Marchand, L. & de Ajuriaguerra, J. (1948): *Epilepsies: leurs formes cliniques, leurs traitements.* Paris: Desclée de Brouwer.

Michel, A. (1999): *Manifestations faciales dans les crises à point de départ temporal chez les enfants. A propos de cinq cas.* Mémoire pour le Diplôme Interuniversitaire d'Epileptologie. Universités Paris VI et Montpellier.

Mulder, D.W., Daly, D. & Bailey, A.A. (1954): Visceral epilepsy. *Arch. Int. Med.* **93**, 481–493.

Munari, C. & Bancaud, J. (1992): Electroclinical symptomatology of partial seizures of orbital frontal origin. In: *Frontal lobe seizures and epilepsies, Adv. Neurol.,* **57**, eds. P. Chauvel, A.V. Delgado-Escueta, E. Halgren & J. Bancaud, pp. 257–265. New York: Raven Press.

Nashef, L., Walker, F., Allen, P., Sander, J.W.A.S., Shorvon, S.D. & Fish, D.R. (1996): Apnoea and bradycardia during epileptic seizures: relation to sudden death in epilepsy. *J. Neurol. Neurosurg. Psychiatry* **60**, 297–300.

Nelson, D.A. & Ray, C.D. (1968): Respiratory arrest from seizure discharges in limbic system. *Arch. Neurol.* **19**, 199–207.

Oppenheimer, S.M., Gelb, A., Girvin, J.P. & Hachinski, V.C. (1992): Cardio-vascular effect of human insular cortex stimulation. *Neurology* **42**, 1727–1732.

Ostrowski, K., Isnard, J., Ryvlin, P., Guénot, M., Fischer, C. & Mauguière, F. (2000): Functional mapping of the insular cortex: clinical implication in temporal lobe epilepsy. *Epilepsia* **41**, 681–686.

Pampiglione, G. & Falconer, M.A. (1960): Electrical stimulation of the hippocampus in man. In: *Handbook of physiology. Section I: Neurophysiology,* eds. J. Field, H.W. Magoun & V.E. Hall, pp. 1391–1394. Washington: Am. Physiol. Soc. Pub.

Panayiotopoulos, C.P. (1988): Vomiting as an ictal manifestation of epileptic seizures and syndromes. *J. Neurol. Neurosurg. Psychiatry* **51**, 1448–1451.

Penfield, W. (1958): Functional localization in temporal and deep sylvian areas. In: *The human brain and behaviour. Res. Pub. Ass. Nerv. Ment. Dis.,* pp. 210–226. Baltimore: Williams and Wilkins.

Penfield, W. & Faulk, M.E. Jr. (1955): The insula. Further observations on its function. *Brain* **78**, 445–470.

Penfield, W. & Jasper, H. (1954): *Epilepsy and the functional anatomy of the brain.* Boston: Little, Brown.

Penfield, W. & Kristiansen, K. (1951): *Epileptic seizure patterns.* Springfield: C. C. Thomas.

Penfield, W. & Rasmussen, T. (1950): *The cerebral cortex of man. A clinical study of localization and function.* New York: The Macmillan Company.

Penry, J.K., Porter, R.J. & Dreifuss, F.E. (1975): Simultaneous recording of absence seizures with video tape and electroencephalography. A study of 374 seizures in 48 patients. *Brain* **98**, 427–440.

Rathgeb, J.P., Plouin, P., Soufflet, C., Cieuta, C., Chiron, C. & Dulac, O. (1998): Le cas particulier des crises partielles du nourrisson: sémiologie électro-clinique. In: *Epilepsies partielles graves pharmaco-résistantes de l'enfant: stratégies diagnostiques et traitements chirurgicaux,* eds. M. Bureau, P. Kahane & C. Munari, pp. 122–134. Paris: John Libbey Eurotext.

Roze, E., Oubary, P. & Chedru, F. (2000): Status-like recurrent pilo-motor seizures: case report and review of the literature. *J. Neurol. Neurosurg. Psychiatry* **68**, 647–649.

Swartz, B.E. & Delgado-Escueta, A.V. (1987): Complex partial of extra-temporal origin: 'the evidence for'. In: *The epileptic focus. Current problems in epilepsy*, vol. 3, eds. H.G. Wieser, E.J. Speckmann & J.Engel Jr., pp. 137–174. London, Paris: John Libbey.

Talairach, J., Bancaud, J., Geier, S., Bordas-Ferrer, M., Bonis, A., Szikla, G. & Rusu, M. (1973): The cingulate gyrus and human behaviour. *Electroenceph. Clin. Neurophysiol.* **34**, 45–52.

Taylor, J. ed. (1931): Reprint of: *Selected writings of J. H. Jackson. Vol. 1: On epilepsy and epileptiform convulsions*. London: Hodder & Stoughton.

Taylor, D.C. & Lochery, M. (1987): Temporal lobe epilepsy: origin and significance of simple and complex auras. *J. Neurol. Neurosurg. Psychiatry* **50**, 673–681.

Temkin, O. (1945): *The falling sickness*. Baltimore: The Johns Hopkins Press.

Trousseau, A. (1868): De l'épilepsie. In: *Clinique médicale de l'Hôtel-Dieu de Paris*. Vol. 2, 3ème edn., pp. 86–149. Paris: J. B. Baillière et Fils.

Van Buren, J.M. (1958): Some autonomic concomitants of ictal automatisms. A study of temporal lobe attacks. *Brain* **81**, 505–528.

Van Buren, J.M. (1961): Sensory, motor and autonomic effects of mesial temporal stimulation in man. *J. Neurosurg.* **18**, 273–288.

Van Buren, J.M. (1963): The abdominal aura. A study of abdominal sensations occuring in epilepsy and produced by depth stimulation. *Electroenceph. Clin. Neurophysiol.* **15**, 1–19.

Van Buren, J.M. & Ajmone-Marsan, C.M. (1960): A correlation of autonomic and EEG components in temporal lobe epilepsy. *Arch. Neurol.* **3**, 683–703.

Van Buren, J.M., Bucknam C.A. & Pritchard W.L. (1961): Autonomic representation in the human orbitotemporal cortex. *Neurology* **11**, 214–224.

Veilleux, F., Saint-Hilaire, J.M., Giard, N., Turmel, A., Bernier, G.P., Rouleau, I., Mercier, M. & Bouvier, G. (1992): Seizures of the human medial frontal lobe. In: *Frontal lobe seizures and epilepsies, Adv. Neurol.*, **57**, eds. P. Chauvel, A.V. Delgado-Escueta, E. Halgren & J. Bancaud, pp. 245–255. New York: Raven Press.

Wannamaker, B.B. (1985): Autonomic nervous system and epilepsy. *Epilepsia* **26** (Suppl. 1), S31–S39.

Wieser H.G. (1983): *Electro-clinical features of the psychomotor seizure*, vol. I. Stuttgart, London: G. Fischer, Butterworths.

Wieser H.G. (1986): Psychomotor seizures of hippocampal-amygdalar origin. In: *Recent advances in epilepsy*, vol. 3., eds. T.A. Pedley & B.S. Meldrum, pp. 57–79. Edinburgh: Churchill, Livingstone.

Wieser H.G. (1987): The phenomenology of limbic seizures. In: *The epileptic focus. Current problems in epilepsy*, vol. 3, eds. H.G. Wieser, E.J. Speckmann & J.Engel Jr., pp. 113–136. London, Paris: John Libbey.

Wieser, H.G. & Williamson P.D. (1993): Ictal semiology. In: *Surgical treatment of the epilepsies*, 2nd edn., ed. J. Engel Jr., pp. 161–171. New York: Raven Press.

Wieser, H.G., Engel, J. Jr., Williamson, P.D., Babb, T.L. & Gloor, P. (1993): Surgically remediable temporal lobe syndromes. In: *Surgical treatment of the epilepsies*, 2nd edn., ed. J. Engel Jr., pp. 49–63. New York: Raven Press.

Williams, D. (1956): The structure of emotions reflected in epileptic experiences. *Brain* **79**, 29–67.

Williamson, P.D., Spencer, D.D., Spencer, S.S., Novelly, R.A. & Mattson R.H. (1985): Complex partial seizures of frontal lobe origin. *Ann. Neurol.* **18**, 497–504.

Wyllie, E. (1995): Developmental aspects of seizure semiology: problems in identifying localized onset seizures in infants and children. *Epilepsia* **36**, 1170–1172.

Wyllie, E., Chee, M., Granström, M.-L., DelGiudice, E., Estes, M., Comair, Y., Pizzi, M., Kotagal, P., Bourgeois, B. & Lüders, H. (1993): Temporal lobe epilepsy in early childhood. *Epilepsia* **34**, 859–868.

Yamamoto, M., Watanabe, K., Negoro, T., Takaesu, E., Aso, K., Furune, F. & Takahashi, T. (1987): Complex partial seizures in children: ictal manifestations and their relation to clinical course. *Neurology* **37**, 1379–1382.

Chapter 8

Language and speech disturbances in patients with limbic epilepsy

Hans O. Lüders

Cleveland Clinic Foundation, Department of Neurology – S90, 9500 Euclid Avenue, Cleveland, Ohio 44195–5226, USA

Summary

Patients with limbic epilepsy (seizures arising from the limbic system) may have language and/or speech alterations due to activation of the basal temporal language area or Wernicke's language area. This may be manifested as aphasic seizures if the patient is still responsive or may be a contributing factor to the typical 'unresponsiveness' observed in patients with limbic epilepsy. Patients with limbic seizures affecting the dominant hemisphere also frequently have postictal aphasia. Ictal speech, on the other hand, is usually an expression of a limbic epilepsy of the non-dominant hemisphere. Selective activation of the limbic system can produce pure amnestic seizures but usually has no effect on language or speech.

Introduction

Speech and language disturbances are seen frequently in patients with limbic epilepsy. In this chapter we will discuss the type of language and speech disturbances often observed in patients with limbic epilepsy, analyse the pathophysiology of these manifestations and its value for lateralizing or localizing the epileptogenic zone.

Mechanisms for speech disturbances in patients with epilepsy

Speech arrest or slowing elicited by an epileptiform discharge or electrical stimulation of the cortex can be produced by the following mechanisms (Fig.1):

(a) Activation of a positive motor area (Brodmann's areas 4 and 6) (Penfield & Jasper, 1954);

(b) Activation of the primary negative motor area (inferior frontal gyrus just in front of the primary face motor area) or the supplementary negative motor area (in front of the supplementary sensorimotor area) in the dominant or non-dominant hemisphere (Lüders *et al.*, 1992; Lüders *et al.*, 1995; Lüders *et al.*, 1987);

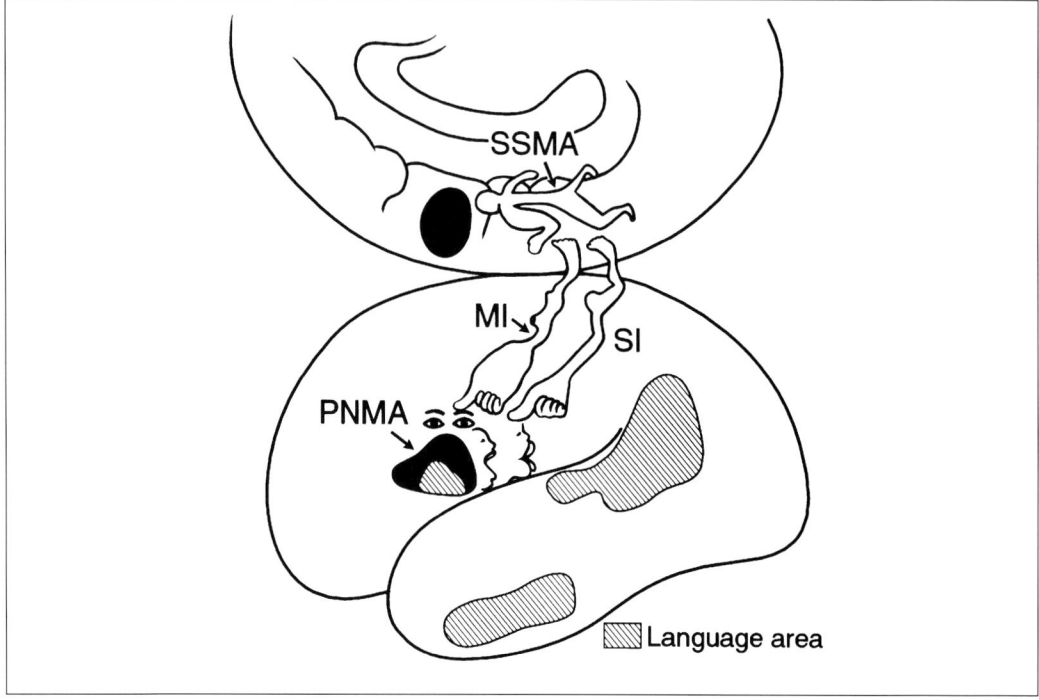

Fig. 1. Diagram of all major eloquent cortical areas.
(1) MI = primary motor cortex; (2) PNMA = primary negative motor area; (3) SI = primary somatosensory area; (4) SSMA = supplementary sensori-motor area.

  (c) Alteration of consciousness or responsiveness elicited by electrical stimulation or the epileptiform discharge;

  (d) Language alteration (Shäffler *et al.*, 1996; Shäffler *et al.*, 1993; Lüders *et al.*, 1991; Shäffler *et al.*, 1994).

It is essential to consider all the mechanisms listed above when electrical stimulation or an epileptiform activity produced a speech or language alteration. In other words, we can only conclude that a patient had a language disturbance if we have excluded all the other three mechanisms that can produce speech alterations.

The speech alteration produced by activation of the primary motor area is easy to recognize and corresponds to what has been identified as anarthria or dysarthria in clinical neurology. It occurs when the electrical stimulation (or the epileptiform discharge) produces an activation of muscles involved in the production of speech (tongue, pharynx, buccal musculature). It is best documented by directly observing the contraction of these muscles during the seizure or during electrical stimulation. It usually occurs when stimulating the primary motor area of the face (Brodmann's areas 4 and 6) (see Fig. 2)

Activation of the negative motor areas (primary or supplementary) produces inability to perform voluntary movements, particularly of the distal segments (hands, mouth, tongue). Activation of a negative motor area also frequently produces speech arrest because of inability to move the muscles involved in the production of speech (pharynx, tongue, lips) (Penfield & Jasper, 1954;

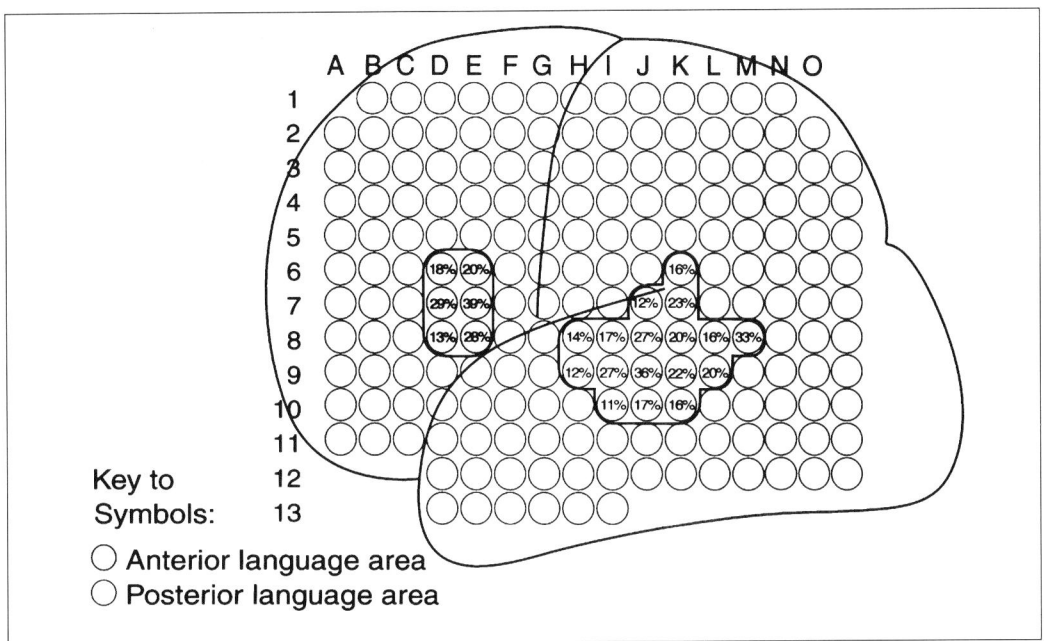

Fig. 2. Diagram showing the electrode positions in the left lateral convexity at which electrical stimulation elicited language deficits in more than 10 per cent of the time (Shäffler et al., 1996).

Lüders *et al.*, 1992; Lüders *et al.*, 1995; Lüders *et al.*, 1987). Penfield & Roberts (1959) reported on the existence of a language area (so called 'superior language area') located in the supplementary sensorimotor area. In our stimulation studies we were unable to produce any language disturbances (Lüders *et al.*, 1992; Lüders *et al.*, 1995; Lüders *et al.*, 1987) when stimulating this area. However, just in front of the supplementary sensorimotor area we identified a supplementary negative motor area which when stimulated usually produces speech arrest. It is likely that the 'superior speech area' identified by Penfield & Roberts (1959) actually corresponds to this supplementary negative motor area.

Epileptiform cortical activation frequently produces alteration of consciousness during which the patient becomes more or less unresponsive and, therefore, speech and language cannot be tested. Similar alterations of consciousness may be triggered by electrical stimulation when it triggers an afterdischarge or an actual EEG seizure.

Alterations of speech or language which are not produced by any of the three mechanisms discussed above are attributed to activation (epileptiform or due to electrical stimulation) of a language area.

Cortical language areas

Electrical stimulation has identified the following three cortical areas that can produce alterations of language functions (Shäffler *et al.*, 1996; Shäffler *et al.*, 1993; Lüders *et al.*, 1991; Shäffler *et al.*, 1994) (Fig. 1).

(1) Anterior language area: this area is located in the dominant hemisphere in the inferior

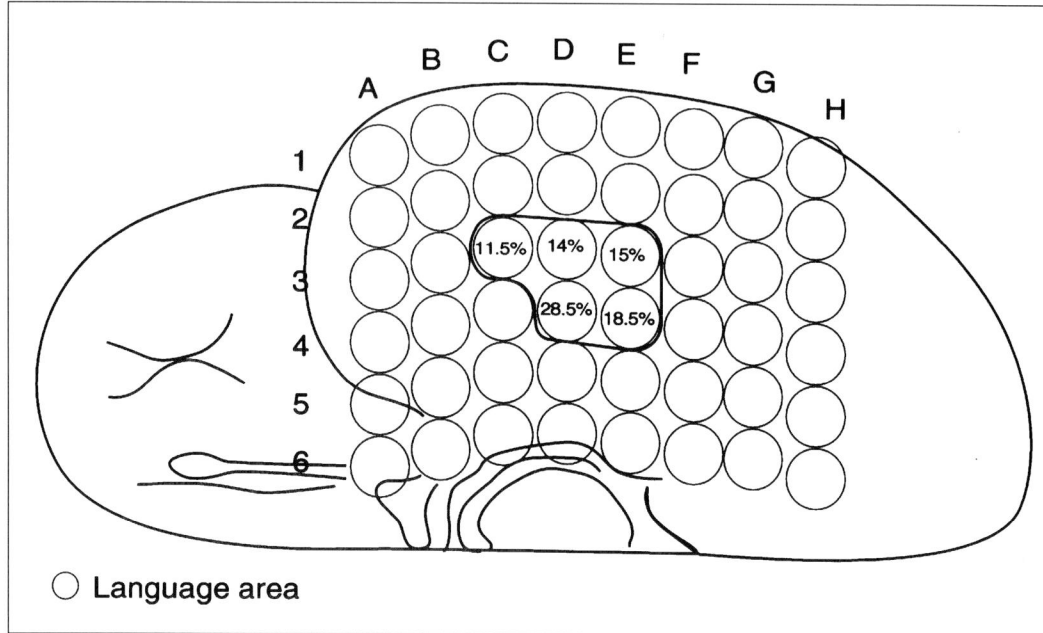

Fig. 3. Diagram showing the electrode positions in the basal temporal cortex at which electrical stimulation elicited language deficits for more than 10 per cent of the time.

frontal gyrus immediately in front of the primary motor area of the face (Brodmann's areas 44, 45);

(2) Posterior language area: this area is located in the dominant hemisphere in the superior temporal gyrus usually posterior to Heschl gyrus and also posterior with respect to the point where the central sulcus meets the Sylvian Fissure. It may include part of the supramarginal or angular gyrus (Brodmann's areas 21, 22, 39, 40);

(3) The basal temporal language area: this area is located in the dominant hemisphere in the fusiform gyrus (Brodmann area 20).

Figures 2 and 3 show the electrode positions that most frequently produced language alteration when stimulated electrically (Shäffler et al., 1996). The effect of electrical stimulation is a function of the stimulus parameters (stimulus intensity, duration and stimulus frequency). At relatively low stimulus intensities, no language interference can be detected. As the stimulus intensity increases, language interference becomes progressively more intense until global aphasia occurs. At intermediate stimulus intensities the most varied 'aphasic syndromes' can be triggered. The same effect would be expected to occur when language areas are activated by epileptiform discharges. However, the spike-wave form, amplitude or duration is not necessarily a good index of the strength of the stimulus it is delivering on the cortex. In other words, 'relatively prominent' epileptiform discharges may occur in eloquent cortex without producing any positive or negative effects and, therefore, the observation that epileptiform discharges occurred in any cortical area without producing any functional alteration does not lead to the conclusion that that area is non-eloquent.

Limbic epilepsy, limbic seizures and language alterations

In this study, we define *limbic epilepsy* as a disease with an epileptogenic zone in the limbic system, including particularly the hippocampus, the amygdala and the cingulate gyrus. An *epileptogenic zone* is defined as the area of cortex from which clinical seizures originate and whose resection results in seizure freedom. Finally, we define *limbic seizures* as the clinical manifestations of seizures arising from the limbic structures.

As mentioned above, language alterations are seen frequently during limbic seizures. However, electrical stimulation of the limbic system produces no language alterations unless afterdischarges occur. Therefore, it is very likely that all the language alterations observed during limbic seizures are an expression of seizure spread with involvement of one of the language areas located outside the limbic system (see below).

Activation of the limbic system and language alterations

The hippocampus is an essential structure in the formation of anterograde memories. Bilateral destruction of the hippocampus completely abolishes our capacity to form new memories leading to a severe and irreversible anterograde memory deficit (Scoville & Milner, 1957). Patients with bilateral hippocampal lesions, however, still preserve immediate and remote memory, and suffer no language deficits. We would expect also that an inactivation of the hippocampus by an epileptiform discharge would produce similar deficits. Indeed, electrical stimulation of the hippocampus produces no language deficit unless there is an afterdischarge or an electrical seizure involving structures outside the hippocampus. There is also evidence that the clinical semiology seen during mesial temporal seizures is usually an expression of a spread of the seizure outside the hippocampus. An exception are the so called 'pure amnestic seizures', described by Palmini *et al.* (1992) which consist just of short episodes of anterograde amnesia. During the episodes itself the patient is able to speak, and interacts normally with the environment. After the seizure, however, the patient does not recall any of the events that happened during the seizure. Palmini *et al.* (1992) observed that these pure amnestic seizures occurred only when the epileptiform discharge involved more or less selectively both hippocampi or involved one hippocampus while the other hippocampus was already significantly damaged. Summarizing, it seems that amnesia can be due to epileptic discharges limited to the hippocampus. However, language alterations seen in patients with limbic seizures are an expression of seizure spread with involvement of one of the language areas described above.

Language alterations due to seizure spread

Seizure spread to involve any of the language areas described above will result in different degrees of ictal or postictal aphasia. The exact mechanism by which an epileptiform discharge produces language deficits, including complete receptive and expressive aphasia is unknown. However, results of electrical stimulation studies show that electrical stimulation of a language area does not result in positive effects (like production of speech) but exclusively in negative phenomena, most notoriously speech arrest and complete incapacity to understand oral or written language. It is assumed that electrical or epileptiform activation of the language areas leads to depolarization of neurons and, therefore, inability of the neuronal pool within a language area to perform the delicate functions necessary to produce or understand (compare incoming visual or auditory signals with previous language engrams, the so-called 'Wortschatz' (Word Treasury) of Wernicke (Wernicke, 1874). Cortical stimulation of other higher cortical centres also results in similar 'negative' effects. For example, stimulation of the dominant angular gyrus produces the different elements of the Gerstman syndrome (Morris *et al.*, 1984) and stimulation of the negative motor areas, which are most probably involved in the generation of voluntary movements, results in inability to perform distal voluntary movements (Lüders *et al.*, 1992; Lüders *et al.*, 1995; Lüders *et al.*, 1987).

It has been documented that epileptiform activation of the basal temporal language area results in ictal aphasia. We also know that the epileptiform discharge in seizures arising from an hippocampus will usually spread first to the contralateral hippocampus and then into the ipsilateral basal temporal and lateral temporal convexity. Spreading of the seizure to the contralateral temporal neocortex will usually be associated with an alteration of consciousness. Therefore, ictal language alterations tend to occur only when the seizures originate from the language dominant hemisphere and most probably are primarily due to inactivation of the basal temporal area. Later during the seizure, inactivation of the Wernicke's and Broca's areas may participate in the language deficit observed with limbic seizures. In seizures arising from the non-dominant hemisphere, the contralateral language areas are usually only inactivated at a later stage of the seizure, when the patient already has lost consciousness.

There is some evidence that temporal lobe seizures produce a predominantly receptive aphasia whereas frontal lobe seizures (which most probably will lead to aphasias by inactivation of Broca's area) produce primarily a receptive aphasia.

Unfortunately, most patients with limbic seizures will become 'unresponsive' and inattentive during seizures, making detailed language testing impossible.

Language deficits during limbic seizures and alterations of 'consciousness' during limbic seizures

Limbic seizures are associated with an unusual unresponsiveness and confusion with postictal amnesia for the events occurring during the seizure. This state has been identified as 'unconsciousness' even if it is very different from the unconsciousness seen in patients suffering from coma. The mechanisms producing this special state have not been elucidated. However, it seems that it tends to occur more frequently or at least earlier with seizures arising from the left dominant temporal lobe. Patients with left temporal lobe epilepsy reach this state of unresponsiveness almost without exception at the time the patient has ictal automatisms (finger, hand and oro-alimentary automatisms). On the other hand, in almost 10 per cent of patients with right temporal, non-dominant epilepsy, the patients have automatisms *before* there is unresponsiveness (and also frequently before anterograde amnesia occurs) (Ebner *et al.*, 1995). This suggests that this special state of unresponsiveness and confusion may well be related to inactivation of some crucial functions in the left, dominant temporal cortex which tends to be involved in the initial spread of the epileptiform discharge. It is, therefore, tempting to speculate that the unresponsiveness and confusion usually seen at the early stages of limbic seizures is the result of inactivation of the basal temporal language area and perhaps also Wernicke's language area. In addition, the anterograde amnesia, which frequently accompanies this state of unresponsiveness and confusion, could well be the expression of inactivation of both hippocampi. This hypothesis is in good agreement with the early spread of the epileptiform discharge into the contralateral hippocampus and the ipsilateral basal temporal region. The relatively later involvement of the contralateral temporal basal region would explain the interesting occurrence of automatisms without 'loss of consciousness' in patients with right, non-dominant temporal lobe epilepsy (Ebner *et al.*, 1995). The contribution of inactivation of language areas to the special state of 'alteration of consciousness' seen during temporal lobe epilepsy would explain also why it is rare for patients with temporal lobe epilepsy to produce intelligible speech during seizures after the patients loses consciousness ('ictal speech') (Gabr *et al.*, 1989). Ictal speech is seen most frequently during right temporal epilepsy and most probably is an expression of an epileptiform discharge which inactivates both hippocampi but affects the contralateral basal temporal and posterior language areas only incompletely leading to some comprehension deficits but preserved language output. Ictal speech is a sign pointing to a right, non-dominant temporal lobe epilepsy but occasionally it may also occur in dominant left temporal lobe epilepsies.

Language disturbances in patient with cingulate epilepsy

Epileptiform discharges originating in the cingulate (anterior or posterior cingulate) frequently spread to involve the supplementary sensorimotor area (SSMA) during early stages. It would be possible, therefore, that patients suffering from cingulate epilepsy will also have speech arrest due to involvement of the supplementary negative motor area. However, in the series of nine patients with cingulate epilepsy studied at the Cleveland Clinic, none had aphasic seizures or speech arrest during the conscious part of the seizure. This is most probably related to the fact that cingulate seizures originate at a considerable distance from the SSMA and, therefore, when the epileptiform discharge spreads into the SSMA it tends to activate simultaneously the negative and positive motor areas of that region. Simultaneous activation of negative and positive motor areas leads to predominantly positive motor signs which overshadow the negative motor manifestations.

Clinical significance of language disturbances in patients with limbic epilepsy

The following alterations of language which are observed during limbic seizures have lateralizing significance:

(1) Occurrence of automatisms with preservation of comprehensive and expressive language is characteristic of right, non-dominant hippocampal seizures (Ebner *et al.*, 1995).

(2) Clear understandable speech at a time the patient has lost responsiveness and has become amnestic for the seizure (patient unable to recall that he talked during the seizure). This sign is also most often seen with right, non-dominant temporal lobe epilepsy. However, false positives occur (Gabr *et al.*, 1989).

(3) Postictal aphasia. Patients with left, dominant temporal lobe epilepsy not infrequently have a striking postictal aphasia. This aphasia is most probably produced by a mechanism very similar to Todd's paralysis. Only patients who have recovered completely from the seizure and appear attentive to the observer's questions but are aphasic should be considered as having postictal aphasia. In these patients usually a global aphasia occurs initially. Then with time (2–20 min) the patient slowly recovers, understanding the observer's questions better and better, and progressively answering more complex questions. At that time it is frequent also to notice literal paraphasias, echolalia, and perseverations. Postictal aphasia should be clearly differentiated from postictal confusion during which the patient may also not answer any questions but is

inattentive and does not make any efforts to follow the observer's commands. Postictal aphasia, if appropriately diagnosed, is a reliable sign that the patient presents left, dominant lobe temporal lobe epilepsy (Gabr et al., 1989).

Conclusions

Limbic seizures very frequently produce language disturbances. Epileptiform activation limited to the limbic system does not produce any language disturbance. It appears that most if not all the language disturbances seen in patients with limbic epilepsy are an expression of an epileptiform inactivation of the basal temporal and Wernicke's language areas. It is also possible that relatively early inactivation of these language areas contributes, together with amnesia for anterograde events (due to inactivation of both hippocampi), to the unusual state of unresponsiveness and amnesia seen with most temporal lobe seizures. Ictal speech (clearly understandable speech in spite of confusion and anterograde amnesia) is seen significantly more frequently in right, non-dominant temporal lobe epilepsy. Automatisms in spite of preserved language functions and relative responsiveness are a relatively reliable sign pointing to a right, non-dominant limbic epilepsy. On the other hand, postictal aphasia is a reliable sign of a left, dominant temporal lobe epilepsy.

References

Ebner, A., Dinner, D.S., Noachtar, S. & Lüders, H. (1995): Automatisms with preserved responsiveness: a lateralizing sign in psychomotor seizures. *Neurology* **45**, 61–64.

Gabr, M., Lüders, H., Dinner, D., Morris, H. & Wyllie, E. (1989): Speech manifestations in lateralization of temporal lobe seizures. *Ann. Neurol.* **25**, 82–87.

Lüders, H.O. (1992): In: *Epilepsy surgery,* ed. H.O. Lüders, p. 854. New York: Raven Press.

Lüders, H., Lesser, R.P., Morris, H.H., Dinner, D.S. & Hahn, J. (1987): Negative motor responses elicited by stimulation of the human cortex. *Adv. Epileptol.* **16**, 229–231.

Lüders, H., Lesser, R.P., Hahn, J., Dinner, D.S., Morris, H.H., Wyllie, E. & Godoy, J. (1991): Basal temporal language area. *Brain* **114**, 743–754.

Lüders, H.O., Lesser, R.P., Dinner, D.S., *et al.* (1992): A negative motor response elicited by electrical stimulation of the human frontal cortex. In: *Advances in neurology,* eds. P. Chauvel, A.V. Delgado-Escueta *et al.*, vol. 57, pp. 149-157. New York: Raven Press.

Lüders, H.O., Dinner, D.S., Morris, H.H., Wyllie, E. & Comair, Y.G. (1995): Cortical electrical stimulation in humans: the negative motor areas. In: *Advances in neurology: negative motor phenomena,* vol. 67, pp. 115–130. Lippincott-Raven Publishers.

Morris, H.H., Lüders, H., Lesser, R.P., Dinner, D.S. & Hahn, J. (1984): Transient neuro-psychological abnormalities (including Gerstmann's Syndrome) during cortical stimulation. *Neurology* **34**, 877–883.

Palmini, Al., Gloor, P. & Jones-Gotman, M. (1992): Pure amnestic seizures in temporal lobe epilepsy. Definition, clinical symptomatology and functional anatomical considerations. *Brain* **115** (Pt3), 749–769.

Penfield, W. & Jasper, H. (1954): *Epilepsy and the functional anatomy of the human brain,* p. 896. Boston: Little, Brown & Company.

Penfield, W. & Roberts, L. (1959): *Speech and brain mechanisms,* p. 279. New Jersey: Princeton University Press.

Scoville, W.B. & Milner, B. (1957): Loss of recent memory after bilateral hippocampal lesions. *J. Neurol. Neurosurg. Psychiatry* **20**, 11–21.

Schäffler, L., Lüders, H.O., Dinner, D.S., Lesser, R.P. & Chelune, G.J. (1993): Comprehension deficits elicited by electrical stimulation of Broca's area. *Brain* **116**, 695–715.

Schäffler, L., Lüders, H., Morris, H. & Wyllie, E. (1994): Anatomic distribution of cortical language sites in the basal temporal language area in patients with left temporal lobe epilepsy. *Epilepsia* **35,** 525–528.

Shäffler, L., Lüders, H.O. & Beck, G.J. (1996): Quantitative comparison of language deficits produced by extraoperative electrical stimulation of Broca's Wernicke's, and basal temporal language areas. *Epilepsia* **37**(5), 463–475.

Wernicke, C. (1874): *Der aphasiche Symptomencomplex*, p. 72. Breslau: Max Cohen and Weigert.

Chapter 9

Motor automatisms in limbic seizures

Arnaud Biraben*, Delphine Taussig†, Serge Belliard*, Eric Seigneuret‡ and Jean-Marie Scarabin‡

*Service de Neurologie, CHU Pontchaillou, Rennes, France; †Service d'Explorations Fonctionnelles, CHU Pontchaillou, Rennes, France; ‡Service de Neurochirurgie, CHU Pontchaillou, Rue Henri Le Guilloux, 35033 Rennes, France

Summary

The first definition of automatism, proposed by Jackson (1875), described motor activities in unconscious subjects resulting from a dysfunction of the centres controlling motricity. It is now recognized that such automatisms can occur in conscious subjects. Classically a distinction is made between automatisms occurring during epileptic seizures involving a cerebral structure, and post-ictal automatisms resulting from brain disorganization. Certain authors also distinguish 'de novo' automatisms occurring in response to internal solicitation and automatisms related to external solicitation or pursuit of ongoing activity. Motor automatisms can be described according to their clinical presentation:

– Oro-alimentary automatisms, where early discharge in the amygdala, and almost always in the anterior Ammon's horn is observed on stereoelectroencephalography (SEEG) recordings. Oro-alimentary automatisms appear to be related to a disruption of the subcortical systems connected to the amygdala structures.

– Simple gesture automatisms involving exploratory activities such as touching, grasping, rubbing or picking and which originate in the temporal or orbito-frontal lobes. These automatisms should be distinguished from reactions to seizure-related sensations or secretions. They could result from a loss of the limbic system's inhibitory effect against attraction to exterior stimuli situated in the immediate pericorporal vicinity.

– Verbal automatisms are stereotypic utterances, whether comprehensible or not. In our experience they are related to activity in the temporal neocortex of the dominant hemisphere.

– Complex automatisms are intense activities such as pedalling movements and are often attributed to activity in the medial orbito-frontal and medial frontal regions. We have observed this type of automatisms in seizures with a temporal then a frontal discharge or in seizures limited to the temporal lobe, either in association with or in reaction to strong emotions such as fear. The underlying mechanism might be related to a disorganized limbic system which leads to defective control of motor activity or to an abnormal response to external or internal solicitations. It is difficult to draw a line between complex automatisms and forced activity.

Definitions

The first definition of automatism was proposed by Jackson who wanted to describe the signs observed during and after epileptic seizures. 'It is convenient to have one name for all kinds of doings after epileptic fits ... They have one common character, they are automatic; they are done unconsciously and the agent is irresponsible. Hence, I use the term mental automatism ... The mental automatism results, I consider, from overaction of lower nervous centres because the highest or controlling centres have been thus put out of use' (Jackson, 1875). When Feindel & Penfield described temporal lobe automatisms, they also referred to unconscious patients and did not distinguish between different types of activity or behaviour (Feindel & Penfield, 1954). Gloor considered that purposeful voluntary motor behaviour, performed by an unresponsive patient with no memory of what he has done, is an automatism (Gloor, 1986). Loiseau & Jallon defined automatism as any involuntary motor activity occurring during an epileptic seizure irrespective of the state of consciousness (Loiseau & Jallon, 1990). We retain this latter definition.

Classically, automatisms occurring during seizures apparently related to hyperactivity of a given brain structure are distinguished from automatisms occurring after seizures subsequent to brain disorganization. Penry & Dreyfuss examined absences and distinguished '*de novo*' automatisms produced in response to internal solicitation, and automatisms related to external stimulation or pursuit of an ongoing activity which are certainly greatly affected by memory (Penry & Dreyfuss, 1969).

Certain types of automatic activities can be termed 'reactional'. Simple reactional automatisms accompanying temporal lobe seizures, such as nose scratching or eye rubbing, can be related to sensations or secretions occurring during the seizure, favoured by declining consciousness; the same type of reaction occurs when a subject moves a hand to the stomach area when feeling an epigastric sensation. Complex reactional automatisms, such as flight, aggressive behaviour, grasping or facial expressions, can, in our experience, also be related to what the patient feels, although the consciousness or memory disorders accompanying seizures sometimes preclude formal proof. Activities in the limbic, particularly the amygdala, and orbito-frontal structures participate in the genesis or expression of these emotions (Gloor, 1997). It is often difficult to draw a line between reactional automatism and 'true' complex automatism (see below).

Several types of automatisms may occur together during a given seizure. The Sainte-Anne experience demonstrates that automatic or involuntary activity does not always imply a given localization. Inversely, certain specific activities, examined over the time-course of the seizure, would suggest the involvement of a particular structure (Bancaud, 1987). Two pathogenic hypotheses have been put forward: the 'layer' theory and the 'parallel' theory. According to the 'layer' hypothesis, a lower motor centre is 'freed' from the controlling influence of higher centres. In the 'parallel' hypothesis, there would be an imbalance between 'external' sensorial and 'internal' influences controlling motor activity.

We will describe separately oro-alimentary automatisms, simple gesture automatisms, verbal automatisms and complex automatisms.

Oro-alimentary automatisms

Clinically, chewing movements and other oral manifestations such as movements of the lips and tongue unrelated to deglutition should be distinguished from 'viscero-vegetative' movements

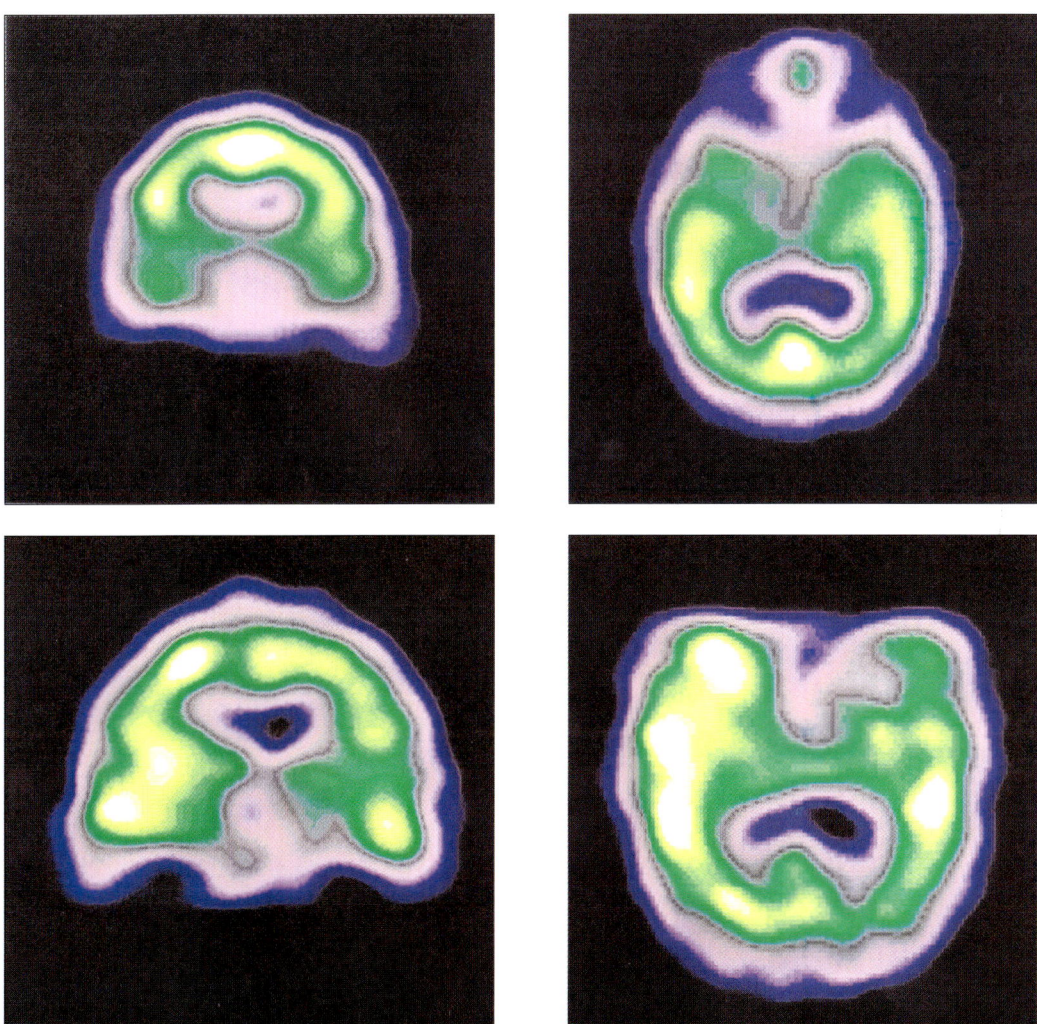

Fig. 1. Ictal single photon emission computed tomography (SPECT) of a patient with chewing as main clinical feature of right internal temporal seizure.
1a: Interictal SPECT (upper).
1b: Ictal SPECT (lower).

such as deglutition, spitting, lip licking, and degustation which implicate the participation of suprasylvian regions. Chewing and oral movements are related to an early discharge in the amygdala and almost always in the anterior Ammon's horn, as Munari et al. (1979) demonstrated with stereoelectroencephalography (SEEG) recordings. These authors studied spontaneous or provoked seizures in 27 patients with chewing movements and observed that they occurred within 5 s of an amygdala discharge in all 27 patients and with activity in the anterior Ammon's horn in 25 (Murani et al., 1979). Chewing movements can occur without loss of consciousness (only one patient had an initial loss of consciousness in Munari's series). We also observed one patient with a lesion of the right amygdala (latter identified as a ganglioglioma) whose seizures were almost exclusively chewing movements after an ascending epigastric

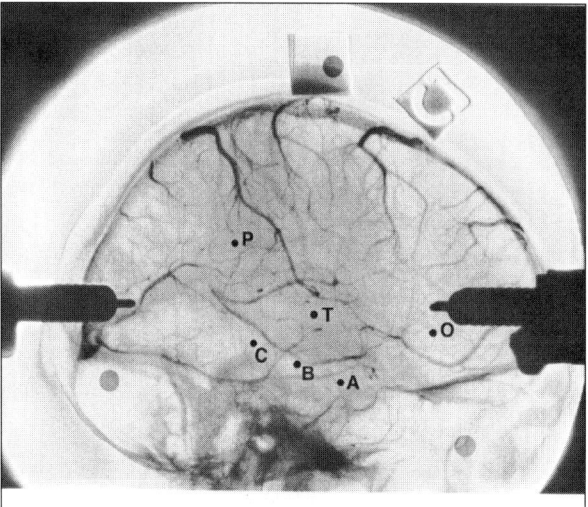

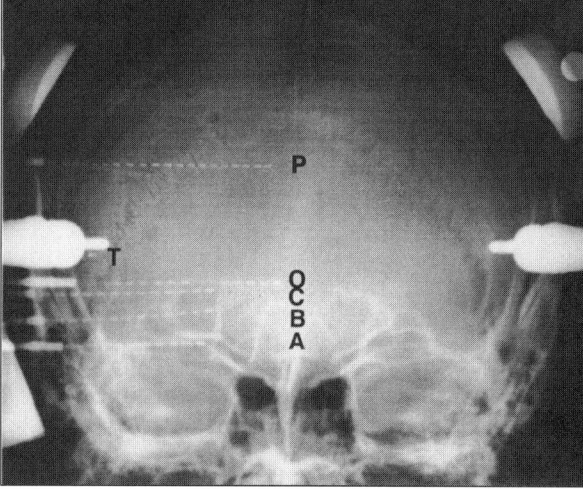

Fig. 2. Complex oro alimentary automatisms in right temporal medial seizure.
2.a: X-ray of the skull during depth electrodes recording showing the implantation
Top: profile view. Bottom: front view.

sensation; the subject had complete amnesia of the episode. On the EEG recording, the background rhythm of the right anterior temporal region was disrupted before a series of spikes occurred in the same territory. Ictal SPECT demonstrated a characteristic temporal pattern (Fig. 1). The patient was cured by temporal lobectomy (seizure-free at 3.5 year follow-up). The underlying pathophysiological mechanism would be related to a disorganization of the subcortical systems linked to the amygdala structures. Kaada (1951) demonstrated that chewing movements are produced in the cat, the monkey and the dog by stimulating the rostal piriform cortex and the amygdala, independently of the motor cortex. There is no direct projection of the amygdala on to the motor cortex (Amaral, 1990), but the amygdala circuits are connected with the brain stem neurons implicated in the integration of the mastication motor programme (Nakamura & Kubo, 1978). Although the inhibitory role of the amygdala remains to be proven, the most likely hypothesis is that the chewing seizure results from disinhibition of the amygdala's control over these brain stem structures.

In frontal seizures, the chewing movements are less characteristic and do not occur so precociously. They are often short-lived, not particularly rhythmic and are often observed after seizures terminate. Chewing may be seen in some seizures with a frontal origin, possibly in relation with temporal propagation via the anterior cingulate (Geier et al., 1977). Electrical stimulation of the anterior cingulate can produce different types of oral movements such as lip licking, sucking, exploration of the buccal cavity with the tongue, deglutition, or sometimes even chewing (Bancaud et al., 1976).

Oral movements are sometimes difficult to interpret: in one of our patients with a right medial temporal epilepsy, the seizure began by chewing followed some tens of seconds later by a more complex oral activity: the patient started tearing out the pages of a magazine and tried to eat them. At this moment, the spikes had reached the orbito-frontal region (Fig. 2). Clinically, the

Chapter 9   Motor automatisms in limbic seizures

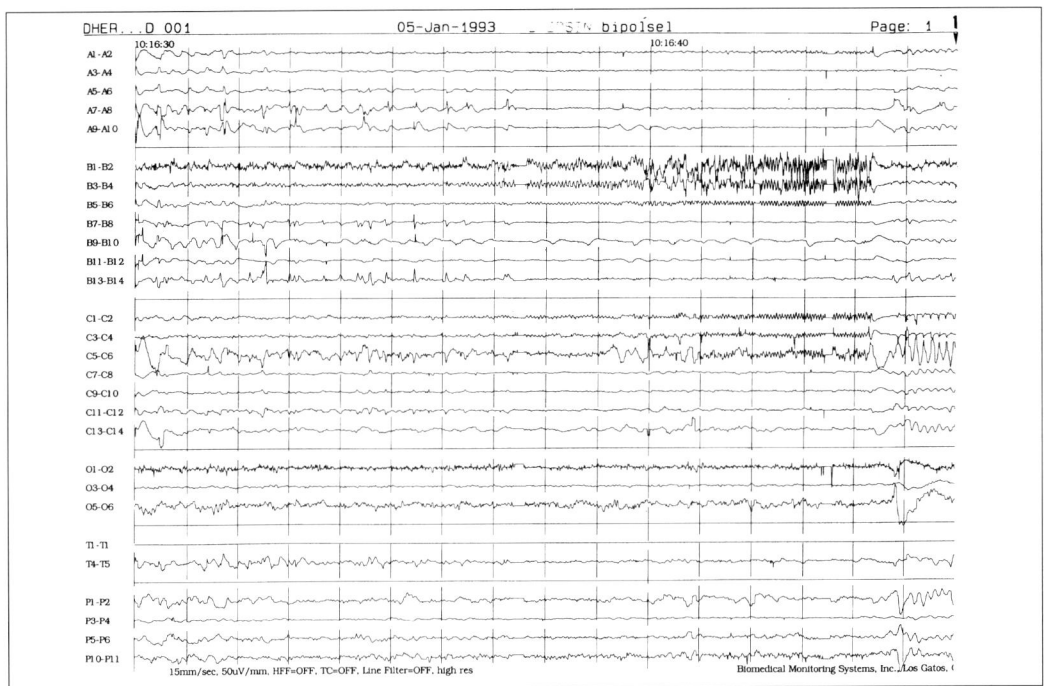

Fig. 2b. Seizure. 1: Onset of chewing.

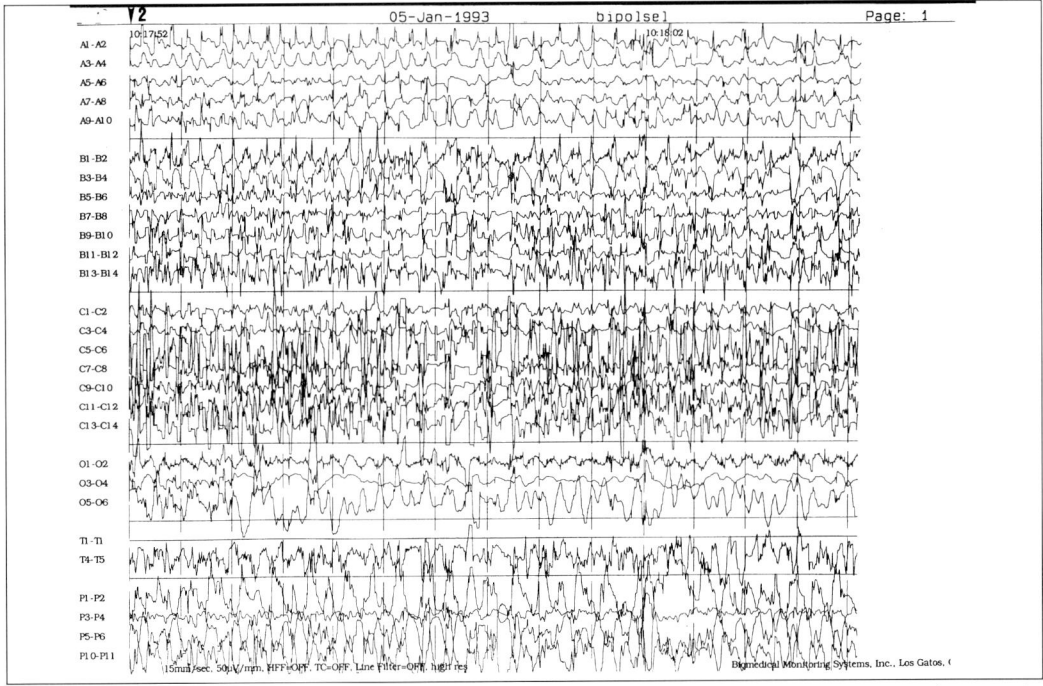

2: Onset some tens of seconds later of a more complex oral activity: the patient starts tearing out the pages of a magazine and tries to eat them.

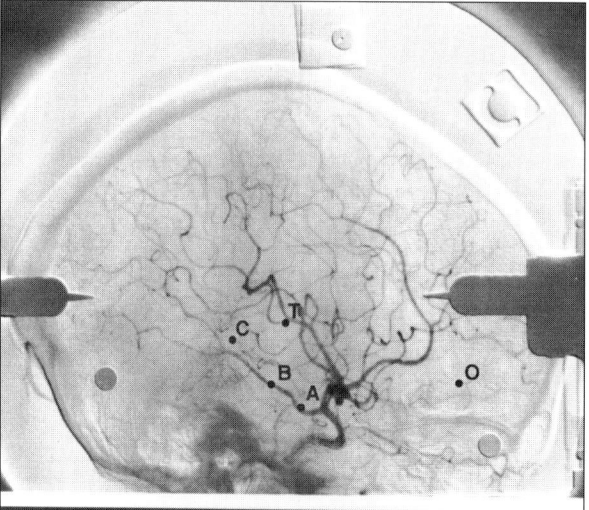

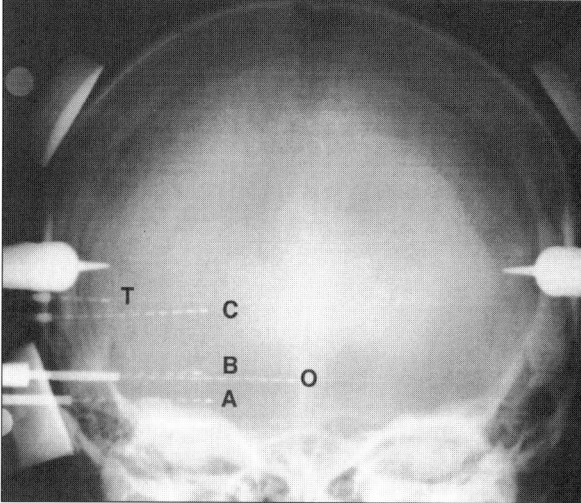

Fig. 3. Simple gesture automatisms.
3a: X-ray of the skull during depth electrode recording showing the implantation.
Top: profile view. Bottom: front view. Seizure induced by stimulation of right amygdala (5 s, 50 Hz, 1.5 mA).

distinction is not clear, but the secondary eating behaviour may be a more complex 'mastication' phenomenon. Perhaps disinhibition of a more archaic behaviour would be a more likely explanation. In this hypothesis, instead of being secondary to subcortical disorganization related to the discharge in the amygdala, the oral activity would be the expression of circuits implicating the frontal lobe.

Simple gesture automatisms

Simple gesture automatisms involve exploratory activities: the individual repeatedly touches, grasps, rubs or picks at him/herself and the immediate environment. Unilateral automatisms most often involve the upper limb homolateral to the discharge; bilateral forms are nevertheless often reported (Quesney, 1986). Automatisms homolateral to the discharge can be associated with contralateral dystonia (Kotagal et al., 1989). Such automatisms are not induced by electrical stimulation of Ammon's horn or the amygdala when the post-discharge remains within these structures (Bancaud et al., 1966). In our experience, we have also found that this type of automatism is not observed when ictal discharges are limited to the medial temporal structures. We reviewed the spontaneous or electrically triggered seizures in 10 patients with medial temporal epilepsy proven by intracerebral recordings and who were explored by SEEG using the anatomo-electroclinical method described by Talairach & Bancaud (Talairach et al., 1974) with electrodes implanted in the temporal lobe and at least one orbito frontal electrode. Among the seven patients who exhibited simple gesture automatisms, the automatisms occurred a few seconds after the onset of slow waves in the orbital cortex (Fig. 3).

This type of automatism can also be observed in orbito-frontal seizures. We have seen this in one patient whose seizures were characterized by an elementary motor behaviour comparable to that observed in temporal seizures; the patient rubbed his pyjama with his hand and made no other movements. The atypical element was the sudden onset of the seizure which began

Chapter 9 Motor automatisms in limbic seizures

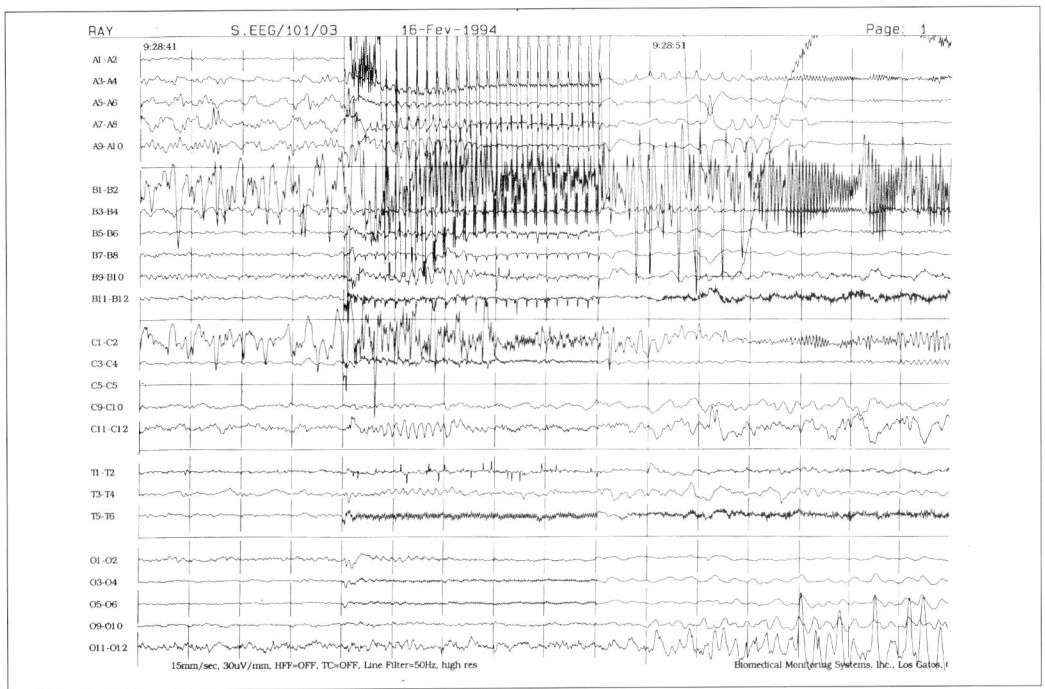

Fig. 3b. Seizure induced by stimulation of right amygdala (15 s, 50 Hz, 1 mA).

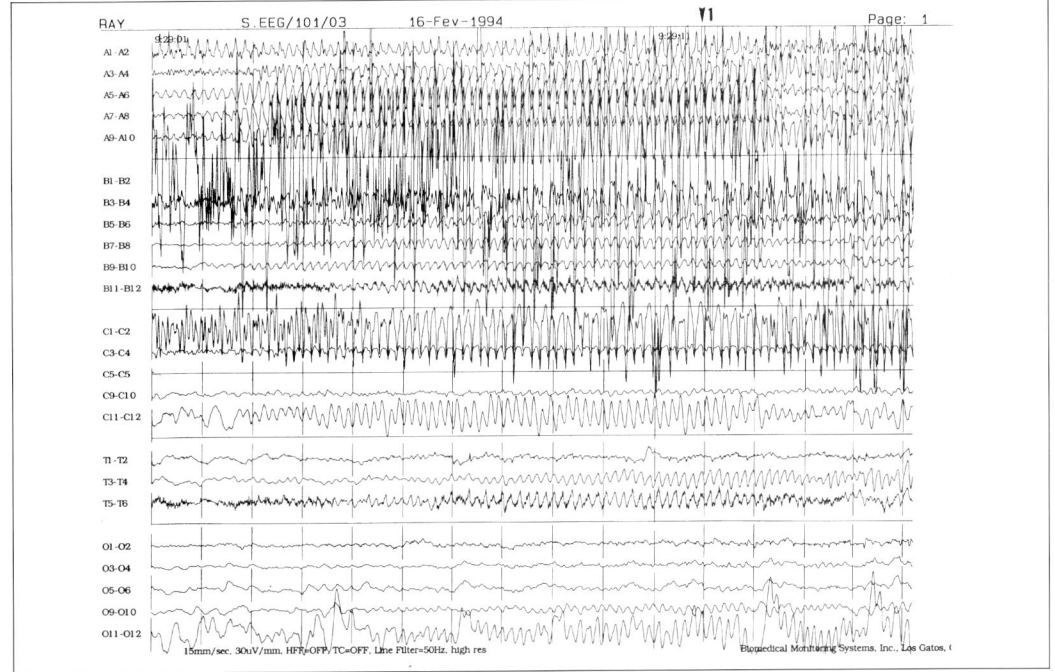

Fig. 3b. 1: Simple automatism of left hand.

95

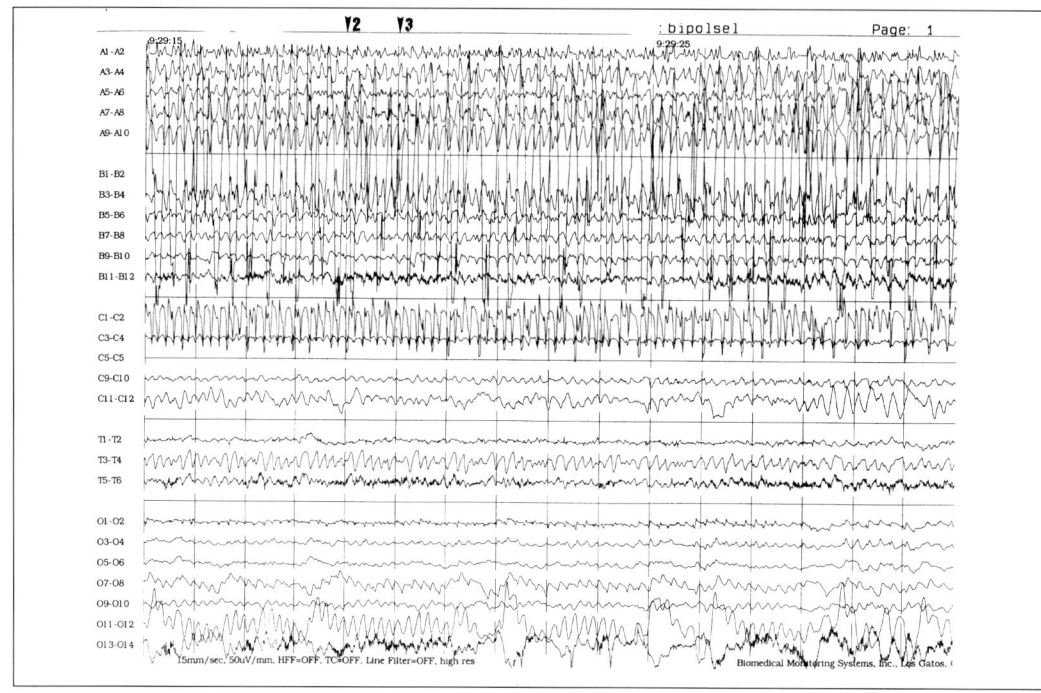

Fig. 3b. 2: Chewing. 3: Grips and grasps the doctor's hand.

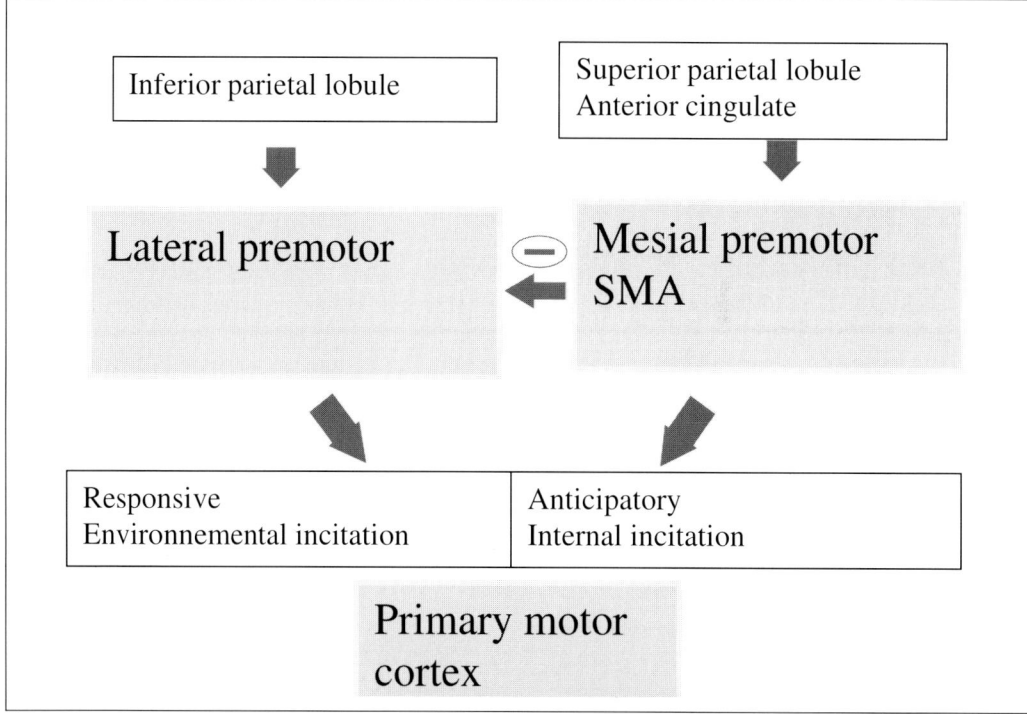

Fig. 4. Prefrontal connections in primate (from Goldman-Rakic, 1995).

without any prior subjective manifestation. The SEEG temporo-frontal recording confirmed the frontal focus of these seizures. Orbito-frontal cortectomy cured this patient who has been symptom-free for 7 years.

Bancaud et al. reported electrical stimulation of the cingulate in 83 patients and observed different types of effects. The most characteristic effect was an elementary motor activity found in 70 per cent of the patients (rubbing, lint picking, kneading, crumpling, scratching, pinching, grasping) (Bancaud et al., 1976). More elaborate motor activity is however observed in some cases. In addition, the high intensity of the stimulation would suggest that more distant structures are recruited.

The symptomatology of these automatisms is somewhat similar to the alien or 'capricious' hand described by Poncet et al. (Poncet et al., 1994) which is attracted to stimuli lying in the close vicinity. This compulsive eupraxic gesture is poorly controlled and related to a lesion of the medial portion of the frontal lobe and the corpus callosum (Goldberg et al., 1981). Grasping and manipulating objects situated in the pericorporal space could be attributed to an imbalance between the activating lateral premotor system and an inhibitory medial premotor system induced by the seizure. Since the work reported by Goldberg (1985), it can be accepted that the premotor ventrolateral system, connected to the secondary retrorolandic senso-

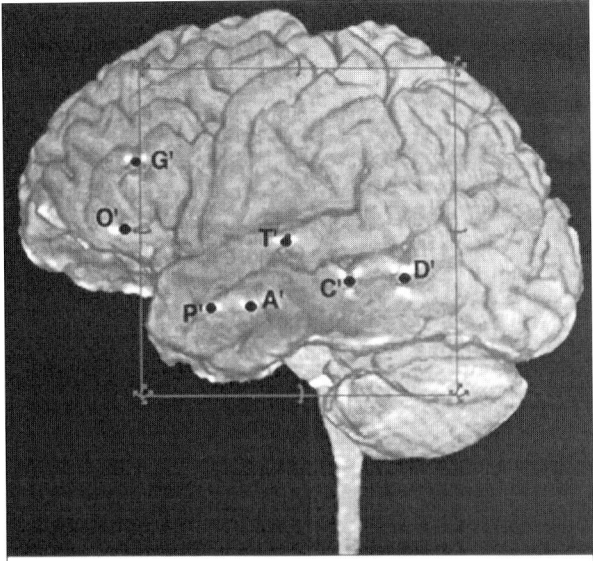

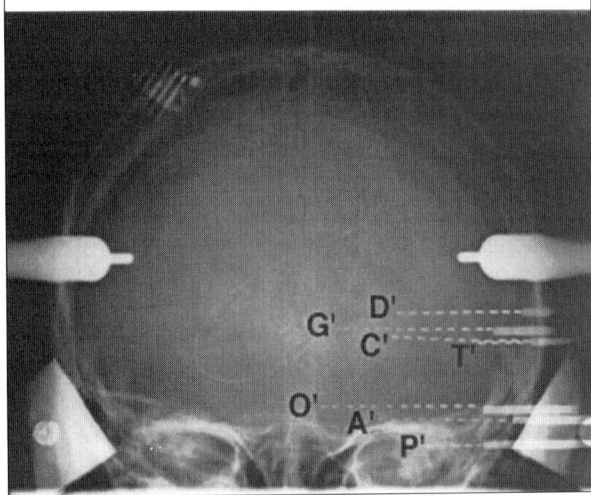

Fig. 5a. Pedalling movement associated with fear in left temporal lobe seizure.
Top: lateral view of the depth electrodes implantation on the patient's 3D MRI.
Bottom: X-ray of the skull during depth electrodes recording showing the implantation.

rial regions, plays a role in the 'reactive motricity' of grasping and manipulating objects in the near environment. 'Grasping' neurons have been mapped in F5 (Sakata et al., 1997). This lateral premotor system would be controlled by inhibitory regulation from the medial premotor system, particularly the supplementary motor area (SMA). The SMA is strongly connected to limbic structures and would be implicated in 'projective motricity', related to internal intentionality (Fig. 4).

LIMBIC SEIZURES IN CHILDREN

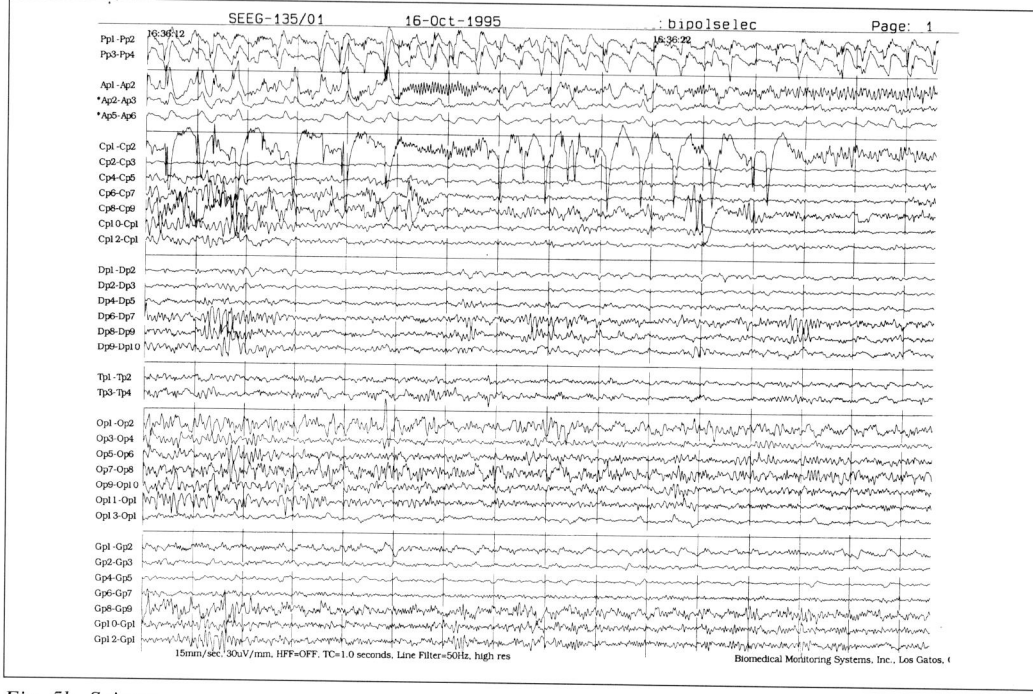

Fig. 5b. Seizure.

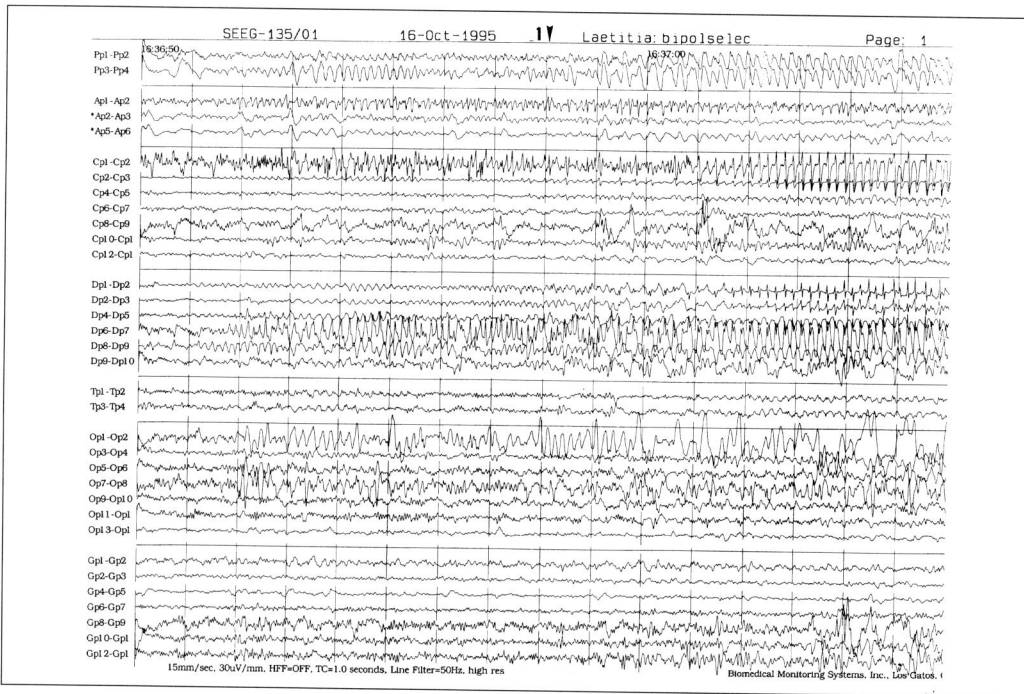

Fig. 5b. 1: The patient is still, and begins complaining of abdominal pain.

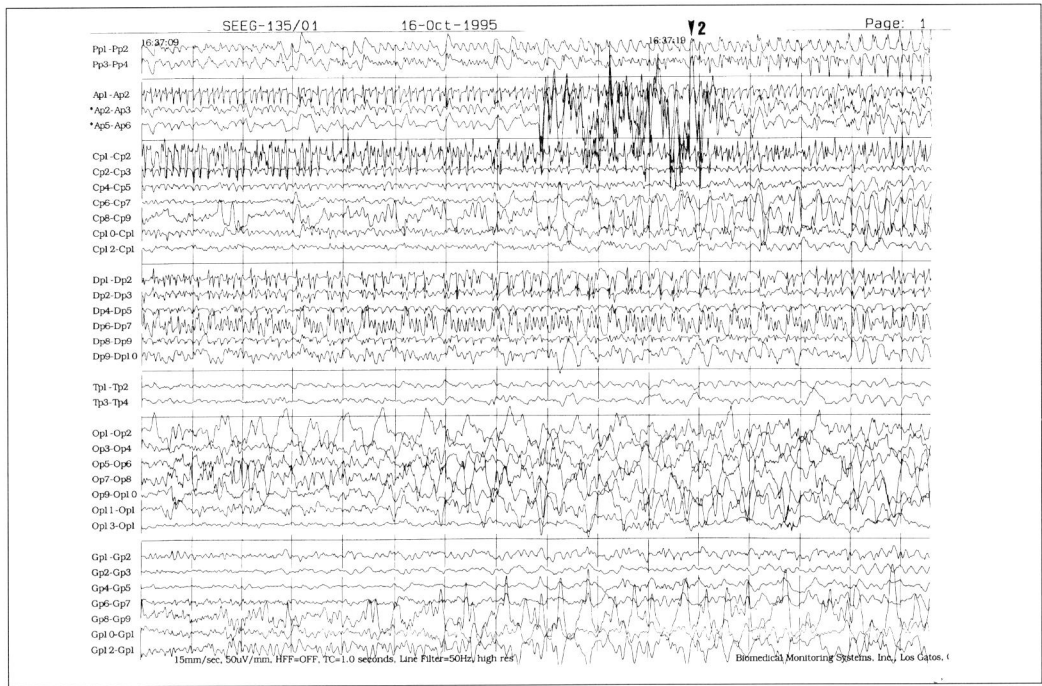

Fig. 5b. 2: Agitation with leg beating, the patient screaming 'I am afraid'.

Verbal automatisms

We confine this term to verbal activity occurring during seizures, whether the utterance is comprehensible or not. Verbal automatisms can be stereotypic and appear to follow a pre-established motor scheme as in one patient where ictal activity in the fusiform gyrus was documented by SEEG. The same non-word was repeated at each seizure and could be reproduced by electrical stimulation of the left fusiform gyrus while the patient was conscious. The patient would then ask 'what did I say?' (Devière *et al.*, 1997). Verbal automatisms can also appear as 'random' utterances and differ from one seizure to the next, but only if the discharge is located in the lateral temporal cortex of the dominant hemisphere (Bancaud, 1987; Devière *et al.*, 1997). For this reason, such types of automatisms are not considered to be found in limbic seizures.

Complex automatisms

Complex automatisms with intense bilateral agitation such as a pedalling movement are often attributed to activation of the medial orbito-frontal and medial frontal regions (Williamson, 1995). We have observed such activities during SEEG explorations in patients with temporal seizures and a secondary discharge of spikes extending to the frontal lobe. We have also seen them in temporal lobe seizures in association with (or in reaction to?) strong emotions such as fear (Taussig *et al.*, 1998) (Fig. 5). This behaviour is also observed in the post-seizure period of frontal or temporofrontal epilepsy and is frequently modulated by the surroundings (presence of observers, particular situation or circumstances). It is difficult to explain the origin of such automatisms. Perhaps a disorganization of the limbic system produces a defect in motor activity control or an abnormal response to external or internal solicitations.

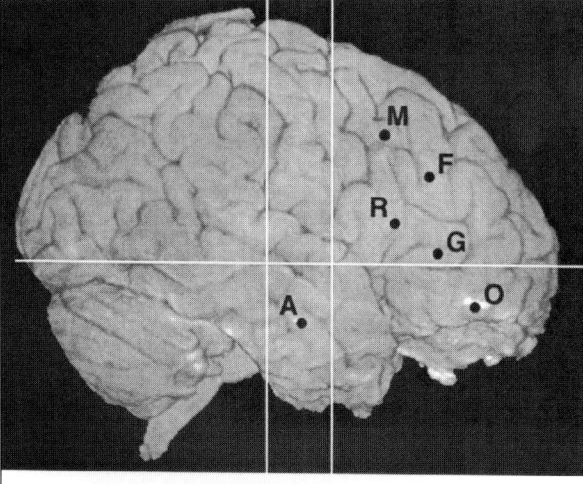

Distinguishing between automatisms and forced activity is a difficult task, particularly for complex automatisms classically attributed to the frontal lobe. For example, in a 13-year-old patient with SEEG-proven right orbito-frontal epilepsy related to a ganglioglioma, the documented seizures mostly involved a highly elaborated apparently automatic stereotypic behaviour which varied little from one seizure to another. After an initial phase of immobility, the child folded his hands together and hooted like an owl while the discharge terminated or persisted uniquely in the lateral temporal cortex (Fig. 6). This behaviour had not been observed during seizures a few month previously. Actually, the child had just learned how to make this sound and had been practising for days, without attaining the performance level reached during seizures. In this case, we do not consider this to be a verbal automatism but rather an internal context-dependent forced action.

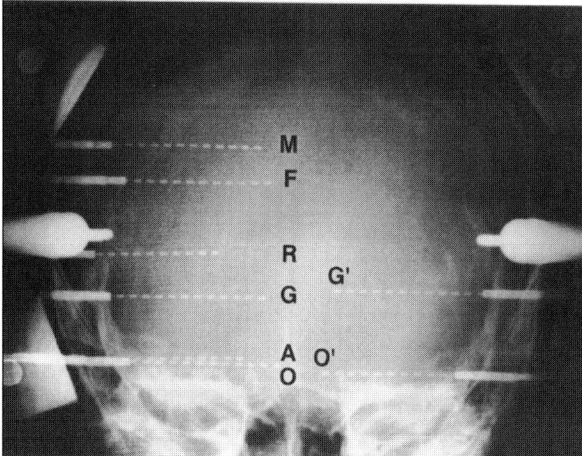

Fig. 6a. Complex automatisms in right orbito-frontal seizure.
Top: lateral view of the depth electrodes implantation on the patient's 3D MRI.
Bottom: X-ray of the skull during depth electrodes recording showing the implantation.

Conclusions

The nosological framework of automatisms remains to be fully established. In our opinion, ictal automatisms should only refer to involuntary activity which is very difficult to modulate and which occurs during the time-course of an electroencephalographic discharge, excluding reactional motor activities as well as dystonia and posture.

Oral chewing automatisms are highly localized and related to a sometimes unique discharge in the amygdala, implicating subcortical structures. The distinction with other types of oral movements is a fundamental notion because such activities can have a frontal or more posterior suprasylvian origin.

In our experience, simple gesture automatisms are not seen during discharges limited to the temporolimbic structures. They may occur subsequent to orbito-frontal perturbation seen as a rapid discharge or slow waves. Thus the limbic system is not responsible for automatisms except via cortico-subcortical or cortico-cortical circuits.

Chapter 9   Motor automatisms in limbic seizures

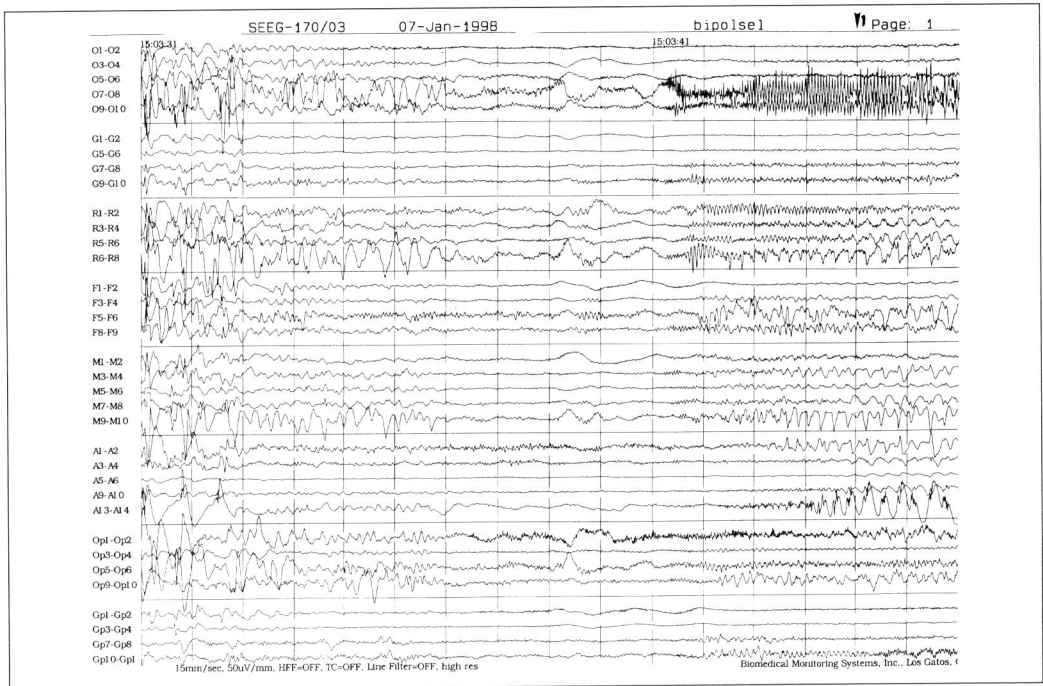

Fig. 6b. 1: Stops hyperventilation and remains still and mute.

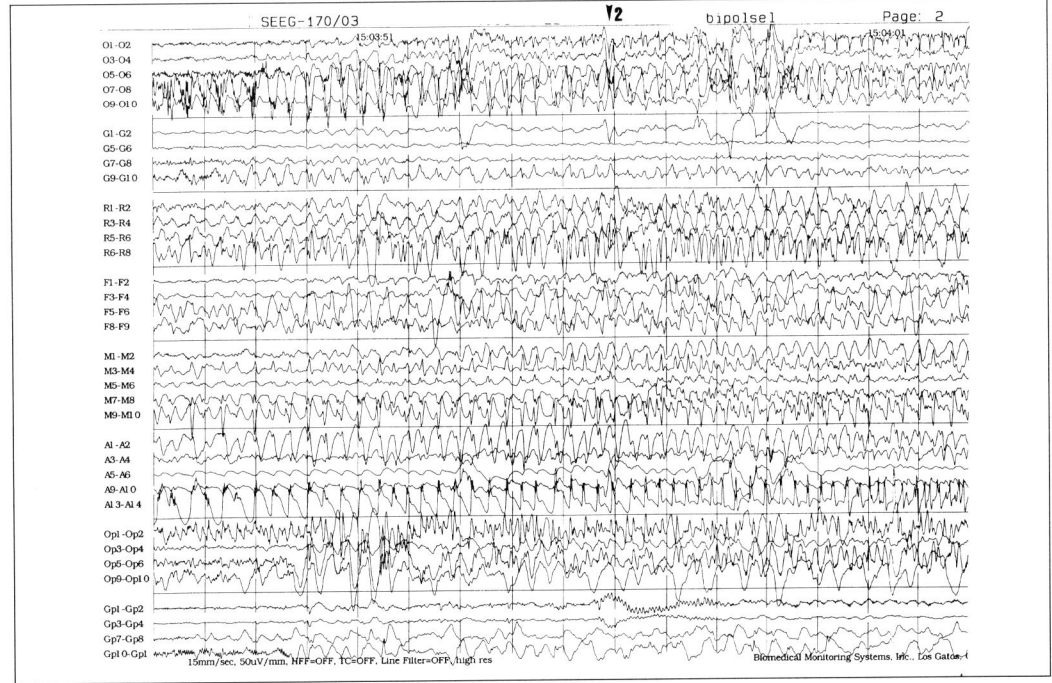

Fig. 6b. 2: The child folds his hands together and hoots like an owl.

For us, the complex motor activities observed during seizures can be classified into three categories: reactional actions (fear, flight …), forced action, and true automatisms. The distinction between these three categories is, however, quite difficult. It would appear that context and environment could affect the activities in the first two categories, emphasizing the importance of recording several seizures and interacting with the patient during the seizures.

References

Amaral, D. (1990): Amygdaloid cortical interconnections in the primate brain. In: *Learning and memory: discussions in neuroscience*, eds. L. Squire & M. Mishkin, pp. 24–32. Amsterdam: Elsevier Science.

Bancaud, J. (1987): Sémiologie clinique des crises d'origine temporale. *Rev. Neurol.* **143**, 392–400.

Bancaud, J., Talairach, J., Morel, P. & Bresson, M. (1966): La corne d'Ammon et le noyau amygdalien: effets cliniques et électriques de leur stimulation chez l'homme. *Rev. Neurol.* **115**, 329–351.

Bancaud, J., Talairach, J., Geier, S., Bonis, A., Trottier, S. & Manrique, M. (1976): Manifestations comportementales induites par la stimulation électrique du gyrus cingulaire antérieur chez l'homme. *Rev. Neurol.* **132**, 705–724.

Devière, F., Vignal, J.-P., Biraben, A. & Chauvel, P. (1997): Automatisme verbal ou jargon ictal? *Epilepsies* **9**, 149–152.

Feindel, W. & Penfield, W. (1954): Localization of discharge in temporal lobe automatism. *Arch. Neurol. Psych.* **72**, 605–630.

Geier, S., Bancaud, J., Talairach, J., Bonis, A., Szikla, G. & Enjelvin, M. (1977): The seizures of frontal lobe epilepsy. A study of clinical manifestations. *Neurology* **27**, 951–958.

Gloor, P. (1986): Consciousness as a neurological concept in epileptology: a critical review. *Epilepsia* **27**, S14–S26.

Gloor, P. (1997): *The temporal lobe and limbic system*. New York: Oxford University Press.

Goldberg, G. (1985): Supplementary motor area stucture and function: review and hypotheses. *Behav. Brain Sci.* **8**, 567–616.

Goldberg, G., Mayer, N. & Toglia, J. (1981): Medial frontal cortex infarction and the alien hand sign. *Arch. Neurol.* **38**, 683–686.

Goldman-Rakic, P.S. (1995): Anatomical and functional circuits in prefrontal cortex of nonhuman primates. *Adv. Neurol.* **66**, 51–65.

Jackson. J. (1875): On temporary mental disorders after epileptic paroxysms. *West Riding Lunatic Asylum Medical Reports* **5**, 105–129.

Kaada, B. (1951): Somato-motor, autonomic and electrocorticographic responses to electrical stimulation of 'rhinencephalic' and other structures in primates, cats and dog. *Acta Physiol. Scand.* **24**, 1–285.

Kotagal, P., Lüders, H., Morris, H.H., Dineer, D., Wyllie, E., Godoy, J. & Rothner, A. (1989): Dystonic posturing in complex partial seizures of temporal lobe onset: a new lateralizing sign. *Neurology* **36**, 196–201.

Loiseau, P. & Jallon, P. (1990): *Dictionnaire analytique d'épileptologie clinique*. Paris: John Libbey Eurotext.

Munari, C., Bancaud, J., Bonis, A., Buser, P., Talairach, J., Szikla, G. et al. (1979): Rôle du noyau amygdalien dans la survenue de manifestations oro-alimentaires au cours des crsies épileptiques chez l'homme. *Rev. EEG Neurophysiol.* **9**, 236–240.

Nakamura, Y. & Kubo, Y. (1978): Masticatory rhythm in intracellular potential of trigeminal motoneurons induced by stimulation of orbital cortex and amygdala in cats. *Brain Res.* **148**, 504–509.

Penry, J. & Dreyfuss, F. (1969): Automatisms associated with the absence of Petit Mal epilepsy. *Arch. Neurol.* **21**, 142–149.

Poncet, M., Etcharry-Bouyx, F. & Ceccaldi, M. (1994): Dyspraxie diagonistique et main capricieuse. Deux comportements gestuels anormaux distincts. In: *L'apraxie*, eds. D. Le Gall & G. Aubin, pp. 148–159. Marseille: Solal.

Quesney, L. (1986): Clinical and EEG features of complex partial seizures of temporal lobe origin. *Epilepsia* **27,** S27–S45.

Sakata, H., Taira, M., Kusunoki, M., Muraat, A. & Tanaka, Y. (1997): The TINS lecture. The parietal association cortex in depth perception and visual control of hand action. *Trends Neurosci.* **8,** 350–357.

Talairach, J., Bancaud, J., Szikla, G., Bonis, A., Geier, S. & Védrenne, C. (1974): Approche nouvelle de la neurochirurgie de l'épilepsie. Méthodologie stéréotaxique et résultats thérapeutiques. *Neurochirurgie* **20,** 1–249.

Taussig, D., Biraben, A., Thomas, P., Scarabin, J.M., Vignal, J.-P. & Chauvel, P. (1998): Fear as the main feature of epileptic seizures. *Epilepsia* **39** (Suppl. 2), 123.

Williamson, P.D. (1995): Frontal lobe epilepsy. Some clinical characteristics. *Adv. Neurol.* **66,** 127–152.

Chapter 10

Postural disturbances and changes in facial expression during temporo-limbic seizures in children

Elisabeth Landré, Baris Turak, Francine Chassoux, Dominique Chagot,
Jean-Paul Gagnepain and Jean-Paul Chodkiewicz

Centre Hospitalier Sainte-Anne, Service de Neurochirurgie, 1 rue Cabanis, 75014 Paris, France

Summary

This report is based on a series of 11 children (seven boys and four girls) aged 3½ to 15 years (average 10) who underwent stereo-EEG evaluation followed by surgical treatment for mesial temporal epilepsy in the Department of Neurosurgery at the Sainte Anne Hospital.

In nine cases the epilepsy was symptomatic of brain tumour (seven DNT's and two gangliogliomas) and hippocampal atrophy was present in the remaining two (one with an HHE syndrome).

The seizure semiology of all discharges clearly starting in the mesial lobe, as demonstrated by video-SEEG recording, were analysed with particular regard to changes in facial expression and postural disturbances.

(1) In all cases a change in facial expression was noted at the very beginning of the seizure. In five children this was an appearance of fright with, for four of them, accompanying subjective manifestations. In six children expression was motionless, with associated subjective manifestations in four. This motionless expression was all that could be objectively noted in the two cases with brief seizures where the ictal discharge remained within amygdalo-hippocampal structures.

(2) Postural changes occurred in only five cases:

— In three children bilateral extension, elevation and abduction of the upper limbs with forward flexion of the head was observed. This was seen during brief seizures with rapid discharge spread to the frontal lobe.

— Two children presented dystonic posturing of the upper limb contralateral to the epileptic discharge. These were seizures of more than 1 min duration where the medial temporal discharge spread secondarily to the temporal pole and the temporal neocortex.

Introduction

Between 1970 and 1996, 57 children with severe partial epilepsy underwent depth electrode (SEEG) evaluation followed by surgical treatment at the Sainte Anne Hospital. Twenty-four of these children had temporal epilepsy including 11 cases (seven boys and four girls) of mesial temporal epilepsy. All 11 children have now been free from seizures for at least 2 years after having an anterior and medial corticectomy. Anatomo-electroclinical correlations established by SEEG were retrospectively analysed in these cases with regard to ictal postural disturbances and changes in facial expression. We report on our observations and discuss the location of these signs occurring during mesial temporal seizures.

Material and methods

In this series of 11 children we reviewed the ictal semiology of the seizures associated with a medial temporal lobe discharge on SEEG recording. Age varied between 3½ and 15 (average 10) with an average duration of epilepsy of 7 years (range: 1–13 years). In all cases the neurological examination was normal. Nine children had symptomatic epilepsy: seven dysembryoplastic neuroepithelial tumours, and two gangliogliomas. There were two cases of hippocampal atrophy (including one HHE syndrome).

All underwent video-EEG recording, a stereotaxic mapping procedure (with arteriography and MRI) and stereoelectroencephalographic exploration according to the methodology established for presurgical evaluation of partial epilepsy (Bancaud et al., 1965) as applicable to children (Broglin et al., 1991; Landré et al., 1998; Kahane et al., 1998). The essentially temporal lobe exploration was completed by extratemporal electrodes in nine cases (in the hemisphere dominant for speech in three cases). As a result of these investigations all 11 children underwent anterior temporal and medial corticectomies and have now been seizure free for at least 2 years.

Results

Seizure duration varied between 10 s and 1 min 30 s. Seizure semiology included changes in facial expression in all cases, associated in eight cases with a neurovegetative aura in the form of abdominal pain followed by loss of contact. Oro-alimentary automatisms (seven cases), gestural automatisms (eight cases), and postural changes (five cases) were then observed. Later urination in three cases and salivation in three cases were noted.

Changes in facial expression at ictal onset consisted of a frightened appearance in five children and a motionless expression in six. Of these children eight reported initial subjective manifestations: abdominal pain in seven and one dreamy state. In two children seizure semiology was limited to arrest of facial expression: these were brief seizures in which the discharges remained within amygdalo-hipppocampal structures.

Postural changes were observed in five cases:

- In three children they consisted of a bilateral extension and elevation of the upper limbs with forward flexion of the head. This semiology was noted during short seizures with rapid discharge spread to the frontal lobe.

- Two children presented with dystonic posturing of the upper limb contralateral to the discharge associated with gestural automatisms of the ipsilateral upper limb. These were seizures of more than 1 min duration with secondary spread of the medial temporal discharge to the temporal pole and temporal neocortex.

The following five examples illustrate this series:

Chapter 10   Postural disturbances and changes in facial expression during temporo-limbic seizures

Example 1. A 12-year-old child with epilepsy since the age of 1½ years

The semiology consisted of an initial subjective manifestation in the form of abdominal pain, with oro-alimentary automatisms, a frightened expression, followed by loss of contact, gestural automatisms, mydriasis and flushing. MRI demonstrated left hippocampal atrophy. The SEEG investigation consisted of six electrodes in the left temporal lobe (Fig. 1). A seizure with the usual semiology was recorded on SEEG (Fig. 2). The discharge starts in the amygdalo-hippocampal region: electrodes A'1-B'1-C'1, in the form of a rapid, low amplitude discharge which gradually increases in amplitude. This is the stage when the child reports the seizure. Then, when the child becomes unresponsive, the discharge has spread to the temporal neocortex.

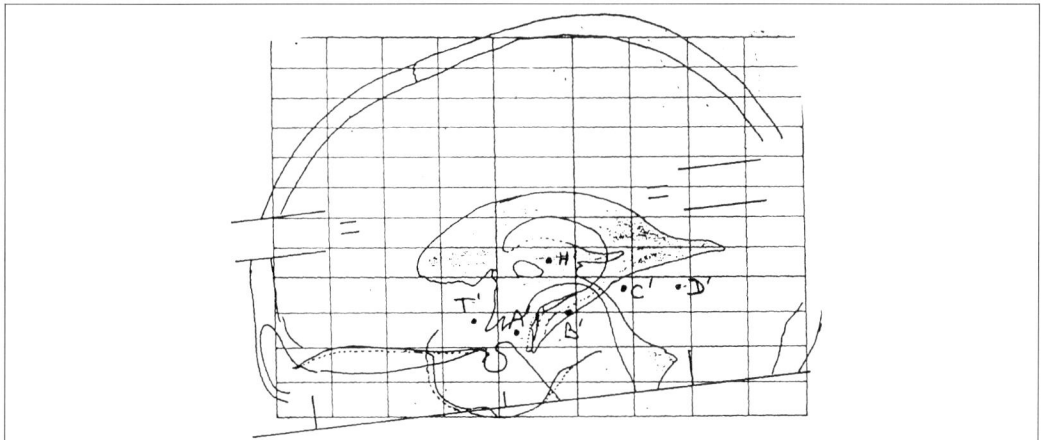

Fig. 1. Example 1: Location of electrodes in left temporal lobe.

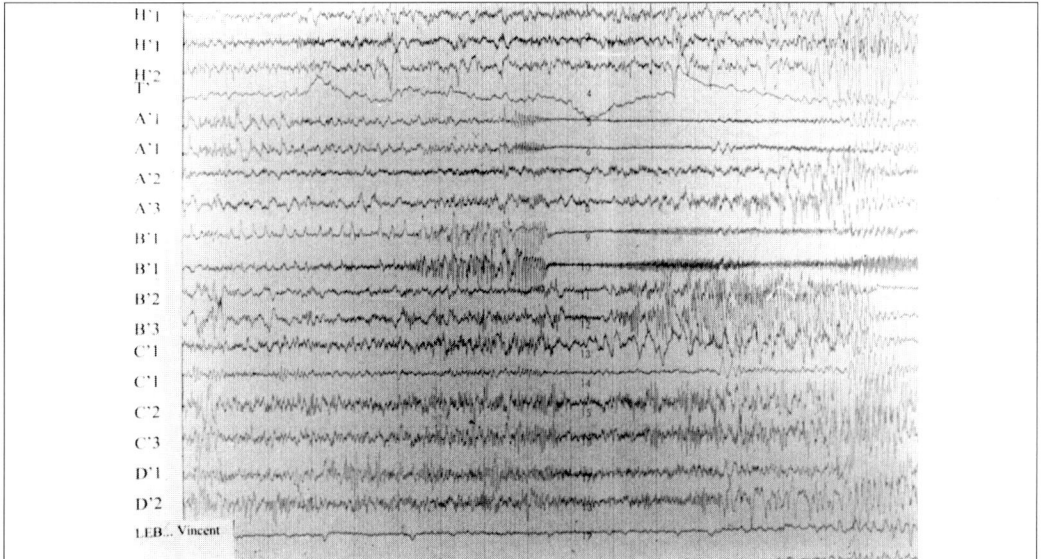

Fig. 2. Example 1: SEEG seizure recording: Discharge in amygdalohippocampal region, electrodes A'1, B'1, C'1 (abdominal pain – oro-alimentary automatisms), spread to the temporal neocortex, electrodes A'2, A'3, B'2, B'3, C'2, C'3 and then D' (loss of contact – gestual automatisms).

Example 2. An 8-year-old child with epilepsy since the age of 7 years

The semiology consisted of initial subjective manifestations in the form of abdominal pain, an expression of fear, followed by unresponsiveness, a groan, gestural automatisms, oro-alimentary automatisms, flushing then pallor. MRI demonstrated a right anterior and medial temporal lesion which subsequently turned out to be a dysembryoplastic neuroepithelial tumour. Because of the spread of the ictal discharge recorded on video-EEG, the SEEG investigation consisted of a temporal lobe exploration with two electrodes in the frontal lobe (Fig. 3). During the interictal phase the spikes were limited to the medial temporal and temporal polar regions: electrodes A1-B1-C1, and P1-P2. The frontal electrodes showed slow activity and some slow spikes. The seizure begins with a change in facial expression, a frightened look, with the

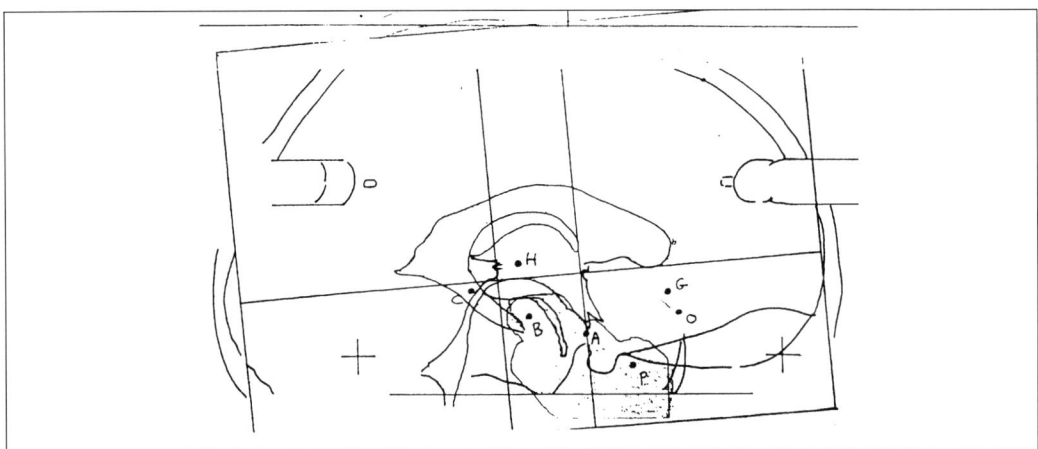

Fig. 3. Example 2: Location of electrodes in temporal and frontal right lobes.

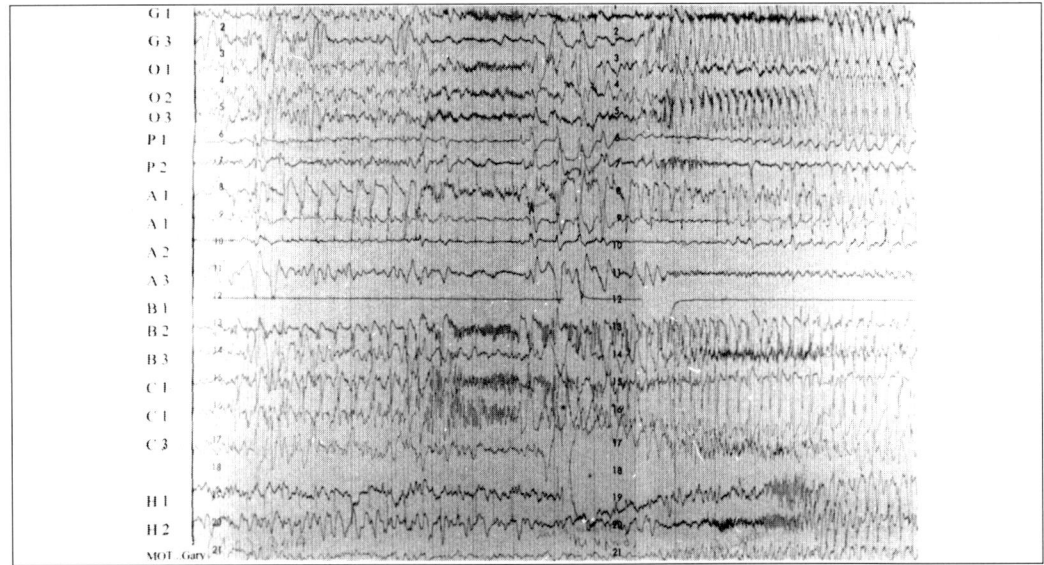

Fig. 4. Example 2: SEEG seizure recording: discharge on medial temporal electrode A1 (frightened look), spreads on temporal and frontal electrodes (loss of contact – oro-alimentary and gestural automatisms).

discharge appearing on electrode A1 and remaining temporal for 12 s before spreading to the temporal pole and frontal electrodes then, secondarily, to the temporal neocortex when the loss of contact and other objective manifestations occur (Fig. 4).

Example 3. A 3½-year-old child epileptic since the age of 2½ years

The semiology of the brief seizures, of 10 s duration, consisted in a change of facial expression, either as the only manifestation or in association with a forward flexion of the head and the abduction and elevation of both upper limbs.

MRI demonstrated a left medial temporal lesion which subsequently proved to be a dysembryoplastic neuroepithelial tumour. The SEEG consisted essentially of a temporal lobe explo-

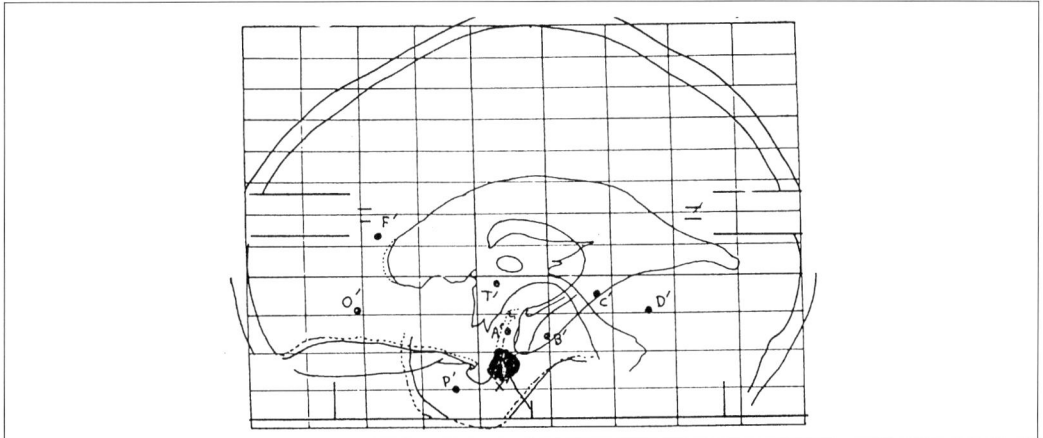

Fig. 5. Example 3: Location of electrodes in temporal and frontal left temporal lobes.

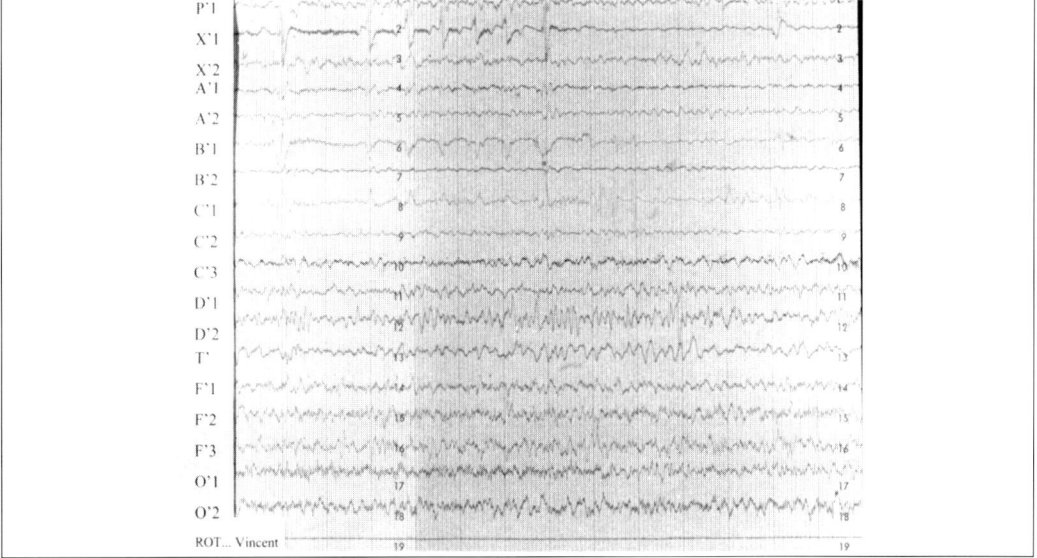

Fig. 6. Example 3: SEEG seizure recording: Ictal discharge on medial temporal structures electrodes A'1, B'1, C'1, X'1 (change in facial expression).

LIMBIC SEIZURES IN CHILDREN

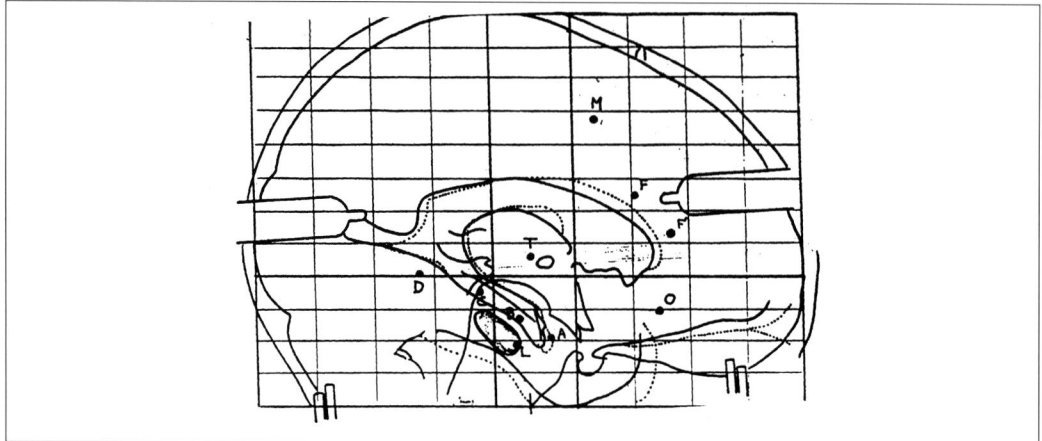

Fig. 7. Example 4: Location of electrodes in temporal and frontal right lobes and one electrode (F') in frontal left lobe.

ration with two electrodes in the frontal lobe because of the semiology accompanying the discharges recorded on video-EEG (Fig. 5). Two seizures clinically limited to a change in facial expression were recorded. The ictal discharges during the 12 s seizures involved only the medial temporal structures: electrodes A'1-B'1-C'1 and X'1 inside the lesion (Fig. 6).

Example 4. An 8-year-old child with epilepsy since the age of 1 year

Ictal semiology consisted of a motionless facial expression, disturbances of contact, and posturing with forward flexion of the head and elevation and abduction of both upper limbs. MRI demonstrated a right medial temporal lesion which subsequently proved to be a dysembryoplastic neuroepithelial tumour. Taking into account this semiology and the widespread discharges recorded on video-EEG, SEEG investigation included six electrodes in the temporal lobe and three electrodes in the frontal lobe on

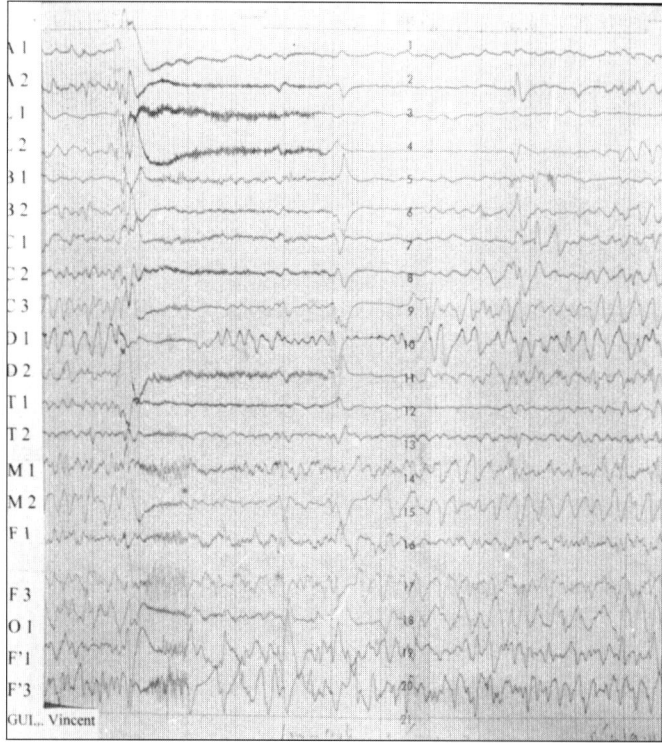

Fig. 8. Example 4: SEEG seizure recording: brief ictal discharge involving all the temporal and frontal electrodes (motionless facial expression, loss of contact, posturing with forward flexion of the head and elevation and abduction of both upper limbs).

the right side and one electrode in the left frontal lobe (Fig. 7). One seizure with the usual semiology was recorded: the brief 10 s ictal discharge is very widespread involving all the temporal and frontal electrodes but is more tonic in the medial temporal region (Fig. 8). A second seizure limited to a motionless expression was recorded after intrarectal injection of valium and this time the discharge was more limited and predominated on the medial temporal electrodes A1-L-B1 and C1 (Fig. 9).

Example 5. A 15-year-old child with seizures since the age of 2 years

Seizure semiology consisted of a subjective manifestation in the form of a rising epigastric feeling, a motionless expression, loss of contact, oro-alimentary automatisms, gestural automatisms of the right hand and posturing of the left hand. MRI showed a partially cystic right medial anterior lesion which turned out to be a ganglioglioma. The SEEG consisted of six temporal and one fronto-orbital electrodes (Fig. 10). The ictal discharge begins as a long paroxysm of rhythmic slow paced spikes while the patient reports a feeling in the abdomen and oroalimentary automatisms have already begun, and when loss of contact occurs the discharge takes on a fast, low amplitude aspect gaining the temporal pole and neocortex. When the dystonic attitude of the left hand appears, the discharge has already spread to all temporal electrodes (Fig. 11). This posture is associated with simple automatisms of the right hand.

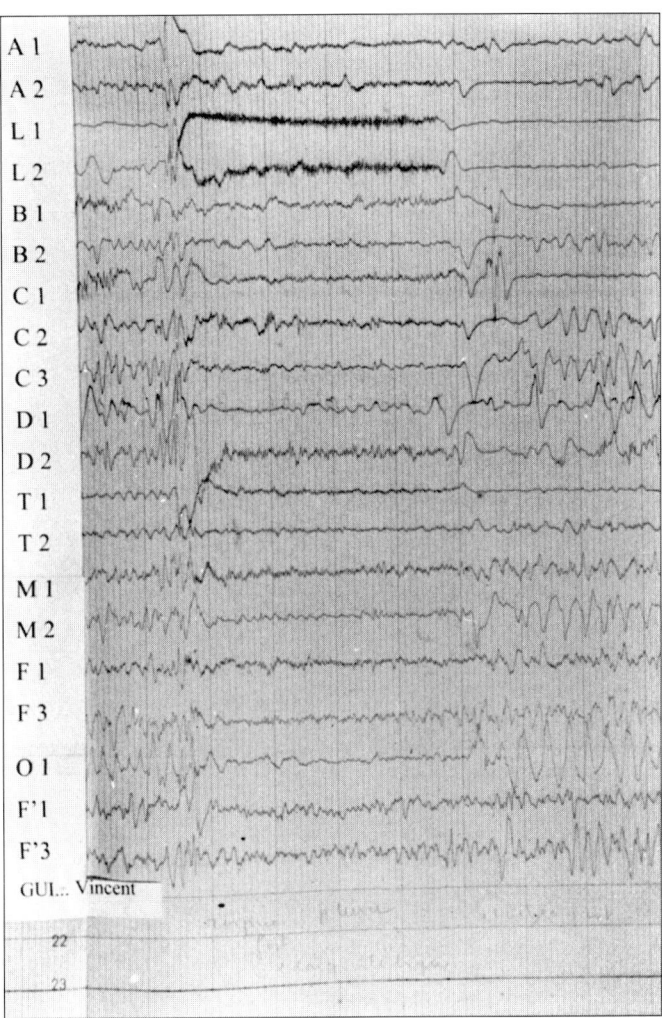

Fig. 9. Example 4: SEEG seizure recording after intrarectal injection of valium: discharge on medial temporal electrodes A1, L, B1, C1 (motionless expression).

Commentary

Changes in facial expression are classically considered as being part of temporal lobe seizures. (Bancaud & Talairach, 1991) We have observed this sign to be the initial manifestation of medial temporal lobe seizures in all 11 children of this series. In children this may reflect subjective manifestations, especially distressing or painful abdominal feelings (Wyllie *et al.*, 1993). The facial expression is then mostly a frightened look, sometimes associated with oro-alimentary automatisms while consciousness is maintained (Examples 1 and 2). The corresponding ictal discharge on SEEG remains restricted to mesial temporal structures. However, a motionless expression, with or without staring, may be the only component of seizure semiology (Wyllie *et al.*, 1993). Two children in our series presented this type of seizure with SEEG correlations showing a brief discharge strictly limited to the amygdalo-hippocampal region

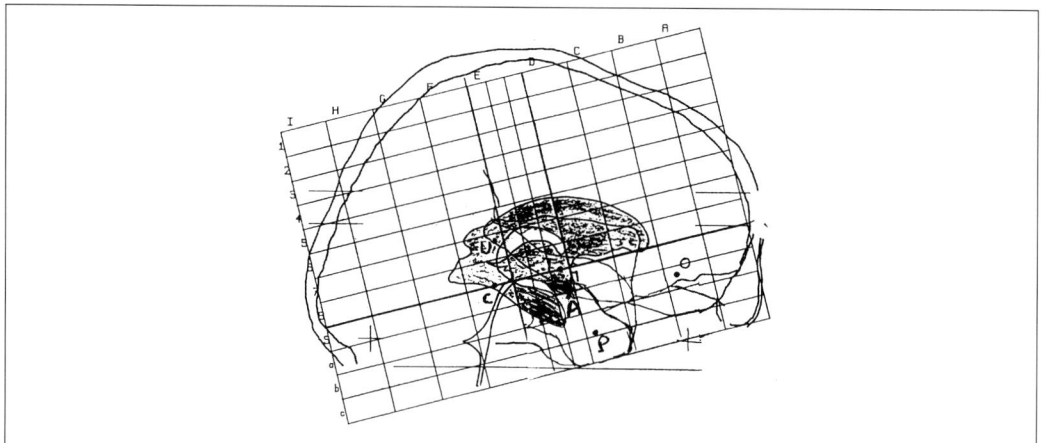

Fig. 10. Example 5: Location of electrodes in temporal and frontal right lobe.

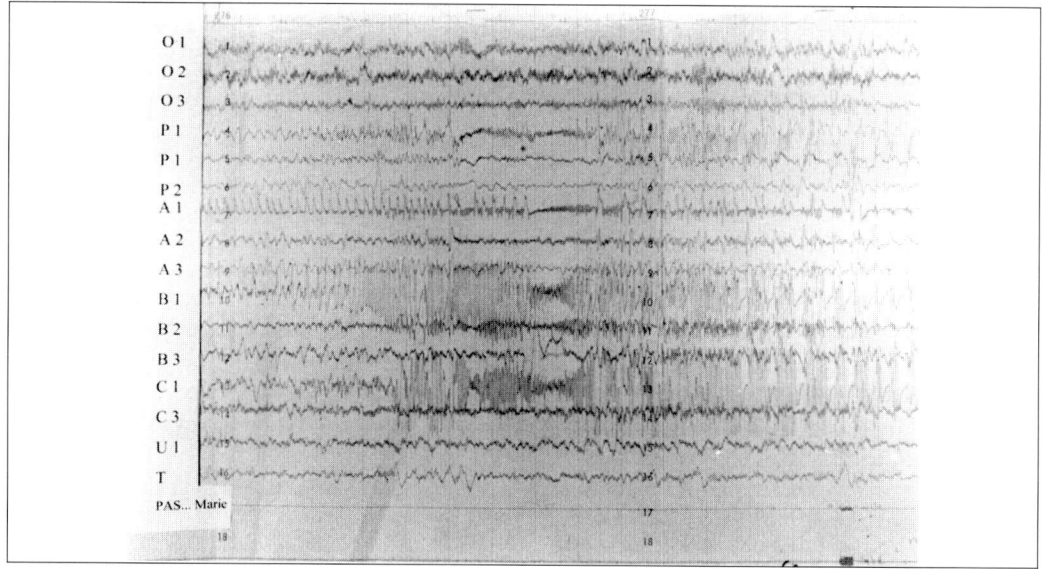

Fig. 11. Example 5: SEEG seizure recording: discharge begins as rhythmic slow spikes appear on medial temporal electrode A1 (feeling in the abdomen and oro-alimentary automatisms), the discharges gaining the temporal pole and neocortex (loss of contact) then spreading to all temporal electrodes (dystonic attitude of the left hand, gestual automatisms of right hand).

(Example 3). In these two cases the lack of reported subjective manifestations was perhaps due to age as they were the youngest (age 3 and 5 years) children in this series (Landré et al., 1998). Of the 11 children in this series two presented a dystonic attitude of the upper limb contralateral to the EEG discharge during seizures. This sign has largely been reported and discussed in the literature on medial temporal lobe seizures (Kotagal et al., 1989a; O'Brien et al., 1996; Gil-Nagel & Risinger, 1997; Bleasel et al., 1997; Serles et al., 1998). Depending on the reported series, this postural change, always involving the upper limb contralateral to the discharge, was seen in 35–52 per cent of medial temporal lobe seizures.

The dystonic attitude involved the distal part of the upper limb, the elbow being sometimes slightly flexed, the wrist rotated, and the fingers spread and extended. The other upper limb often presented simple gestural automatisms. From the semiological point of view this attitude was quite different from the tonic posture of extratemporal seizures (arising during discharges of the parietal and premotor regions). In temporal lobe seizures dystonic posturing never occurred during the early stages but only secondary to loss of contact and corresponded to an extratemporal spread of the amygdalo-hippocampal discharge (Kotagal et al., 1989a, b; Bennet et al., 1989). In our two cases this sign corresponded on SEEG to an already widespread discharge across the temporal neocortex, secondarily gaining frontal regions (Example 5). However, in each of these two cases there was only one extratemporal, fronto-orbital, electrode. The hypothesis of a spread to subcortical structures, either by direct connections or via the supplementary area has been discussed (Kotagal et al., 1989a, b; Bennet et al., 1989). Ictal SPECT analysis of temporal seizures by Newton et al. in 1992 suggests that basal ganglia may play a role in the physiology of this dystonic attitude. Recently, Dupont et al. in 1998, using FDG positron emission tomography, find an interictal hypometabolism in the striatal region of patients with medial temporal lobe epilepsy and ictal dystonic posturing.

In three of our children the postural changes observed during medial temporal lobe seizures involved the body axis with sudden forward flexion of the head and the arms thrown out upwards and proximally abducted, associated with a change in facial expression. In all cases seizures were brief. This type of seizure takes on the semiology of frontal lobe seizures (Bancaud & Talairach, 1992). In the three cases of this series the medial temporal ictal discharge recorded on SEEG appeared very rapidly or simultaneously on the frontal electrodes. The anatomo-electroclinical correlations obtained in Example 4 illustrate this clearly. During the first seizure, comprised of a motionless facial expression, loss of contact and postural changes involving the body axis and the upper limbs, the discharge is widespread appearing over temporal and frontal areas; after an injection of valium clinical semiology is limited to a motionless facial expression corresponding to a discharge remaining wholly within medial temporal structures.

Conclusion

In children initial temporo-limbic seizure semiology includes changes in facial expression, usually associated with subjective manifestations. However in younger children these subjective manifestations are rarely reported. In short seizures a simple motionless facial expression may be the only sign, and corresponds to a discharge remaining within amygdalo-hippocampal structures.

On the other hand postural disturbances reflect spread of the amygdalo-hippocampal discharge to extratemporal areas. A dystonic attitude of the upper limb contralateral to the ictal discharge appears to indicate spread to subcortical structures. A sudden forward flexion of the head with extension, elevation and proximal abduction of the two upper limbs would imply ictal discharge spread to frontal regions.

References

Bancaud, J. & Talairach, J. (1991): Séméiologie clinique des crises du lobe temporal. In: *Crises épileptiques et épilepsies du lobe temporal*. Tome II. Documentation médicale Labaz.

Bancaud, J. & Talairach, J. (1992): Clinical semiology of frontal lobe seizures. In: *Frontal lobe seizures and epilepsies, Advances in neurology*, vol. 57, eds. P. Chauvel, A.V. Delgado-Escueta, E. Halgren & J. Bancaud, pp. 3–58. New York: Raven Press.

Bancaud, J., Talairach, J., Bonis, A., Schaub, C., Szikla, G., Morel, P. & Bordas-Ferrer, M. (1965): *La stéréo-électro-encéphalographie dans l'épilepsie. Informations neuro-physio-pathologiques apportées par l'investigation fonctionnelle stéréotaxique*. Paris: Masson.

Bennett, D., Ristanovic, R., Morrell, F. & Goetz, C. (1989): Dystonic posturing in temporal lobe seizures. *Neurology* **39**, 1270–1271.

Bleasel, A., Kotagal, P., Kankirawatana, P. & Rybicki, L. (1997): Lateralizing value and semiology of ictal limb posturing and version in temporal lobe and extratemporal epilepsy. *Epilepsia* **38**, 168–174.

Broglin, D., Landré, E., Chauvel, P., Munari, C., Trottier, S., Chodkiewicz, J.P., Bancaud, J. & Talairach, J. (1991): Epilepsy surgery in adolescent and children: stereotactic preoperative evaluation and results. *Epilepsia* **32** (Suppl. 1), 21.

Dupont, S., Semah, F., Baulac, M. & Samson, Y. (1998): The underlying pathophysiology of ictal dystonia in temporal lobe epilepsy. An FDG-positron emission tomography study. *Neurology* **51**, 1289–1292.

Gil-Nagel, A. & Risinger, M.W. (1997): Ictal semiology in versus extrahippocampal temporal lobe epilepsy. *Brain* **120**, 183–192.

Kahane, P., Hoffmann, D., Francione, S., Tassi, L., Di Leo, M., Benabid, A.L. & Munari, C. (1998): La stéréo-électro-encéphalographie chez l'enfant: outil diagnostique et préchirurgical. In: *Epilepsies partielles graves pharmaco-résistantes de l'enfant. Statégies diagnostiques et traitements chirurgicaux*, eds. M. Bureau, P. Kahane & C. Munari, pp. 135–151. London: John Libbey Eurotext.

Kotagal, P., Lüders, H., Morris, H., Dinner, D.S., Wyllie, E., Godoy, J. & Rothner, A.D. (1989a): Dystonic posturing in complex partial seizures of temporal lobe onset: a new lateralizing sign. *Neurology* **39**, 196–201.

Kotagal, P., Lüders, H., Morris, H., Dinner, D.S., Wyllie, E., Godoy, J. & Rothner, A.D. (1989b): Dystonic posturing in temporal lobe seizures. *Neurology* **39**, 1271–1272.

Landré, E., Turak, B., Chassoux, F., Ghossoub, M., Devaux, B., Chagot, D., Gagnepain, J.P. & Chodkiewicz, J.P. (1998): Enregistrement vidéo-EEG. In: *Epilepsies partielles graves pharmaco-résistantes de l'enfant. Statégies diagnostiques et traitements chirurgicaux*, eds. M. Bureau, P. Kahane & C. Munari, pp. 107–112. London: John Libbey Eurotext.

Newton, M., Berkovic, S., Austin, M., Reutens, D., McKay, W. & Bladin, P. (1992): Dystonia, clinical lateralization, and regional cerebral blood flow changes in temporal lobe seizures. *Neurology* **42**, 371–377.

O'Brien, T.J., Kilpatrick, C., Murrie, V., Vogrin, S., Morris, K. & Cook, M.J. (1996): Temporal lobe epilepsy caused by mesial temporal sclerosis and temporal neocortical lesions. A clinical and electroencephalographic study of 46 pathologically proven cases. *Brain* **119**, 2133–2141.

Serles, W., Pataraia, E., Bacher, J., Olbrich, A., Aull, S., Lehrner, J., Leutmezer, F., Deecke, L. & Baumgartner, C. (1998): Clinical seizure lateralization in mesial temporal lobe epilepsy: differences between patients with unitemporal and bitemporal interictal spikes. *Neurology* **51**, 742–747.

Wyllie, E., Chee, M., Granström, M.L., DelGiudice, E., Estes, M., Comair, Y., Pizzi, M., Kotagal, P., Bourgeois, B. & Lüders, H. (1993): Temporal lobe epilepsy in early childhood. *Epilepsia* **34**, 859–868.

Chapter 11

Perisylvian cortex involvement in seizures affecting the temporal lobe

Philippe Kahane[*†‡], Jean-Claude Huot[*§], Dominique Hoffmann[*], Giorgio Lo Russo[¶], Alim Louis Benabid[*‡] and Claudio Munari[‡¶#]

[*]Neurosciences Department, [†]Physiology Laboratory and [‡]INSERM 318 Research Unit, Centre Hospitalier Universitaire de Grenoble, BP 217, 38043 Grenoble Cedex 09, France; [§]Larrieu Clinic, Pau, France; [¶]Regional Center of Epilepsy Surgery, Niguarda Hospital, Milan, Italy; [#]Department of Neurosurgery, San Martino Hospital, Genoa, Italy

Summary

Perisylvian cortex involvement in seizures affecting the temporal lobe was assessed in 50 partial epileptic patients who underwent stereotactic EEG recordings before surgery. Seizures arose from temporal lobe structures in 33 patients (66 per cent), from temporal and suprasylvian opercular cortices in six (12 per cent), and from widely extended temporal and extra-temporal areas in 11 (22 per cent). Surgical resections were never restricted to the perisylvian cortex.

The superior temporal gyrus (STG) was involved at seizure onset or within the first 5 s in 38 of the 50 studied patients (76 per cent), and the suprasylvian opercular cortex (SSOC) in eight of the 32 patients in whom it was investigated (25 per cent). Hippocampal sclerosis was found in almost 40 per cent of these patients with initial or early perisylvian involvement.

When an adequate removal of the epileptogenic area could be achieved, seizures disappeared in 76 per cent of temporal lobe epilepsies with initial or early involvement of the STG. Late or absence of STG involvement allowed more limited temporal lobe resections which lead to similar good results, i.e. 78 per cent of seizure-free patients. Stereotactic investigation of the perisylvian cortex also proved particularly useful in temporo-perisylvian epilepsies, since all the five patients in whom the whole epileptogenic area could be removed were cured after surgery. Results were much more disappointing in widely extended multilobar epilepsies (success rate: 36.5 per cent) and perisylvian involvement in such cases did not seem to have any prognosis significance.

Introduction

In adults, as in children, several ictal symptoms are particularly suggestive of perisylvian cortex involvement during partial epileptic seizures. On one hand, ictal dysfunction of the superior temporal gyrus (STG) can be suspected when a patient presents auditory illusions and hallucinations, vestibular symptoms, or aphasic disturbances (Penfield & Jasper, 1954;

Smith, 1960; Bancaud, 1987; Bancaud & Talairach, 1991; Munari *et al.*, 1996). On the other hand, facial and pharyngo-laryngeal sensory-motor signs, bilateral dysaesthesia of the genitals, gustatory symptoms or sialorrhea strongly suggest the ictal involvement of the suprasylvian opercular cortex (SSOC) (Penfield & Jasper, 1954; Hausser-Hauw & Bancaud, 1987; Bancaud *et al.*, 1991). In addition, vegetative signs that are classically related to mesio-temporal lobe structures, and notably epigastric aura, can also be produced by ictal discharges arising from the insulo-opercular complex (Penfield & Rasmussen, 1950; Penfield & Jasper, 1954; Penfield, 1958; Bancaud & Talairach, 1991).

When surgical treatment is considered, particular attention must be paid to these ictal clinical phenomena, notably when they occur early during seizures supposed to arise from antero-mesial temporal lobe structures. Indeed, early perisylvian involvement could explain some failures of epilepsy surgery, and particularly those of temporal lobe surgery (Munari *et al.*, 1980).

The aim of this retrospective study was to verify, in seizures involving the temporal lobe, if the stereotactic investigation of the perisylvian cortex was useful for the precise delineation of the epileptogenic area, and consequently for the presurgical prognosis. In that respect, we judged it necessary to have a post-operative follow-up of at least 5 years, since results of epilepsy surgery may evolve significantly with time (Berkovic *et al.*, 1995).

Patients and methods

The patients included in this retrospective study were part of a group of 135 consecutive patients suffering from medically intractable partial epilepsy and operated on at Grenoble Hospital between March 1990 and October 1993. They were selected on the basis of the following criteria: (i) cryptogenic or symptomatic partial epilepsy without evidence of progressive neurological disease (e.g. Rasmussen's encephalitis); (ii) stereotactic intracerebral EEG recordings (stereo-EEG) performed before surgery, with at least one intracerebral electrode investigating the STG; (iii) unilateral partial seizures involving at least mesial and/or lateral temporal lobe structures; (iv) more than 5 years of post-operative follow-up.

Patients

We found 50 patients who met the above selection criteria. They were 28 females and 22 males, whose age at surgery ranged from 4 to 44 years (mean 24). Mean age at seizure onset was 9 years (birth–31). Seizures had begun before the age of 16 years in 82 per cent of the cases (0–5 years: 13 patients; 6–10 years: 16 patients; 11–15 years: 12 patients) and average epilepsy duration was 13 years (2–32).

On the basis of video-stereo-EEG recordings, the origin of seizures proved to be temporal in 33 patients (T, 66 per cent), temporo-perisylvian (i.e. including also the SSOC) in six (TS, 12 per cent), and multilobar including the temporal lobe in 11 (T+, 22 per cent). Seizures arose from the dominant hemisphere for language in nine cases (T: 6; T: 1; T+: 2).

Before surgery, the multidisciplinary team defined the extent of the so-called 'epileptogenic zone' (Talairach & Bancaud, 1966) and the feasibility of its complete removal. Accordingly, a tailored surgical resection was performed in all the patients, among whom three were operated twice due to the incomplete removal of the epileptogenic zone ($n = 1$) or of the underlying lesion ($n = 2$). The resection was restricted to temporal lobe structures in 34 patients, while it included both temporal and extra-temporal areas in the remaining 16 patients.

Pathological examination showed various types of anatomical lesions in 22 cases (44 per cent), which involved the perisylvian cortex in only two patients. These lesions comprised six hamartomas, five dysembryoplasic neuroepithelial tumours, four gangliogliomas, three scars, one xantho-astrocytoma, one cavernoma, one grey matter heterotopia, and one arachnoidian cyst. In addition, an associated hippocampal sclerosis (HcS) was found in three cases (dual pathology). An isolated HcS was found in other 20 patients (40 per cent), and there were no specific histological changes in the remaining eight patients (cryptogenic cases, 16 per cent).

At the last evaluation (October 1998), post-operative follow-up in 47 patients ranged from 5 years 1 month to 8 years 3 months (mean: 6 years 9 months). In the three patients operated twice, reoperations were performed after a mean delay of 3 years 9 months; the mean follow-up period after the second intervention was 3 years 10 months.

Stereo-EEG study

The stereo-EEG study was performed according to a previously described methodology (Bancaud et al., 1965; Talairach et al., 1974; Munari & Bancaud, 1987; Munari et al., 1994). We would like just to stress here that: (i) the number and positions of implanted electrodes varied from one patient to the other, depending on previously acquired clinical, scalp EEG and MRI data; (ii) electrodes were implanted in stereotactic conditions and their placement was assessed using the proportional atlas of Talairach & Tournoux (1988), taking into account the individual anatomical characteristics as assessed by stereotactic and stereoscopic cerebral angiography (Szikla et al., 1977); (iii) video-stereo-EEG recordings were performed in chronic condition under direct clinical control, with reduced medication in a majority of the cases. This allowed us to record spontaneous seizures, and to perform intracerebral electrical stimulation in order to reproduce part or all of the ictal clinical symptomatology and to map functionally eloquent areas (Kahane et al., 1993; Munari et al., 1993).

Ictal involvement of perisylvian areas was assessed on the basis of the most representative seizure recorded in each patient. The STG and/or the SSOC were considered as involved when a fast activity occurred. Patients were thus subdivided into four categories according to the rapidity of perisylvian involvement with respect to discharge onset: (i) initial involvement, i.e. involvement at seizure onset; (ii) early involvement, i.e. within the first 5 s from seizure onset; (iii) late involvement, i.e. after the first 5 s from seizure onset; (iv) no involvement.

Results

Investigation of the perisylvian cortex

A total number of 531 multilead intracerebral electrodes were implanted in the 50 studied patients (mean: 10.6 per patient), among which 130 investigated the perisylvian cortex at different levels (Fig. 1).

The STG was the only perisylvian area investigated in 18 patients (STG group). It was explored at different sites (anterior part, mid part, posterior part) by means of 24 electrodes, depending on patient's characteristics. In addition, other temporal and extratemporal areas were evaluated by means of 124 electrodes. Figure 1a shows a typical example of a predominantly temporal stereo-EEG investigation including the STG.

In 32 patients (PS group), 106 electrodes explored both the STG (anterior, mid and/or posterior part) and the SSOC (frontal, central and/or parietal operculum). Other temporal and extra-tem-

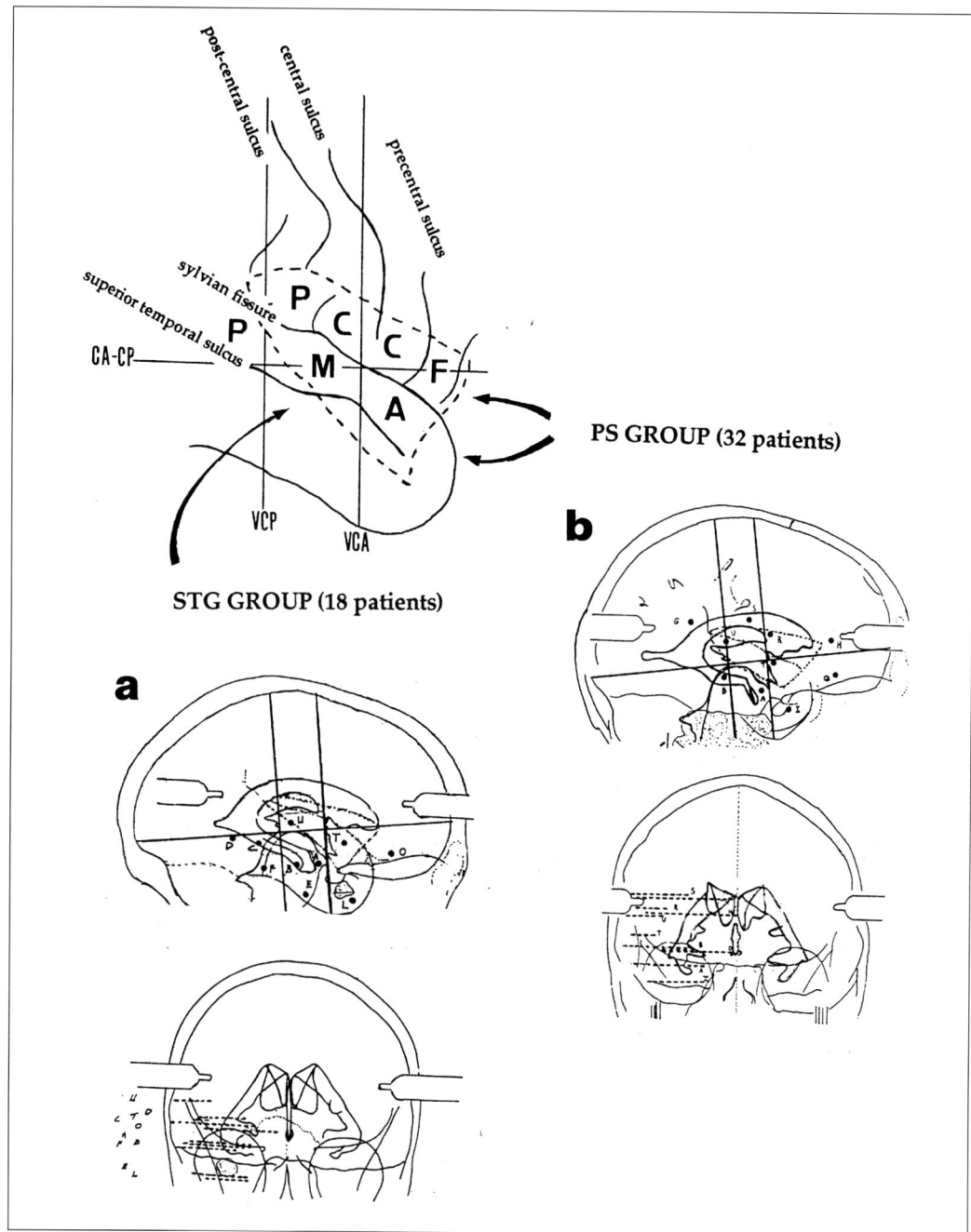

Fig. 1. Perisylvian cortex investigation.
Both the superior temporal gyrus (STG) and the suprasylvian opercular cortex (SSOC) were explored in 32 patients (see example in Fig. 1b), while the STG was the only perisylvian area investigated in the remaining 18 cases (see example in Fig. 1a).
F: frontal, C: central, P: parietal parts of the SSOC; A: anterior, M: mid, P: posterior parts of the STG; CA-CP: bicommissural line; VCA/VCP: vertical line passing through the anterior/posterior commissure.

poral areas were also evaluated, by means of 277 electrodes. A typical temporo-perisylvian stereo-EEG investigation is shown on Fig. 1b.

Complications directly linked to the stereo-EEG procedure occurred in two patients, and consisted in parietal haematoma in one case, and parietal oedema in another one. Both of these complications were asymptomatic and were observed on CT-scan after electrode removal.

Perisylvian involvement during ictal discharges

Overall, the STG was initially or early involved in 38 out of the 50 studied patients (76 per cent), and the SSOC in eight out of the 32 patients in whom it was investigated (25 per cent). Conversely, the STG was totally spared by the discharges in 7/50 patients (14 per cent), and the SSOC in 19/38 (50 per cent).

STG group (Table 1)

In 13 out of the 18 patients of this group (72 per cent), ictal discharges involved the STG initially or within the first 5 s. In such cases, a HcS was found three times (23 per cent). Other anatomical lesions, when present, were almost always located in the temporal pole (five/six). The only patient whose anatomical lesion was not located within the temporo-polar region exhibited seizures which arose simultaneously from the STG and the lateral aspect of the pole (Fig. 2). The STG was secondarily involved or not involved at all in five patients. A HcS was present in two out these five cases (40 per cent), and other anatomical lesions in three. These latter lesions dit not involve the temporo-polar region.

Table 1. Ictal involvement of the superior temporal gyrus (STG) with respect to seizure onset in the 18 patients of the STG group.
HcS: hippocampal sclerosis; other L: anatomical lesion other than hippocampal sclerosis; TP: lesion located within the temporal pole.

STG involvement			HcS	other L
Initial < 5"	2 11	72 %	3/13 (23%)	6/13 (TP=5)
> 5" = 0	2 3		2/5 (40%)	3/5 (TP=0)

PS group (Table 2)

The STG was involved initially or early on during the seizures in 25 out the 32 patients of this group (78 per cent). Initial or early involvement of the SSOC was rather less frequent (8/32 patients, i.e. 25 per cent), and it was only observed in patients whose seizures involved the STG at onset or within the first 5 s. Late involvement or absence of any involvement of the perisylvian cortex was observed in seven patients (22 per cent). HcS was found with a similar frequency, whatever the rapidity of STG and/or SSOC involvement. Conversely, anatomical lesions located within the temporal pole were only found in patients whose seizures involved the STG at onset or within the first 5 s, without initial or early concomitant involvement of the SSOC.

Table 2. Ictal involvement of the superior temporal gyrus (STG) and the suprasylvian opercular cortex (SSOC) with respect to seizure onset in the 32 patients of the PS group.
HcS: hippocampal sclerosis; other L: anatomical lesion other than hippocampal sclerosis; TP: lesion located within the temporal pole.

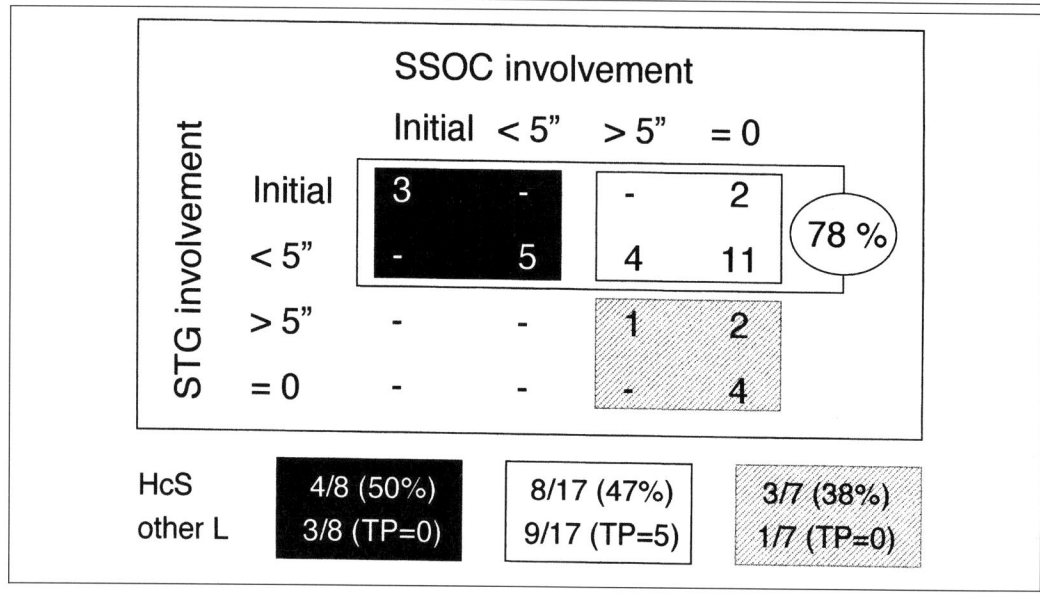

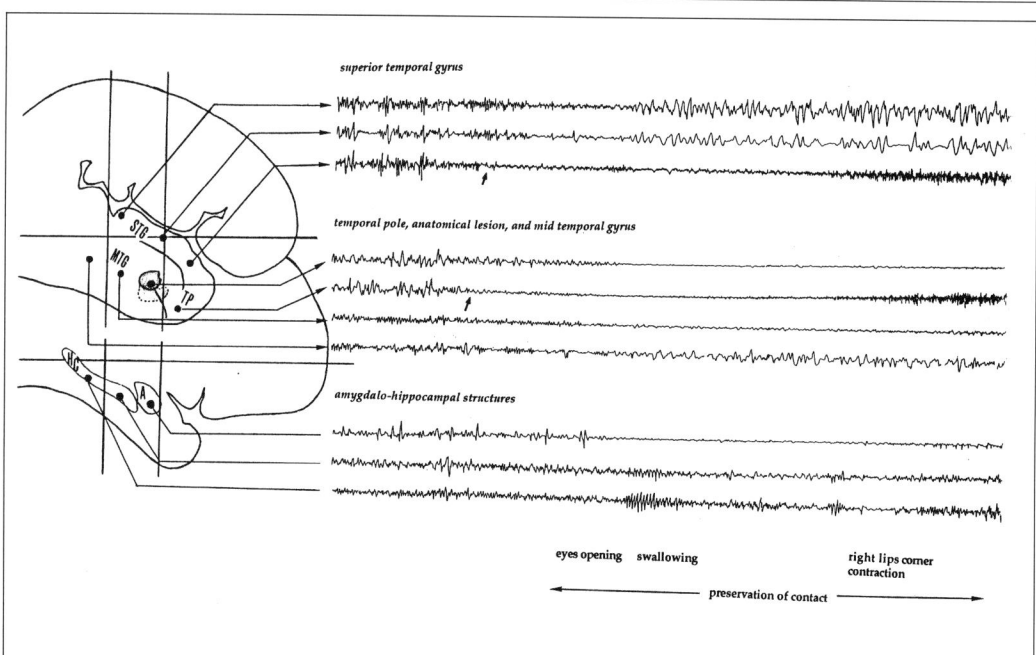

Fig. 2. Stereo-EEG recorded seizure arising simultaneously from the superior temporal gyrus (anterior part) and the lateral aspect of the pole (arrows).
Note that the anatomical lesion (hamartoma), located in the mid temporal gyrus, seems to be involved a few seconds later, and that the hippocampus is spared by the ictal discharge.

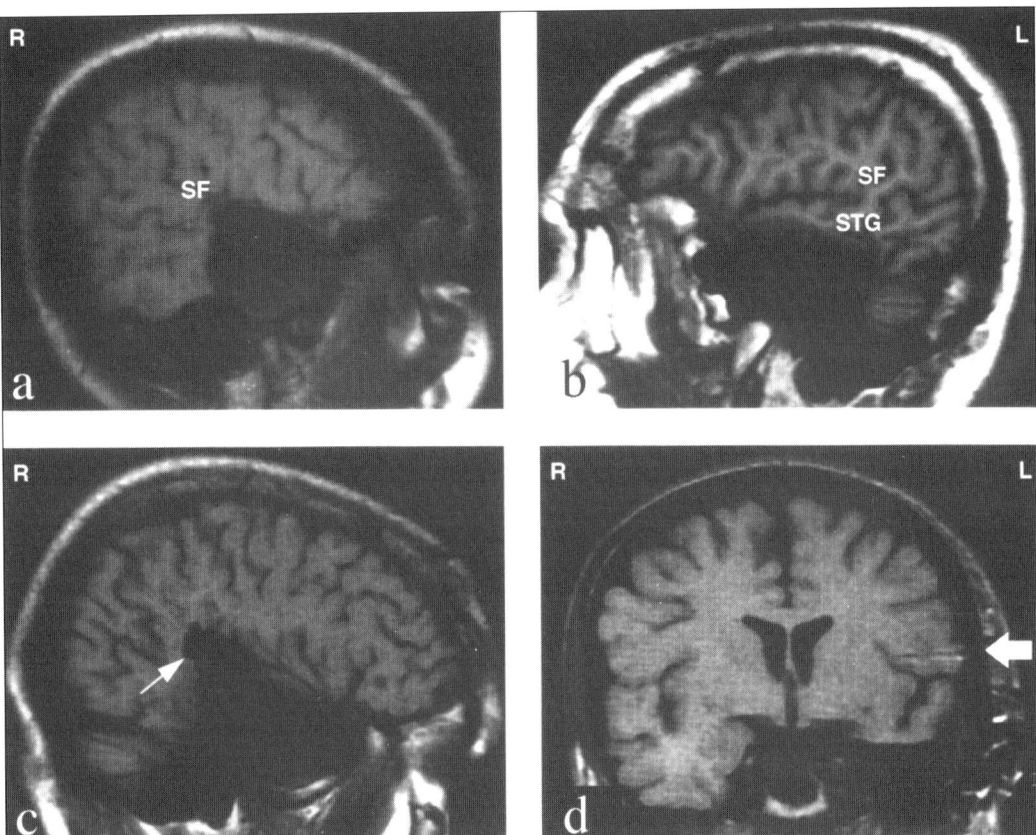

Fig. 3. Examples of surgical resections.
a: right temporal lobectomy including all the superior temporal gyrus.
b: left temporal lobectomy sparing the superior temporal gyrus.
c: right temporo-perisylvian resection, including all the superior temporal gyrus and the parietal operculum (thin arrow).
d: postoperative MRI (left temporal lobectomy sparing the superior temporal gyrus) showing the trace of an electrode which explored the suprasylvian opercular cortex (thick arrow).
R/L: right/left; SF: Sylvian fissure; STG: superior temporal gyrus.

Surgical resection of the perisylvian cortex

Surgical resections were never restricted to the perisylvian cortex alone. Overall, the STG was removed in 37/50 patients (74 per cent), and the SSOC in eight out the 32 patients in whom it was investigated (25 per cent). The extent of the perisylvian cortical resection was guided by stereo-EEG findings, taking into account the anatomical constraints (Fig. 3). In that respect, in the dominant hemisphere for language, removal of the STG, when judged necessary, was always restricted to its anterior part, and the SSOC was never resected. Thus, an adequate resection of the STG was performed in 35 out of the 38 patients in whom it was involved at seizure onset or within the first 5 s, and resection of the SSOC could be achieved in seven out the eight patients in whom it was involved initially or early on. In addition, it was judged necessary in three cases to remove the STG ($n = 2$) or the SSOC ($n = 1$) despite an ictal involvement which occurred more than 5 s after the onset of seizures (see Tables 4 and 5).

Transient neurological deficit directly linked to the removal of the perisylvian cortex was observed in four cases, and consisted in aphasic disturbances ($n = 2$), contralateral facial paresis ($n = 1$), and contralateral sensory deficit of the hand ($n = 1$).

Surgical outcome with respect to epileptic seizures

Surgical results were expressed according to the classification proposed by Engel (1987). Particular attention was paid to patients completely seizure free after surgery (class IA). Surgical results were mainly analysed with respect to the ictal involvement of the perisylvian cortex.

Global results (Table 3)

Overall, 64 per cent of the patients were completely seizure free after surgery. Similar good results were obtained in patients with HcS (IA: 70 per cent) and in patients with other anatomic lesions (IA: 68 per cent). The best results (IA: 83.5 per cent) were obtained in a small group of six patients whose seizures proved to be of temporo-perisylvian origin. Patients with 'pure' temporal lobe epilepsy were cured in almost 70 per cent of the cases, while those suffering from multilobar epilepsy other than temporo-perisylvian epilepsy had clearly a less favourable outcome (IA: 36.5 per cent). Most of these latter had a widely extended fronto-temporal epileptogenic area.

Table 3. Global post-operative results.
Total: total population; HcS: patients with hippocampal sclerosis; other L: patients with anatomical lesion other than hippocampal sclerosis; crypto: cryptogenic cases; T/TS/T+: patients suffering from 'pure' temporal lobe epilepsy/temporo-perisylvian epilepsy/other multilobar epilepsy involving the temporal lobe.

	Total (n=50)	HcS (n=20)	other L (n=22)	crypto (n=8)	T (n=33)	TS (n=6)	T+ (n=11)
IA	32 (64%)	14 (70%)	15 (68%)	3 (37.5%)	23 (69.5%)	5 (83.5%)	4 (36.5%)
IB	6	2	4	-	5	1	-
ID	4	3	1	-	3	-	1
II	2	1	1	-	1	-	1
III	1	-	-	1	-	-	1
IV	5 (10%)	-	1 (4.5%)	4 (50%)	1 (3%)	-	4 (40%)

STG group (Table 4)

Only five out the 13 patients in whom the STG was involved initially or within the first 5 s were cured after surgery, despite an adequate resection of the STG in 12 of these 13 patients. In one patient, the hippocampus was not removed despite its early ictal involvement, due to patient's willingness. Thus, the resection of the epileptogenic area was judged satisfactory in 11 patients, so that unanticipated failures represent 55 per cent of the cases. Better results were obtained in temporal lobe epilepsies when a complete removal of the epileptogenic area could be achieved (IA: 5/8, i.e. 62.5 per cent). Three of the four patients who did not improve after surgery were suffering from fronto-temporal seizures.

The removal of the epileptogenic zone was considered as complete in the five patients with late or no STG involvement during their seizures. Four of them (80 per cent) were seizure-free after surgery, and the STG was spared in all. Three were suffering from temporal lobe seizures, and one from fronto-temporal epilepsy. The remaining patient, whose seizures arose from temporal and fronto-basal cortices, experienced one episode of generalized tonic–clonic seizure during drug withdrawal.

Table 4. Surgical outcome in the 18 patients in whom the superior temporal gyrus (STG) was the only perisylvian area investigated.
Exc+ and Exc- signify that resection of the STG was performed or not, respectively. T/T+: patients suffering from 'pure' temporal lobe epilepsy/multilobar epilepsy other than temporo-perisylvian epilepsy. (a) absence of hippocampal removal due to patient's wishes in one case; (b) absence of STG removal due to anatomical constraints; (c) STG removal despite its late (> 5 s) ictal involvement.

	STG initial or < 5"				STG > 5" or =0			
	Exc+ (n=12)	Exc- (n=1)	T (n=10)	T+ (n=3)	Exc+ (n=1)	Exc- (n=4)	T (n=3)	T+ (n=2)
IA	5	-	5	-	-	4	3	1
IB	3 [a]	1 [b]	4 [a,b]	-	-	-	-	-
ID	-	-	-	-	1 [c]	-	-	1 [c]
II	-	-	-	-	-	-	-	-
III	-	-	-	-	-	-	-	-
IV	4	-	1	3	-	-	-	-

PS group (Table 5)

The STG and the SSOC were involved initially or early on during the ictal discharges in eight patients, of whom five were suffering from temporo-perisylvian seizures, and three from seizures which arose simultaneously from temporal and fronto-basal cortical areas. Six of the seven patients in whom an adequate perisylvian resection could be achieved were seizure free after surgery (85.5 per cent).

The STG was the only perisylvian area involved initially or early on during the seizures in 17 patients. The removal of the epileptogenic area was judged satisfactory in 16 cases (temporal: 13; temporo-perisylvian: one; temporo-frontal: two), of whom 13 were seizure-free after surgery (81 per cent). The STG was not adequately removed in the remaining patient whose seizures arise from mesial and lateral temporal lobe structures, and some generalized tonic–clonic seizures occurred during drug-withdrawal. Overall, particularly good results were obtained in temporal lobe epilepsies when a complete removal of the epileptogenic area could be achieved (IA: 11/13, i.e. 84.5 per cent).

The extent of the resection was considered as complete in all the seven patients in whom perisylvian areas were not involved at seizure onset or within the first 5 s. Four of the six patients who were suffering from temporal lobe seizures were seizure free after surgery (67 per cent). The remaining patient had a widely extended fronto-temporal epileptogenic zone, and seizures persisted despite two operations.

Table 5. Surgical outcome in the 32 patients in whom both the superior temporal gyrus (STG) and the suprasylvian opercular cortex (SSOC) were investigated.
Exc+ and Exc– signify that resection of the infra and/or suprasylvian cortex was performed or not, respectively. T/TS/T+: patients suffering from 'pure' temporal lobe epilepsy/temporo-perisylvian epilepsy/other multilobar epilepsy involving the temporal lobe. (a) inadequate STG resection and absence of SSOC removal, due to anatomical constraints; (b) SSOC removal despite its late (> 5 s) ictal involvement in one patient; (c) inadequate resection of the STG; (d) STG removal despite its late (> 5 s) ictal involvement.

	STG initial or < 5" & SSOC initial or < 5"				STG initial or < 5" & SSOC > 5" or =0					STG > 5" or =0 & SSOC > 5" or =0			
	Exc+ (n=7)	Exc– (n=1)	TS (n=5)	T+ (n=3)	Exc+ (n=16)	Exc– (n=1)	T (n=14)	TS (n=1)	T+ (n=2)	Exc+ (n=1)	Exc– (n=6)	T (n=6)	T+ (n=1)
IA	6	–	4	2	13[b]	–	11	1[b]	1	–	4	4	–
IB	–	1[a]	1[a]	–	1	–	1	–	–	–	–	–	–
ID	–	–	–	–	1	1[c]	2[c]	–	–	–	1	1	–
II	1	–	–	1	–	–	–	–	–	1[d]	–	1[d]	–
III	–	–	–	–	–	–	–	–	–	–	1	–	1
IV	–	–	–	–	1	–	–	–	1	–	–	–	–

Discussion

In patients suffering from severe drug-resistant partial epilepsy, surgical treatment allows good results in a high percentage of cases (Engel et al., 1993). Usually, the outcome is expressed as a function of the type of surgical act performed or according to a lobar classification of the epilepsy, so that the possibility that the 'epileptogenic zone' (Talairach & Bancaud, 1966) can spread beyond the anatomical limits of a lobe is rarely considered (Munari et al., 1995), except in the case of multilobar resections, when proposed as alternative therapy for hemispherectomy. Furthermore, it often remains unclear how the presurgical investigations are utilized for defining the limits of the cortical excision, that is to say the precise origin of seizures. This is notably true in the so-called temporal lobe epilepsies, for which more or less standardized surgical procedures are proposed, i.e. anterior temporal lobectomy (Falconer, 1967), selective amygdalo-hippocampectomy (Wieser & Yasargil, 1982) and neocortical resections (Hardiman et al., 1988). As a matter of fact, surgical failures are mainly discussed according to preoperative MRI findings (Berkovic et al., 1995) and/or the completeness of the causative lesion excision (Awad et al., 1991), the amount of hippocampal or amygadalar tissue resected (Siegel et al., 1990; Feindel & Rasmussen, 1991; Rasmussen & Feindel, 1991; Goldring et al., 1992), or the bilateral origin of seizures (Adam et al., 1997). Whether, how and why the superior temporal gyrus (STG) is removed – or not – has rarely been discussed (Munari et al., 1995), and the hypothesis that the epileptogenic area can include the suprasylvian opercular cortex has almost never been considered (Munari et al., 1980).

Our data suggest that in patients suffering from epileptic seizures affecting the temporal lobe, ictal involvement of the perisylvian cortex is far from uncommon, even when MRI indicates Ammon's horn sclerosis. In 'pure' temporal lobe epilepsies (TLE), an initial or early ictal involvement of the STG was found in 73 per cent of the cases (24/33), including nine of the 12

TLE with HcS and all the 10 TLE associated with a temporo-polar lesion. This latter finding might suggest that seizures involving the temporal pole have a particular trend to quickly propagate to the STG. An initial or early involvement of the STG was also frequently observed in seizures of multilobar origin (14/17, i.e. 82.5 per cent), often in association with an initial or early involvement of the SSOC (8/14). This simultaneous involvement of both infra- and suprasylvian cortical areas was mainly encountered in a particular form of multilobar epilepsy we named temporo-perisylvian epilepsy. Interestingly, four of the six patients suffering from this type of seizures had a HcS, thus underlining that complex epileptogenic networks can be associated with hippocampal atrophy.

When a complete removal of what was defined as the epileptogenic zone could be achieved (46/50 patients), seizures were eliminated in 69.5 per cent of the cases. In TLE with initial or early involvement of the STG, seizures disapperead after surgery in 76 per cent of patients in whom the removal of the epileptogenic area was judged satisfactory. This success rate even reached 84.5 per cent of the cases when it had been verified that the SSOC did not participate in the genesis of seizures. In TLE patients whose seizures did not involve the STG at onset or within the first 5 s, more limited temporal lobe resection led to similar good results, i.e. 78 per cent of seizure-free patients. This usefulness of stereotactic EEG investigation of the perisylvian cortex was also demonstrated for temporo-perisylvian epilepsies, since all the five patients in whom the whole epileptogenic area could be removed were cured after surgery. By contrast, multilobar resections other than temporo-perisylvian resections led to much more disappointing results (IA = 36.5 per cent), possibly due to the large extent of the epileptogenic zone which often included both frontal and temporal cortices. In such cases, whether the perisylvian cortex was involved or not during the ictal discharges did not seem to have any prognostic significance.

In seizures involving the temporal lobe, lack of appreciation of seizure spread patterns can be responsible for incorrect topographic diagnoses, and consequently for failures of standardized temporal lobe resections. In that respect, particular attention must be paid to clinical seizure characteristics, the examination of which helps to identify patients in whom intracerebral recordings are mandatory. In addition, analysis of ictal clinical symptomatology indicate the possible region of seizure origin and spread, so that electrode placement can be tailored and the risk for sampling errors reduced. In these conditions, it becomes possible in each individual patient not only to delineate the amount of cortex which must be resected, but also to formulate a preoperative prognosis.

References

Adam, C., Clémenceau, S., Semah, F., Hasboun, D., Samson, S., Dormont, D., Samson, Y., Philippon, J. & Baulac, M. (1997): Stratégie d'évaluation et résultats chirurgicaux dans l'épilepsie de la face médiale du lobe temporal. *Rev. Neurol.* **153** (11), 641–651.

Awad, I.A., Rosenfeld, J., Ahl, J., Hahn, J.F. & Lüders, H. (1991): Intractable epilepsy and structural lesions of the brain: mapping, resections strategies, and seizure outcome. *Epilepsia* **32**, 179–186.

Bancaud, J. (1987): Sémiologie clinique des crises épileptiques d'origine temporale. *Rev. Neurol.* **143**, 392–400.

Bancaud, J. & Talairach, J. (1991): Sémiologie clinique des crises du lobe temporal (méthodologie et investigations SEEG de 233 malades). In: *Crises épileptiques et épilepsies du lobe temporal*, vol. II. Gentilly: Documentation médicale Labaz.

Bancaud, J., Talairach, J., Bonis, A., Schaub, C., Szikla, G., Morel, P. & Bordas-Ferer, M. (1965): *La stéréo-électroencéphalographie dans l'épilepsie. Informations neurophysiopathologiques apportées par l'investigation fonctionnelle stéréotaxique.* Paris: Masson.

Bancaud, J., Talairach, J., Munari, C., Giallonardo, T. & Brunet, P. (1991): Introduction à l'étude clinique des crises rétro-rolandiques. *Can. J. Neurol. Sci.* **18**, 566–569.

Berkovic, S.F., McIntosh, A.M., Kalnins, R.M., Jackson, G.D., Fabinyi, G.C., Brazenor, G.A., Bladin, P.F. & Hopper, J.L. (1995): Preoperative MRI predicts outcome of temporal lobectomy: an actuarial analysis. *Neurology* **45**, 1358–1363.

Engel, J., Jr (1987): Outcome with respect to epileptic seizures. In: *Surgical treatment of the epilepsies*, ed. J. Engel, Jr., pp. 553–571. New York: Raven Press.

Engel, J., Jr., Van Ness, P.C., Rasmussen, T. & Ojemann, L.M. (1993): Outcome with respect to epileptic seizures. In: *Surgical treatment of the epilepsies*, 2nd edn., ed. J. Engel, Jr., pp. 609–621. New York: Raven Press.

Falconer, M.A. (1967): Surgical treatment of temporal lobe epilepsy. *N. Z. Med. J.* **66**, 539–544.

Feindel, W. & Rasmussen, T. (1991): Temporal lobectomy with amygdalectomy and minimal hippocampal resection: a review of 100 cases. *Can. J. Neurol. Sci.* **19**, 603–605.

Goldring, S., Edwards, I., Haring, G.W. & Bernard, K.L. (1992): Results of anterior temporal lobectomy that spares the amygdala in patients with complex partial seizures. *J. Neurosurg.* **77**, 185–193.

Hardiman, O., Burke, T., Phillips, J., Murphy, S., O'Moore, B., Staunton, H. & Farrel, M.A. (1988): Microdysgenesis in resected temporal neocortex: incidence and clinical significance in focal epilepsy. *Neurology* **38**, 1041–1047.

Hausser-Hauw, C. & Bancaud, J. (1987): Gustatory hallucinations in epileptic seizures. Electrophysiological, clinical and anatomical correlates. *Brain* **110**, 339–359.

Kahane, P., Tassi, L., Francione, S., Hoffmann, D., Lo Russo, G. & Munari, C. (1993): Manifestations électro-cliniques induites par la stimulation électrique intra-cérébrale par 'chocs' dans les épilepsies temporales. *Neurophysiol. Clin.* **22**, 305–326.

Munari, C. & Bancaud, J. (1987): The role of stereo-electro-encephalography (SEEG) in the evaluation of partial epileptic patients. In: *The epilepsies*, eds. R.J. Porter & P.L. Morselli, pp. 267–306. London: Butterworths.

Munari, C., Talairach, J., Bonis, A., Szikla, G. & Bancaud, J. (1980): Differential diagnosis between temporal and 'perisylvian' epilepsy on a surgical perspective. *Acta Neurochir.* **30** (Suppl.), 97–101.

Munari, C., Kahane, P., Tassi, L., Francione, S., Hoffmann, D., Lo Russo, G. & Benabid, A.L. (1993): Intracerebral low frequency electrical stimulation: a new tool for the definition of the 'epileptogenic area'? *Acta Neurochir.* **58** (Suppl.), 181–185.

Munari, C., Hoffmann, D., Francione, S., Kahane, P., Tassi, L., Lo Russo, G. & Benabid, A.L. (1994): Stereo-electroencephalography methodology: advantages and limits. *Acta Neurol. Scand.* **152** (Suppl.), 56–67.

Munari, C., Francione, S., Kahane, P., Hoffmann, D., Tassi, L., Lo Russo, G. & Benabid, A.L. (1995): Multilobar resections for the control of epilepsy. In: *Operative neurosurgical techniques*, 3rd edition, vol. 2, eds. H.H. Schmidek & W.J. Sweet, pp. 1323–1335. Philadelphia: W.B. Saunders Company.

Munari, C., Berta, E., Minotti, L., Di Leo, M., Hoffmann, D., Tassi, L., Kahane, P., Lo Russo, G. & Francione, S. (1996): Contribution to the identification of 'vestibular' cortex in man: a stereoEEG study. In: *Le cortex vestibulaire*, eds. M. Collar, M. Jeannerod M & Y. Christen, pp. 49–53. Paris: Irvinn.

Penfield, W. (1958). Functional localization in temporal and deep sylvian areas. *Res. Ass. Nerv. Ment. Dis.* **36**, 210–226.

Penfield, W. & Jasper, H. (1954): *Epilepsy and the functional anatomy of the human brain.* Boston: Little, Brown and Company.

Penfield, W. & Rasmussen, T. (1950): *The cerebral cortex of man.* New York: Macmillan.

Rasmussen, T. & Feindel, W. (1991): Temporal lobectomy: review of 100 cases with hippocampectomy. *Can. J. Neurol. Sci.* **18,** 601–602.

Siegel, A.M., Wieser, H.G., Wichmann, W. & Yasargil, M.G. (1990): Relationships between MR-imaged total amount of tissue removed, resection scores of specific mediobasal subcompartments and clinical outcome following selective amygdalohippocampectomy. *Epilepsy Res.* **6,** 56–65.

Smith, B.H. (1960): Vestibular disturbances in epilepsy. *Neurology* **10,** 465–469.

Szikla, G., Bouvier, G., Hori, T. & Petrov, V. (1977): *Angiography of the human brain cortex. Atlas of vascular patterns and stereotactic cortical localization.* Heidelberg: Springer.

Talairach, J. & Bancaud, J. (1966): Lesions, irritative zone and epileptogenic focus. *Confin. Neurol.* **27,** 91–94.

Talairach, J. & Tournoux, P. (1988): *Co-planar stereotaxic atlas of the human brain.* Stuttgart: Georg Thieme Verlag.

Talairach, J., Bancaud, J., Szikla, G., Bonis, A. & Geier, S. (1974): Approche nouvelle de la neurochirurgie de l'épilepsie. Méthodologie stéréotaxique et résultats thérapeutiques. *Neurochirurgie* **20,** 1–240.

Wieser, H.G. & Yasargil, M.G. (1982): Selective amygdalohippocampectomy as a surgical treatment of mesiobasal limbic epilepsy. *Surg. Neurol.* **17,** 445–447.

Chapter 12

Mesio-temporal seizures

Jean Isnard

Department of Functional Neurology and Epileptology, Hôpital Neurologique, 69 Boulevard Pinel, 69003 Lyon, France

Summary

Mesio-temporal lobe epilepsy (MTLE) designates the clinical syndrome associated with the development of a critical discharge in the temporal limbic structures of the brain (hippocampus and para-hippocampal gyrus) and the amygdalar nucleus (AN). Simply stated, these seizures begin by the perception of an undefinable diffuse discomfort sometimes associated with a sudden stop of activity. Then early onset of marked neurovegetative manifestations occurs, in the form of a sensation of a rising mediosternal constriction of the chest, as well as other types of manifestations: cardio-vascular (tachycardia), respiratory (polypnea), and vasomotor (reddening of the face). These manifestations are readily accompanied by oral automatic behaviour (chewing movements) and by twitching of the upper limbs (atonic posture of the upper limb of the opposite-side temporal lobe affected by the discharge). The patient usually experiences bewilderment or confusion. There is typically no loss of contact, at least initially.

The critical discharge which develops with the amygdalo-hippocampic structures (AHS) disturbs the multiple circuits controlling the temporal structures and explains the complexity and the richness of the MTLE syndrome. One of the most important circuits connects the AHS to the insular structure. Its role in the viscero-vegetative functions and the organization of affective life suggests that the insular cortex could play a central role in the origin of MTLE clinical symptoms. Recent SEEG explorations seem to confirm that the restrictive label MTLE could be replaced by insulo-mesio-temporal lobe epilepsy.

Notion of partial seizure

The clinical presentation of partial epileptic seizures results from disturbances brought about by the onset and spread of a critical local discharge in a limited sector of the cerebral cortex and its functionally related subcortical areas. Two predefined conditions must be met for this relation to be clearly established:

(i) the discharge site must be identified by intracranial EEG;

(ii) the removal of the epileptic focus thus defined leads to the disappearance of seizures.

Thus, mesio temporal lobe epilepsy (MTLE) means partial epileptic seizures whose clinical presentation conveys the development of a critical electric discharge within the mesio temporal lobe structures: hippocampus, para hippocampal gyrus and amygdalar nucleus (AN).

Clinical semiology

Temporal lobe epilepsy is the most fully described form of partial epilepsy, by widespread consensus. The description of mesio temporal seizures has benefited from the everyday use of synchronized video-EEG recordings providing detailed and *a posteriori* analysis of the clinical symptomatology of seizures. This work, conducted intensively over the last decade, has provided not only the definition of a universally recognized clinical pattern of TLEs, but also the improvement of knowledge on the anatomical-electrical-clinical correlations which serve to determine different subtypes of TLE in relation to the location of the epileptic focus within the temporal lobe. This method's limitations appear in the attempts to evaluate the correlations statistically by considering the clinical event no longer on the scale of a syndrome but rather on that of the symptom and consequently hide the localizing value of seizures (Manford et al., 1996). To be relevant, clinical analysis should attempt to describe critical symptoms, i.e. the chronological progression of symptoms during a seizure.

Between the pitfalls of oversimplification and absolute exhaustiveness, we can provide a general framework for the clinical description of mesio-temporal onset seizures using descriptions based on large numbers of patients (Bancaud, 1987; Wieser, 1981; Delgado Escueta et al., 1982). A major problem in defining the MTLE syndrome has been validation of whether seizures were truly mesial temporal in origin. Several recent publications respond to this criticism with the argument that the analysis of clinical behaviour demonstrated during seizures is carried out on series of patients in whom the origin of mesio-temporal seizure was established with intracranial EEG recording and confirmed by cure after mesial temporal resection (Kotagal et al., 1995; Williamson et al., 1998).

Broadly speaking, these seizures often begin by stereotypical subjective manifestations, the onset of which can occur during full consciousness and remain isolated for a period of a few seconds to 1–2 min. These manifestations, often called aura, can be described as a sensation of epigastric heaviness which often rises from the abdomen to the chest or throat. Occasionally the symptoms are more difficult to describe and are reported as a sensation of undefinable nonlocalized discomfort which can be associated with a sudden stop of activity.

These signs are often associated with several types of neurovegatative manifestations: cardiovascular (tachycardia), respiratory (polypnea), vasomotor (facial reddening); they can also be associated with nonreactive mydriasis beginning upon loss of consciousness.

These manifestations are easily accompanied by automatic behaviour. That is a complex behaviour that resembles normal body movement. They are often stereotypical, associated with consciousness impairment, and the patient usually has no memory of the event. However, in 10 per cent of cases, the behaviour appears as repetitive and seemingly purposeful acts; onset is without loss of consciousness (Ebner et al., 1995). This is the case for automatic mouth movements such as chewing, when the critical discharge remains localized in the amygdaloid nucleus and the anterior part of the hippocampus of a single temporal lobe (Munari et al., 1982). In more than 60 per cent of cases we also see automatic rhythmic tapping or manipulation of an object, usually in the upper limb on the same side of the epileptic focal site and often associated with an atonic aspect of the opposite upper limb (contralateral to the epileptogenic focus).

Typically, consciousness is preserved initially and is perceived as intense, followed a few seconds later by consciousness impairment with complete loss of contact with the surroundings. Partial reestablishment can follow with the patient reactive to stimulation or demonstrating eye tracking behaviour (Kotagal, 1999). For thorough evaluation, these symptoms require the presence of an experienced doctor, capable of examining the patient during a seizure. This will encourage accurate interpretation of these alterations of consciousness: a single nonreactive behaviour can signify a perceptive deficit, cognitive impairment, affective disturbances, amnesia problems, or voluntary movements (Gloor, 1986).

Temporal seizures are also characterized by memory impairment over the period of the seizure but also the 1–2 min preceding the beginning of the seizure. This deficit is probably linked to the diffusion of the epileptic discharge to the opposite-side hippocampus. Once again, the presence of a qualified examiner allows questioning of the patient immediately at the end of the seizure, at a time when he is still capable of reporting critical subjective perceptions, the memory of which will disappear within a few minutes.

Other categories of symptoms are sometimes reported: language impairment; hallucinatory or illusionary, sensory or psychic phenomena; manifestations of chewing, smacking of lips, or of hypersalivation; dysaesthesia or hemifacial convulsions, etc. These signs typically express the diffusion of the critical discharge outside the mesio-temporal area toward the rest of the temporal lobe or toward the extratemporal zones. In all cases, these manifestations are not within the domain of mesio-temporal seizures.

Electroencephalographic (EEG) semiology

The organization of critical discharges in the AH system has been studied with SEEG techniques by Bancaud et al. (1965) and then by Wieser (1981). Despite over 35 years of retrospection, the rules governing the interpretation of invasive EEG recordings are imprecise, though the highest level of codification exists for MTLE exploration. The major limitation of intracranial recording stems from the constraints in spatial sampling. Intracranial electrodes measure the EEG activity of a cortical sector limited to the zone of contact. These electrodes can ignore the activity of a focal site only a few millimeters away. When they do record a critical discharge, it is impossible to claim with certainty that this discharge truly has its origin in the targeted site and that it is not, on the contrary, a signal spread from a more distant source. This constraint must be taken into consideration when establishing electroclinical correlations whose purpose is to evaluate the localizing value of critical symptoms.

Intercritical activity

Many irregularities can be observed. The slow waves are often more frequent at the beginning of exploration because of implant trauma and will progressively subside 2 or 3 days after implantation. Multifocal points are often observed and can be present independently on the hippocampus, the temporal pole, and the temporal neocortex. Several morphologies can also be observed. The localizing value of these irregularities is difficult to determine because, once again, the linear analysis of the intracranial EEG does not provide sufficient evidence to claim whether a recorded point is generated from the collection site or from a diffused point (Spencer & Spencer, 1994).

Ictal activity

Contrary to intercritical activity, the critical discharge of MTLE follows a very stable pattern of high localizing value (Fig. 1). Initial modifications are often seen on only one or two tracks

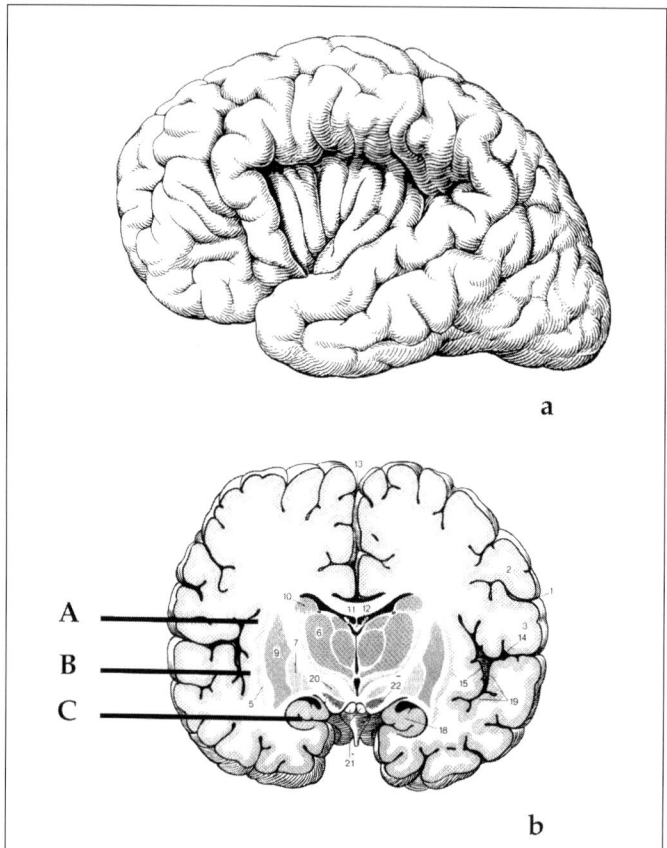

Fig. 1. Continuous depth electrode recorded EEG segments showing spontaneous ictal onset with periodic spiking in the right hippocampus, followed by low voltage fast activity in the same region with spread to the right amygdala and neo cortical regions.
(a): Lateral view of the brain. The insular lobe can be seen, the opercules being drawn aside.
(b): Diagram showing stereotactically implanted trans-opercular electrodes. Electrode A reaches the antero-superior part of the insula, electrode B the antero-inferior part of the insula and electrode C the hippocampus and the anterior part of the medial temporal gyrus.

(pathways). This is conveyed either by a low voltage fast activity or by periodical single-shaped high-amplitude slow activity with possible repetition over a period of a few seconds to a few minutes before rapid discharge begins (King & Spencer, 1995). When the discharge originates in the hippocampus, its frequency varies between 10 and 15 Hz whereas when it originates both in the hippocampus and the external surface of the temporal lobe, the frequency is much higher, around 35 Hz (Javidan et al., 1992). Twenty to 50 per cent of MTLE seizures originate exclusively in the hippocampus, 5–10 per cent exclusively in the amygdoloid nucleus. In the other cases the initial discharge is more diffuse on the inside surface of the temporal lobe (Spencer et al., 1993).

Spreading patterns

Spreading patterns are more systematic in MTLEs than in other epileptic syndromes. Starting from the amygdalo-hippocampal structure, the discharge most systematically spreads toward the posterior cinguli but does not, however, reach Brodmann's area 34 (Wieser, 1981). In 60 per cent of cases the internal temporal discharge spreads to the pole and the external face of the temporal lobe and from there toward the frontal lobe (in particular its orbital face) or the opposite-side temporal lobe. In 30 per cent of cases the discharge spreads first to the opposite-side hippocampus before extending to the external face of the temporal lobe or spreading in the other lobe. Finally, in the 10 per cent of remaining cases, the internal temporal discharge spreads at the same time to the opposite-side hippocampus and to the same-side neocortex (Spencer et al., 1987).

The organization of MTLE critical discharges is so characteristic that invasive exploration is mostly not justified for identification purposes. Scalp recordings or semi-invasive recordings

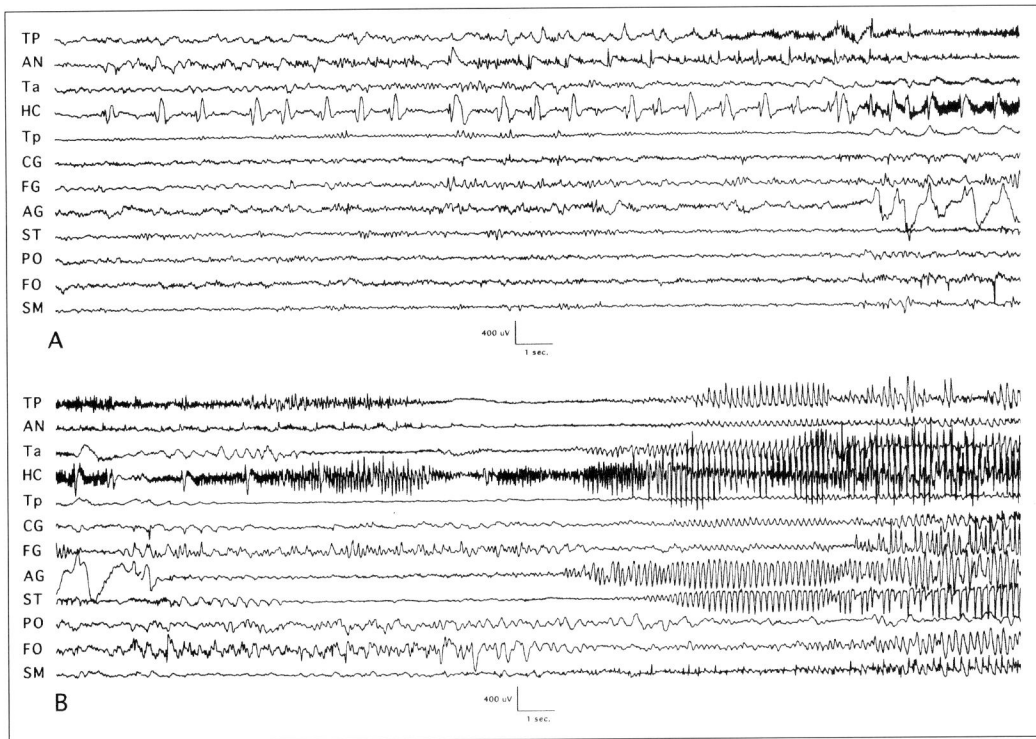

Fig. 2. SEEG recordings of a temporo-mesial seizure: rythmic spike-waves are recorded in the hippocampus for a few seconds before the occurrence of a recruiting fast discharge that can be seen simultaneously in the amygdalar nucleus, the temporal pole and the hippocampus. The discharge is localized to these structures for about 10 s and then evolves into a low voltage fast activity which progressively spreads to all temporal lobe structures explored.
TP: temporal pole, AN: amygdalar nucleus, Ta: anterior part of the medial temporal gyrus, HC: hippocampus, Tp: posterior part of the medial temporal gyrus, CG: cingular gyrus, FG: fusiform gyrus, AG: angular gyrus, ST: superior temporal gyrus, PO: parietal operculum, FO: frontal operculum, SM: supra marginal gyrus.

with sphenoidal electrodes often allow observation of low voltage fast acts localized in the temporal electrodes. Recordings with foramen ovale electrodes are an intermediary solution used by many hospitals (Wieser & Moser, 1988). They provide the advantage of EEG recording of the inner face of the temporal lobes without the constraints of SEEG exploration or craniectomy.

Are temporo-mesial seizures of temporal origin?

Intracranial EEG recordings have established the relation between the development of a critical discharge in the mesio-temporal structures and the onset of MTLE syndrome, but nothing substantiates a claim for a causal link between the two events. The symptoms observed can be linked to disturbances located away from the temporal lobe, either by a trans-synaptic direct excitation effect or, on the other hand, by the removal of an inhibitor of the temporal lobe on areas located at a distance. The persistence of subjective visceral signs following surgical treatment of certain types of seizures labelled mesio-temporal, even after extensive temporal

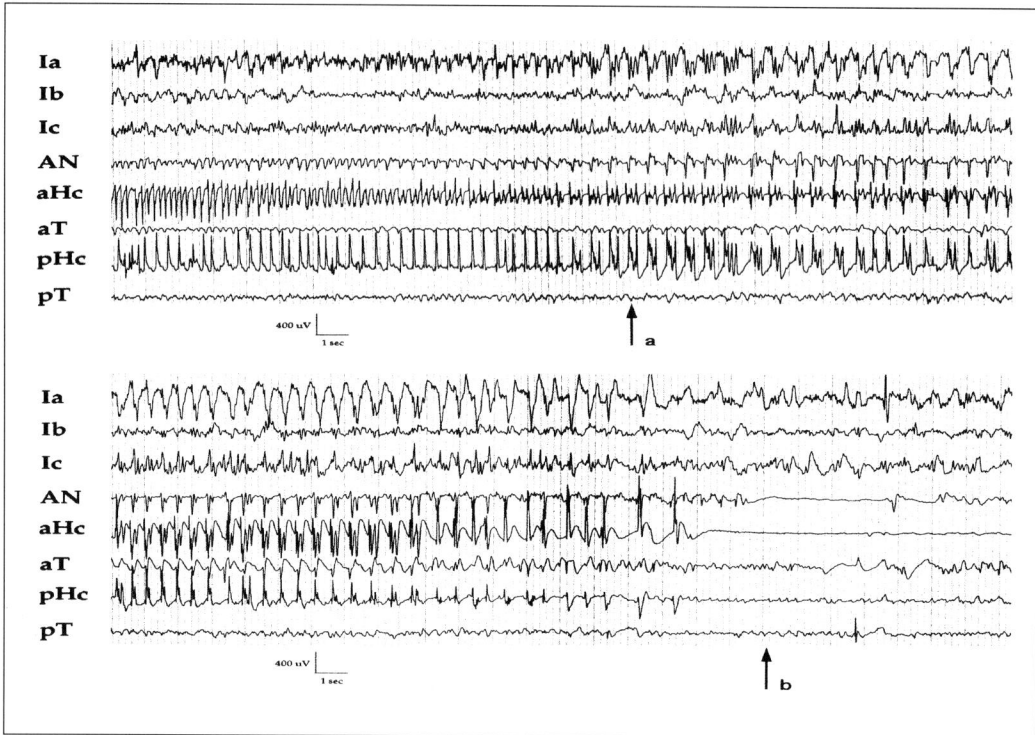

Fig. 3. SEEG recordings of a patient with MTLE. Long asymptomatic discharges of spikes are recorded on the hippocampus. When these spikes spread to the insular cortex, the patient reports his usual aura with nausea and abdominal pain (arrow a). Symptoms disappear when the discharge ceases (arrow b). Ia: antero-superior insular cortex, Ib: posterior insular cortex, Ic: antero-inferior insular cortex, AN: amygdalar nucleus, aHc: anterior hippocampus, pHc: posterior hippocampus, aT: anterior part of the superior temporal gyrus, pT: posterior part of the superior temporal gyrus.

lobectomies, suggests that extratemporal structures intervene in the origin of the symptoms of these seizures. Yet one of the cortical structures most richly connected to the amygdalo-hippocampal structures is the insular lobe (Mesulam & Mufson, 1985). Its intervention in temporal partial epilepsies has often been mentioned but never been demonstrated. This hypothesis is based to a large extent on the results of preoperative electric stimulations of the insular lobe (IL) carried out by Penfield at the beginning of the 1950s on a group of patients suffering from temporal epilepsy (Penfield & Faulk, 1955). Not only were the symptoms mentioned similar to those observed during temporal seizures (viscero-sensitive, vegetative, chewing activities) but in addition patients often described them as identical to those they perceived during spontaneous seizures. Furthermore, a great deal of research in functional anatomy has emphasized the role of the insula viscero-sensitive and motor functions, as well as vegetative and oral functions. It is precisely these categories of symptoms which are observed during temporal seizures.

The SEEG technique records three areas at the same time: the mesio-temporal, the neocortex, and the insular cortex (Fig. 2). In one patient, we were able to record long discharges of polyspikes extending asymptomatically only in the right hippocampus over a period of several minutes. On the other hand, when this discharge diffused to the insular cortex, the patient indicated a perception of her usual aura of thoracic oppression. This preliminary result suggests that the critical discharge, as long as it remains localized in the hippocampus, produces no symptoms, but that the mesio-temporal symptomatology appears when the insular lobe is implicated by this discharge. This hypothesis requires confirmation by other recordings of the insula during presurgical evaluation of TLE. If it proves to be exact, it could explain in part the surgical treatment failures in temporal lobe epilepsies, since today 30 per cent of these patients are not totally free of seizures, even after an extensive temporal lobectomy.

References

Bancaud J. (1987): Sémiologie clinique des crises épileptiques d'origine temporale. *Rev. Neurol.* **143,** 392–400.

Bancaud, J., Talairach, J., Bonis, A., Schaub, C., Szikla, G., Morel, P. & Bordas-Ferrer, P. (1965): *La stéréo-électroencéphalographie dans l'épilepsie.* Paris: Masson.

Delgado-Escueta, A.V., Bascal, F.E. & Treiman, D.M. (1982): Complex partial seizures on closed-circuit television and EEG: a study of 691 attacks in 79 patients. *Ann. Neurol.* **11,** 292–300.

Ebner, A., Dinner, D.S., Noachtar, S. & Lüders, H. (1995): Automatisms with preserved responsiveness: a lateralizing sign in psychomotor seizures. *Neurology* **45,** 61–64.

Gloor, P. (1986): Consciousness as a neurological concept in epileptology: a critical review. *Epilepsia* **27** (Suppl. 2), S14–S26.

Javidan, M., Katz, A., Tran, T., Pacia, S., Spencer, D.D. & Spencer, S.S. (1992): Frequency characteristics of neocortical and hippocampal onset seizures. *Epilepsia* **33,** S58–S58.

King, D. & Spencer, S. (1995): Invasive electroencephalography in mesial temporal lobe epilepsy. *J. Clin. Neurophysiol.* **12,** 32–45.

Kotagal, P. (1999): Seizure semiology of mesial temporal lobe epilepsy. In: *The epilepsies. Etiologies and prevention*, eds. P. Kotagal & H.O. Lüders, pp. 141–148. San Diego: Academic Press.

Kotagal, P., Lüders, H., Williams, G., Nichols, T. & McPherson, J. (1995): Psychomotor seizures of temporal lobe onset: analysis of symptom clusters ans sequences. *Epilepsy Res.* **20,** 49–67

Manford, M., Fish D.R. & Shorvon, S.D. (1996): An analysis of clinical seizure patterns and their localizing value in frontal and temporal lobe epilepsies. *Brain* **119,** 17–40.

Mesulam, M.M. & Mufson E.J. (1985): The insula of Reil in man and monkey. Architectonics, connectivity, and function. In: *Cerebral Cortex*, vol. 4, ed. Peter A. Jones, pp. 179–226. New York: Plenum Press.

Munari, C., Stoffels, C., Bossi, L. & Brunet, P. (1982): Partial seizures with elementary or complex symptomatology: a valid classification for temporal lobe seizures? In: *Advances in epileptology: XIIIth Epilepsy International Symposium,* eds. H. Akimoto, H. Kazamatsuri, M. Seino & A.A. Ward, Jr., pp. 25–27. New York: Raven Press.

Penfield, W. & Faulk, M.E., Jr. (1955): The insula: further observations on its functions. *Brain* **78,** 445–470.

Spencer, S.S. & Spencer, D.D. (1994): Entorhinal-hippocampal interactions in mesial temporal lobe epilepsy. *Epilepsia* **35,** 721–727.

Spencer, S.S., Williamson, P.D., Spencer, D.D. & Mattson, R.H. (1987): Human hippocampal seizure spread studied by depth and subdural recording: the hippocampal commissure. *Epilepsia* **28,** 479–489.

Spencer, S.S., So, N.K., Engel, J., Williamson, P.D., Levesque, M.F. & Spencer, D.D. (1993): Depth electrodes. In: *Surgical treatment of the epilepsies*, ed. J.J. Engel, pp. 359–376. New York: Raven Press.

Wieser, H.G. (1981): *Electroclinical features of the psychomotor seizure*. London: Butterworths.

Wieser, H.G. & Moser, S. (1988): Improved multipolar foramen ovale electrode monitoring. *J. Epilepsy* **1,** 13–22

Williamson , P.D., Thadani, V.D., French, J.A., Darcey, T.M., Mattson, R.H., Spencer, S.S. & Spencer, D.D. (1998): Medical temporal lobe epilepsy: videotape analysis of objective clinical seizure characteristics. *Epilepsia* **39,** 1182–1188.

Chapter 13

Symptoms differentiating 'temporal' and 'frontal' complex partial seizures

Claudio Munari*, Roberto Mai*, Laura Tassi*, Stefano Francione*, Giorgio Lo Russo*, Lorella Minotti† and Philippe Kahane†

*Centro Chirurgia dell'Epilessia 'C. Munari', Ospedale Niguarda Ca' Granda, Piazza Ospedale Maggiore 3, 20162 Milan, Italy; †Neurophysiopathologie de l'Epilepsie, CHU Grenoble, France

Summary

This study aims to verify if the impairment of contact (IC) allows the differentiation of temporal from frontal partial seizures and, if early subjective and objective clinical manifestations are systematically different in frontal and temporal partial seizures. The early clinical semiology is tentatively correlated with the cortical areas initially involved by the ictal discharge, as well as with the type, duration and spreading modalities of the discharge.

In order to be useful, a clinical classification must be clear and simple. The proposed terms should have an unequivocal meaning, thus allowing easy and unambiguous scientific communication among clinical researchers. Moreover, in patients with partial seizures, who are candidates for surgical treatment of severe epilepsy, the identification of clinical signs and symptoms with a clear localizing value can be extremely helpful. Only pre-ictal examination and questioning of the patient entitle the observer to affirm an impairment of contact which is far from being constant, in temporal as well as in frontal lobe seizures, in spite of appearances.

The term 'complex' partial seizures is completely devoid of any localizing value, since an impairment of contact can occur in every kind of partial seizure (frontal and temporal but also parietal and occipital), being related to the intensity, duration and extent of the ictal discharge. Therefore, its use does not seem useful for defining the seizures of surgical candidates. It is probably much more helpful to try and identify those clinical signs and symptoms that, isolated or in a given chronological syndromic association, allow the formulation of a correct hypothesis on the location of the epileptogenic area.

Introduction

The first comprehensive evaluation of a patient with partial epilepsy must include several stages, each one yielding relevant information to try to identify, though still tentatively, the cortical area supposedly responsible for the ictal discharges. Therefore, the identification of this area, called 'epileptogenic zone', rests upon anatomo-electroclinical correlations which differ from one patient to the other (Munari et al., 1994; Munari et al., 1996b).

The patient's clinical history must then be examined (Williamson & Spencer, 1986) by a careful inquiry with both the patient and the relatives, with special attention to timing of onset for each clinical symptom and sign, neurological examination, neuropsychological assessment and, in certain cases, psychiatric evaluation. Complementary diagnostic procedures, such as visual field examination, or functional procedures such as SPECT or PET, may yield additional information.

Neuroimaging techniques (MRI and brain CT scan) may identify a possible structural lesion, which in turn should be characterized by signal features, location, extent and relationship with contiguous cerebral areas. It is especially important to verify how the anatomical lesion may be related to the cortical areas responsible for the organization of ictal discharges.

Neurophysiological examinations performed in the course of the disease (mostly consisting of interictal EEG monitoring) may yield information about the localization of interictal abnormalities (slow waves and spikes).

At this point it could already be possible to advance some hypothesis about the localization of the epileptogenic zone by carefully correlating clinical, neurophysiological and anatomical data.

If the patient proves to be refractory to medical treatment, and presurgical evaluation is deemed feasible, further investigations may be necessary.

Among these the least invasive is certainly the recording of clinical ictal events by video-EEG. Of course, while performing video-EEG the patient must be kept under close clinical surveillance in order to be questioned and examined during seizures.

The data obtained from video-EEG can be sufficient to assess the extent of the epileptogenic zone and to take the decision to proceed to surgery, but in some instances more extensive information may be required. If this is the case, invasive studies will be necessary. In our centre this implies performance of stereo-electro-encephalography (stereo-EEG), i.e. implantation of intracerebral electrodes, adapted to the individual patient in such a way as to allow focusing on a well circumscribed area of the brain identified according to the anatomo-electroclinical data specific to that patient (Munari et al., 1994). Thus, a wealth of information is made available to the epileptologist and, in most cases, this allows accurate localization of the epileptogenic zone.

Following the above remarks, reviewing the criteria proposed by the International Classification to differentiate temporal lobe seizures from seizures originating in the frontal lobe, we realize that things are much more complex than envisaged by any classification (Commission on Classification, 1989). As a matter of fact, the classification of clinical ictal symptoms, both subjective and objective, though essential in a clinical perspective, does not account for the complexity of a seizure and, mostly, for the observation that, even in the same patient, seizures are only exceptionally monosymptomatic. In fact, subjective symptoms are most often multiple, characterized by a timing sequence, and it is extremely rare to observe one isolated symptom even for the shortest and most limited subjective feeling. We face the same problem, if not greater, when considering the objective manifestations, which overlap with each other, although an individual and repetitive pattern can usually be defined in each patient.

Given the above observations, it appears that among complex partial seizures the differentiation between frontal seizures and seizures originating in the temporal lobe is particularly demanding (Kramer et al., 1997; Munari et al., 1981; Swartz et al., 1991). However, on the basis of data from the literature and our personal experience with stereo-EEG, we will try to assess whether significant differences exist between the two types of seizures and how to identify them.

Methodological approach

Basic features

For many years literature studies have tried to discriminate between seizures originating in the frontal lobe and those originating in the temporal lobe, keeping in mind that temporal seizures are by far the most frequent and best known, also because of the high number of patients evaluated for surgical treatment (surgically treated temporal epilepsies account for almost 70 per cent of all cases). Therefore, recordings of temporal seizures (both video-EEG and invasive procedures) are considerably more frequent than for frontal ones. Moreover, the issue is further complicated by the fact that the complex structure and the specific functions of the frontal lobe are far from being clarified.

It is generally held that some features differentiate these types of seizures (Fig. 1) (Ajmone Marsan & Goldhammer, 1973; Bancaud & Talairach, 1992; Chauvel *et al.*, 1995; Geier *et al.*, 1977; Laskowitz *et al.*, 1995; Rasmussen, 1983; Wieser & Hajek, 1995; Williamson *et al.*, 1985).

Among these, it is worth mentioning a higher ictal frequency of frontal seizures, with more frequent occurrence of status epilepticus and secondarily generalized seizures. Falls are present almost only in frontal seizures, while being extremely rare in temporal ones.

Frontal seizure duration is usually shorter than for temporal seizures. Post ictal confusion is usually less severe and prolonged than in temporal lobe seizures.

Subjective disturbances at onset are considered prevalent in temporal lobe seizures (Bancaud & Talairach, 1991). However, when accurately questioned a high percentage of patients with frontal seizures report subjective feelings, which are usually briefer and more 'complex', so that they are often difficult to report even by scrupulous patients (Williamson *et al.*, 1985). To the epileptologists' dismay, epigastric subjective discomfort may be present in frontal lobe seizures

ICTAL MANIFESTATIONS
General Characteristics

Temporal	Frontal
Seizures in cluster at intervals or randomly.	Frequent seizures, often in cluster
	Especially nocturnal
Duration > 1 min	Brief seizures
Recovery is gradual	Sudden onset and offset
Marked post-ictal confusion	Slight post-ictal confusion
Simple & complex partial	Frequent generalized seizures
Typically initial "sensations"	Rare warning, usually indefinite
Gradual clouding of consciousness	Early loss of contact
	Frequent status epilepticus
Interictal EEG well-localizing	Interictal & ictal EEG (useful?)

Fig. 1.

as well as in temporal seizures. In these cases the timing of associated signs and symptoms may be of great significance.

The issue of the usefulness of the EEG is still a matter of debate because, notwithstanding its widely recognized reliability in temporal lobe seizures, its role in frontal seizures is greatly diminished, it being claimed that neither interictal nor ictal abnormalities would allow localization or even lateralization (Bancaud & Talairach, 1992; Quesney, 1992; Quesney et al., 1995; Williamson et al., 1986).

Actually, especially for ictal recordings, if we look for a low voltage fast discharge and closely correlate the onset of clinical manifestations with electrical changes, localization is much more feasible than expected. Clearly, as the seizure proceeds, the speed of diffusion and bilateral spreading of frontal ictal discharges makes the task much more difficult.

When the issue of ictal clinical semiology is faced, things become complicated. The frontal lobe has been basically differentiated into several areas, each assumed to be homogeneous as to ictal clinical symptomatology and anatomo-neurophysiological features. Unfortunately, authors differ about the classification of functional areas, although the great majority of them would agree about the following (Lüders, 1996; Munari et al., 1995; Munari et al., 1996a; Tharp, 1972; Van Buren et al., 1961; Wieser & Hajek, 1995):

- orbitary lobe;
- intermediate mesial frontal cortex;
- supplementary motor area;
- cingulate gyrus;
- frontal pole;
- dorso-lateral cortex;
- motor or rolandic cortex.

The authors assign different ictal signs and symptoms (Figs. 2–7) to each region, albeit with some overlapping between them.

Thus, for instance, oculocephalic deviation could be related to involvement of the supplementary motor area or the frontal dorso-lateral cortex or the intermediate mesial cortex as well.

ORBITARY LOBE

- autonomic
- gestural automatisms
- "timic" modifications
- hunger and thirst
- olfactory hallucinations
- enuresis
- bradycardia
- motor signs
- no manifestations

Fig. 2.

Chapter 13 Symptoms differentiating 'temporal' and 'frontal' complex partial seizures

---

INTERMEDIATE MESIAL COR

- loss of contact
- speech arrest
- gestural automatisms
- oculocephalic deviation
- autonomic
- tonic
- secondary generalization

Fig. 3.

SUPPLEMENTARY MOTOR AREA

- vocalization
- postural manifestation (often asymmetric)
- bimanual and "bipedal" activities
- trunk anteflexion
- vocal and respiratory modification
- contralateral head and eyes deviation
- often without loss of contact
- oral activity

Fig. 4.

CINGULATE GYRUS

- awakening
- "integrated" movements
- buccal movements
- bipedal movements
- hand ->mouth movement
- "thymic" alterations
- autonomic
- visual hallucinations
- incomplete loss of contact
- archaic complex motor behaviour

Fig. 5.

FRONTOPOLAR CORTEX

- "pseudoabsences"

- motor negative

- secondary generalization

Fig. 6.

DORSO-LATERAL CORTEX

- staring

- contralateral head and eyes deviation

- gestural automatisms

Fig. 7.

Therefore, only the retrieval of the precise timing sequence of onset of symptoms related to ictal electrical changes allows the identification of the true cortical area responsible for the seizure.

Subjective disturbances

We tried to classify the different subjective manifestations according to the most likely presentation in temporal seizures compared to frontal lobe seizures (Fig. 8).

It is widely, albeit wrongly, held that in frontal seizures subjective disturbances are rare or even absent. In fact, they occur very often but most of the time they are reported only after they have finished, unlike temporal seizures in which the patient has the time and the opportunity to report them while still experiencing them.

Feelings of epigastric discomfort, usually attributed to discharges in the temporal lobe, are well represented in frontal seizures also. However, it is true that ascending epigastric feelings (to the throat or the face) are in fact present in the great majority of cases in temporal seizures.

Even olfactory hallucinations (once associated to so-called 'uncinate seizures'), considered typical of temporal, and especially mesial, seizures, nowadays are recognized as pertaining also

---
ICTAL MANIFESTATIONS

Subjective Sensations

Mostly Temporal	Both	Mostly Frontal
Rising epigastric	Epigastric	
	Gustatory	Forced thinking
Psychic (experiential, illusions of comparison)	Visual	
	Olfactory	
	Autonomic	
Auditory	Cephalic	
	Fear, anxiety	
	Vertiginous	Somatosensory
	"Sexual seizures"	

Fig. 8.

Chapter 13 Symptoms differentiating 'temporal' and 'frontal' complex partial seizures

```
                    ICTAL MANIFESTATIONS

                  Neurovegetative modifications

     Mostly Temporal        Both              Mostly Frontal

                        Tachycardia
                                Bradycardia

                        Respiratory modif.
                        Flushing
                        Mydriasis
                        Visceral
                                         Enuresis
                                         Salivation
```

Fig. 9.

to frontal lobe seizures (particularly those originating in the orbitary lobe) (Bancaud & Talairach, 1991).

Surely we can ascribe psychic manifestations of *déjà vu*, *déjà vécu*, and dreamy state to the temporal lobe, while auditory changes (illusions and hallucinations) are related to discharges involving the first temporal gyrus (Bancaud & Talairach, 1991). On the other hand, we can take forced thinking and somatosensory disturbances as typical of the frontal lobe, though keeping in mind that bilateral or even unilateral paresthetic manifestations, often limited to the upper limbs (particularly shivering and piloerection) may be part of seizures originating in the mesial and anterior temporal lobe.

As far as neurovegetative manifestations are concerned (Fig. 9), almost all pertain to both lobes except salivation and per-ictal enuresis, which are specific of frontal seizures. Among cardiac changes, tachycardia is slightly prevalent in temporal lobe seizures, bradycardia in frontal (especially basal) seizures.

Automatisms

The significance of automatisms and their possible localization, as well as their possible occurrence concomitantly with loss of contact, are still matter of a great debate (Ebner *et al.*, 1995;

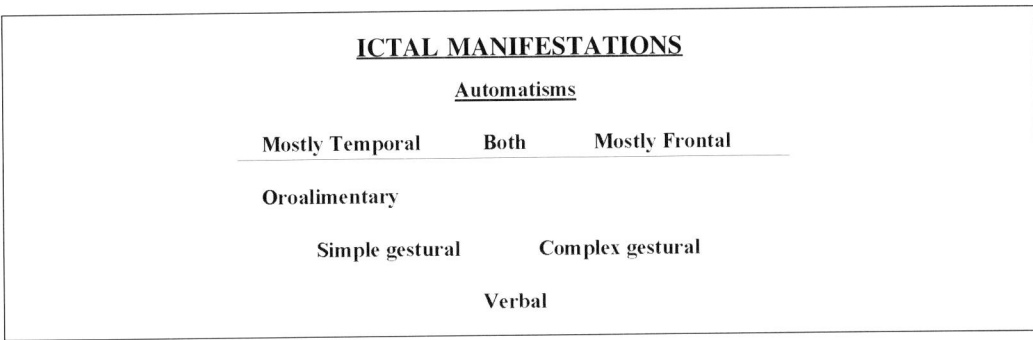

Fig. 10.

```
                        ICTAL MANIFESTATIONS

                          Motor Manifestations

        Mostly Temporal         Both              Mostly Frontal

                                                  Tonic
                                                  Clonic
                                                  Dystonic
                                                  "Negative"
                                Postural
                                Oculocephal
                                                  Rotatory
                                                  Falling

                                Second. General.
```

Fig. 11.

Munari *et al.*, 1980; Munari *et al.*, 1996b). Four types of automatisms have been basically identified: oroalimentary, verbal, simple gestural and complex gestural (Fig. 10). Oroalimentary automatisms (chewing and, less, swallowing) are considered reliable signs of temporal lobe seizures, while the other three types may be present in both lobe seizures. Simple gestural automatisms are commonly considered typical of temporal seizures, while complex ones, which are often forcible and fast and can involve all four limbs, are attributed to frontal seizures.

Motor manifestations

Tonic (in the sense of hypertonic) and clonic changes, which when localized to the limbs can lateralize the ictal discharge, pertain to the primary motor cortex (Fig. 11). On the contrary, when the above changes involve the face, lateralization cannot be ascertained because of the bilateral projection of the motor opercular fibres.

As to dystonic manifestations, they are almost exclusively attributed to frontal seizures, as well as falls, even if the latter are still incompletely understood (modality, type of muscle change, body parts involved, type of associated discharge), due mainly to the limited number of recordings. Motor phenomena such as 'rotatory' seizures and 'negative' manifestations, particularly negative myoclonus, still deserve further investigations.

Secondary generalization is frequent in frontal seizures, present but rare in temporal lobe seizures.

Concluding remarks

Given the fact that syndromes related to frontal lobe seizures are still ill-defined and insufficiently characterized (particularly if compared to what we believe we know about temporal lobe seizures), it appears exceedingly difficult to identify the symptoms differentiating these cortical regions (Lüders, 1996; Munari *et al.*, 1995; Munari *et al.*, 1996a; Tharp, 1972; Van Buren *et al.*, 1961; Wieser & Hajek, 1995).

So far, the clue to a correct localizing diagnosis of the cortical areas responsible for the ictal discharges is still the anatomo-electroclinical correlation, which when correctly performed leads to identification of the epileptogenic zone. The information can sometimes be obtained even without resorting to invasive procedures (i.e. intracerebral electrodes).

The first problem concerning the so called 'complex partial seizures' is the assessment of the patient's consciousness, especially when it is not examined during the ictal episode. In some cases even a careful per-ictal questioning does not allow easy assessment of whether consciousness is fully preserved; then, when it is not possible to interact with the patient we prefer to speak of loss of contact. Certainly, the loss of contact depends on the type of ictal discharge, its extent, its spreading and duration, but not on its site of origin (Munari et al., 1980). Therefore, in temporal lobe seizures, oroalimentary and simple gestural automatisms may be concomitantly present without loss of contact (Ebner et al., 1995), while frontal lobe seizures may be characterized by bilateral motor manifestations without loss of contact.

Although no specific symptoms or signs can be taken as unquestionably pointing to one lobe or the other, we can assume that auditory hallucinations and illusions as well as psychic manifestations (*déjà vu* and dreamy state) pertain to the temporal lobe in addition to oroalimentary automatisms (Bancaud & Talairach, 1991). On the other hand, forced thinking, salivation, per-ictal enuresis and motor changes (hypertonic, clonic) are typical of the frontal lobe.

Beyond these main statements, all the other manifestations, both subjective and objective, do not have a reliable localizing value, unless they are viewed in the perspective of a precise timing sequence of onset in the spontaneous seizures of the individual patient.

Only the careful study of any possible timing sequence of the clinical signs, its correlation with concomitant electrical changes and its relationship with possible anatomical abnormalities can yield a better knowledge and localization of clinical manifestations related to cortical areas which are often still incompletely understood as to their specific anatomo-physiological functions.

References

Ajmone Marsan, C. & Goldhammer, L. (1973): Clinical ictal patterns and electrographic data in cases of partial seizures of frontal-central-parietal origin. In: *Epilepsy: its phenomena in man*, ed. M.A.B. Brazier, pp. 235–258. New York: Academic Press.

Bancaud, J. & Talairach, J. (1991): Séméiologie clinique des crises du lobe temporal (méthodologie et investigations SEEG de 233 malades). In: *Crises épileptiques et épilepsies du lobe temporal*, vol. II, pp. 5–111. Documentation Médicale Labaz.

Bancaud, J. & Talairach, J. (1992): Clinical semiology of frontal lobe seizures. In: *Frontal lobe seizures and epilepsies. Advances in Neurology*, eds. P. Chauvel, A.V. Delgado-Escueta et al., vol. 57, pp. 3–58. New York: Raven Press.

Chauvel, P., Klieman, F., Vignal, J.P., Chodkiewicz, J.P., Talairach, J. & Bancaud, J. (1995): The clinical signs and symptoms of frontal lobe seizures: phenomenology and classification. In: *Epilepsy and the functional anatomy of the frontal lobe*, eds. H.H. Jasper, S. Riggio, P. Goldman-Rakic, pp. 115–126. New York: Raven Press.

Commission on Classification and Terminology of the International League Against Epilepsy (1989): Proposal for revised classification of epilepsies and epileptic syndromes. *Epilepsia* **30**, 389–399.

Ebner, A., Dinner, D.S., Noachtar, S. & Lüders, H. (1995): Automatisms with preserved responsiveness: a lateralizing sign in psychomotor seizures. *Neurology* **45**, 61–64.

Geier, S., Bancaud, J., Talairach, J., Bonis, A., Szikla, G. & Enjelvin, M. (1977): The seizures of frontal lobe epilepsy: a study of clinical manifestations. *Neurology* **27**, 951–958.

Kramer, U., Riviello, J.J. Jr, Carmant, L., Black, P.McL., Madsen, J. & Holmes, G.L. (1997): Clinical characteristics of complex partial seizures: a temporal versus a frontal lobe onset. *Seizure* **6,** 57–61.

Laskowitz, D.T., Sperling, M.R., French, J.A. & O'Connor, M.J. (1995): The syndrome of frontal lobe epilepsy: characteristics and surgical management. *Neurology* **45,** 780–787.

Lüders, H.O. (1996): The supplementary sensorimotor area: an overview. In: *Supplementary sensorimotor area. Advances in Neurology*, vol. 70, ed. H.O. Lüders, pp. 1–16. Philadelphia: Lippincott-Raven.

Munari, C., Bancaud, J., Bonis, A., Stoffels, C., Szikla, G. & Talairach, J. (1980): Impairment of consciousness in temporal lobe seizures: a stereo-electro-encephalographic study. *Advances in Epileptology, XIth Epilepsy International Symposium*, eds. R. Canger, F. Angeleri, J.K. Penry, pp. 111–115. New York: Raven Press.

Munari, C., Stoffels, C. Bossi, L., Bonis, A., Talairach, J. & Bancaud, J. (1981): Automatic activities during frontal and temporal lobe seizures: are they the same? *Advances in Epileptology, XIIIth Epilepsy International Symposium*, eds. M. Dam, L. Gram, J.K. Penry, pp. 287–291. New York: Raven Press.

Munari, C., Hoffmann, D., Francione, S., Kahane, P., Tassi, L., Lo Russo, G. & Benabid, A.L. (1994): Stereo-electroencephalography methodology: advantages and limits. *Acta Neurol. Scand.* **89** (Suppl. 152), 56–67.

Munari, C., Tassi, L., Di Leo, M., Kahane, P., Hoffmann, D., Francione, S. & Quarato, P.P. (1995): Video-Stereo-Electroencephalographic investigation of orbitofrontal cortex: ictal electroclinical patterns. In: *Epilepsy and the functional anatomy of the frontal lobe*, eds. H.H. Jasper, S. Riggio, P. Goldman-Rakic, pp. 273–296. New York: Raven Press.

Munari, C., Quarato, P.P., Di Leo, M., Hoffmann, D., Kahane, P., Tassi, L. & Francione, S. (1996a): Surgical strategies for patients with supplementary motor area epilepsy: the Grenoble experience. In: *Supplementary sensorimotor area, Advances in Neurology*, Vol. 70, ed. H.O. Lüders, pp. 379–404. Philadelphia: Lippincott-Raven.

Munari, C., Cardinale, F., Tassi, L., Mai, R., Colombo, N., Bottini, G., Lo Russo, G. & Francione, S. (1996b): Le epilessie temporali curabili chirugicamente. *Chirurgia Italiana* **48** (6), 1–64.

Quesney, L.P. (1992): Extratemporal epilepsy: clinical presentation preoperative EEG localization and surgical outcome. *Acta Neurol. Scand.* **140,** 81–94.

Quesney, L.P., Cendes, F., Olivier, A., Dubeau, F. & Andermann, F. (1995): Intracranial electroencephalographic investigation in frontal lobe epilepsy. In: *Epilepsy and the functional anatomy of the frontal lobe*, eds. H.H. Jasper, S. Riggio, P. Goldman-Rakic, pp. 243–260. New York: Raven Press.

Rasmussen, T. (1983): Characteristics of a pure culture of frontal lobe epilepsy. *Epilepsia* **24,** 482–493.

Swartz, B.E., Walsh, G.O., Delgado-Escueta, A.V. & Zolo, P. (1991): Surface ictal electroencephalographic patterns in frontal vs temporal lobe epilepsy. *Can. J. Neurol. Sci.* **18,** 649–662.

Tharp, B.R. (1972): Orbital frontal seizures. A unique electroencephalographic and clinical syndrome. *Epilepsia* **13,** 627–642.

Van Buren, J.M., Bucknam, C.A. & Pritchard, W.L. (1961). Autonomic representation in the human orbitotemporal cortex. *Neurology* **11** (2), 214–224.

Wieser, A.G. & Hajek, M. (1995): Frontal lobe epilepsy: compartmentalization, presurgical evaluation and operative results. In: *Epilepsy and the functional anatomy of the frontal lobe*, eds. H.H. Jasper, S. Riggio, P. Goldman-Rakic, pp. 297–320. New York: Raven Press.

Williamson, P.D., Spencer, D.D., Spencer, S.S., Novelly, R.A. & Mattson, R.H. (1985): Complex partial seizures of frontal lobe origin. *Ann. Neurol.* **18,** 497–504.

Williamson, P.D. & Spencer, S.S. (1986): Clinical and EEG features of complex partial seizures of extratemporal origin. *Epilepsia* **27** (Suppl. 2), S46–S63.

Chapter 14

Limbic seizures in children

Christian E. Elger and Guillén Fernández

Department of Epileptology, University of Bonn, Sigmund-Freud-Str. 25, 53105 Bonn, Germany

Summary

Since in the developing nervous system neuronal connections are still in development or even changing, it is not unexpected that seizure semiology in young children differs from the one in older children and adults. It is a well known fact that infantile spasms occur in young children, whereas seizure activity in older children shows phenomena also found in adults.

Already in children suffering from infantile spasms, all kinds of cerebral lesions with different locations are found. Within these groups, small children show infantile spasm-like phenomena during a seizure which is at least supposed to start temporally in the limbic system.

Within the age groups of 1.5 to 6 years, with increasing age the children show arousal reactions like eye opening, body jerking and sitting-up followed by versive movements and/or even tonic–clonic movements of the limbs. In children beyond the age of 6, it is frequently reported that these reactions are often combined with psycho-motor arrest; in some cases a fearful expression can be noticed and some children already point out that they feel a discomfort in the epigastrium. In both age groups single elements like oroalimentory gestural automatisms could be observed; however, in older children they prevailed on the seizure symptomatology.

More complex gestures and automatisms like clapping hands, or beating hands on a blanket, or card shuffling movements were only observed in children over the age of 12. Also their motor phenomena never included tonic or clonic movements asymmetrically, whereas younger children showed a preferential activity on one side. Lateralized signs in all age groups were unilateral clonic movements, which pointed to the contralateral side. Besides this, a reliable finding was a unilateral tonic posturing, which was found predominantly contralateral to the epileptogenic focus. However, ipsilateral tonic movements also occurred. Versive movements had no lateralizing aspects.

As a whole, the phenomena during seizures originating within the limbic system of the temporal lobe in children are unspecific in very young children, and become more and more specific with ongoing age, mimicking the adult phenomena beyond the age of 8.

Complex partial seizures (CPS) of temporal lobe origin in adult patients are well defined and their semiological characteristics are considered important for the determination of the seizure onset zone in patients being evaluated for epilepsy surgery (Bleasel *et al.*, 1997; Gil-Nagel & Risinger, 1997; Fried *et al.*, 1995; Salanova *et al.*, 1999). In children, however, specific clinical features of temporal lobe seizures are not well defined yet, although the number of children referred to epilepsy surgery centres is increasing. Only a few studies analysing seizure features in children have specifically investigated seizures originated within the (medial) temporal lobe. Jayakar & Duchowny (1990) analysed 126 seizures in 26 children aged 12 years or less and reported age-characteristic seizure features: while initial motor phenomena were more common in infants, staring was more common in school-age children. Moreover, temporal lobe seizures tended to be more complex in older children. Wyllie et al. (1993) evaluated 14 children aged 16 months to 12 years who were included in that study after becoming seizure free following temporal lobectomy. They concluded that the symptomatology of temporal lobe seizures in children is similar to that of older patients, except that automatisms tended to be less complex in younger children.

To clarify this topic further, we assessed 83 temporal lobe seizures of 29 children using video and synchronous EEG recordings (Brockhaus & Elger, 1995). Children were selected after they became seizure free following temporal lobe surgery and they were assigned to three groups: (1) preschoolers (age 1.5–6 years), (2) primary school children (age 7–12 years), and (3) adolescents (age 13–16 years). The most frequent initial seizure symptoms in preschool children were a gestural reaction, looking like an arousal reaction (eye opening, body jerking, sitting up), versive movements, and other motor phenomena such as tonic or clonic movements of the limbs. In older children (groups 2 & 3) an arrest reaction was the most frequent initial seizure symptom, hence the disruption of temporal function results in a decrease of behavioural activity like in older patients.

The most frequent behaviours occurring during the course of the seizures in preschoolers were simple motor phenomena and automatisms followed by versive movements, hypermotor activity, and dystonic posturing. The simple motor phenomena were primarily symmetric tonic or clonic movements of the limbs as well as atonic movements like head nodding similar to phenomena seen in infantile spasms. In line with other studies (Acharya et al., 1997), temporal lobe seizures of the youngest children (younger than age 4) were very similar to seizures in children with infantile spasms. They exhibited phenomena like brief head nods and symmetric elevations of the upper limbs. Preschool children exhibited also hypermotor movements and postures similar to behaviours well known from frontal lobe seizures in older patients. Rather simple automatisms such as oroalimentary or gestural ones were frequent in preschool children (~80 per cent) and did not differ in their frequency from those of older children. However, complex automatisms, like clapping hands, beating hands on the blanket, or card shuffling were seen only in children aged eight or older. While preschoolers showed predominantly generalized or bilateral ictal EEG or ECoG activity, older children tended to show more focal seizure onset activity.

Summarizing these findings: (1) temporal lobe seizures in children aged six or older are similar to the ones in grown-up patients, (2) ictal automatisms become more complex with increasing age, and (3) bilateral simple motor phenomena and rather generalized EEG activity in temporal lobe seizures are not uncommon in very young children.

Our clinical and electroencephalographic findings and studies revealed similar frequencies of seizure-free outcome after epilepsy surgery for infants, children, adolescents and adults, and suggest that children should be considered for surgical evaluation at whatever age they manifest severe, intractable, disabling localization-related epilepsy even if ictal symptomatology or EEG does not indicate a focal seizure onset (Wyllie et al., 1998; Gilliam et al., 1997).

References

Acharya, J.N., Wyllie, E., Lüders, H.O., Kotagal, P., Lancman, M. & Coelho, M. (1997): Seizure symptomatology in infants with localization-related epilepsy. *Neurology* **48,** 189–196.

Bleasel, A., Kotagal, P., Kankirawatana, P. & Rybicki, L. (1997): Lateralizing value and semiology of ictal limb posturing and version in temporal lobe and extratemporal epilepsy. *Epilepsia* **38,** 168–174.

Brockhaus, A. & Elger, C.E. (1995): Complex partial seizures of temporal lobe origin in children of different age groups. *Epilepsia* **36,** 1173–1181.

Fried, I., Spencer, D.D. & Spencer, S.S. (1995): The anatomy of epileptic auras: focal pathology and surgical outcome. *J. Neurosurg.* **83,** 60–66.

Gilliam, F., Wyllie, E., Kashden, J., Faught, E., Kotagal, P., Bebin, M., Wise, M., Comair, Y., Morawetz, R. & Kuzniecky, R. (1997): Epilepsy surgery outcome: comprehensive assessment in children. *Neurology* **48,** 1368–1374.

Gil-Nagel, A. & Risinger, M.W. (1997): Ictal semiology in hippocampal versus extrahippocampal temporal lobe epilepsy. *Brain* **120,** 183–192.

Jayakar, P. & Duchowny, M.S. (1990): Complex partial seizures of temporal lobe origin in early childhood. *J. Epilepsy* **3,** 41–45.

Salanova, V., Markand, O. & Worth, R. (1999): Longitudinal follow-up in 145 patients with medically refractory temporal lobe epilepsy treated surgically between 1984 and 1995. *Epilepsia* **40,** 1417–1423.

Wyllie, E. (1998): Surgical treatment of epilepsy in children. *Pediatr. Neurol.* **19,** 179–188.

Wyllie, E., Chee, M., Granstrom, M.L., DelGiudice, E., Estes, M., Comair, Y., Pizzi, M., Kotagal, P., Bourgeois, B. & Lüders, H. (1993): Temporal lobe epilepsy in early childhood. *Epilepsia* **34,** 859–868.

Wyllie, E., Comair, Y.G., Kotagal, P., Bulacio, J., Bingaman, W. & Ruggieri, P. (1998): Seizure outcome after epilepsy surgery in children and adolescents. *Ann. Neurol.* **44,** 740–748.

Chapter 15

Temporal lobe epilepsy in childhood

Christa Pachatz, Raffaella Cusmai and Federico Vigevano

Division of Neurology, Bambino Gesù Children's Hospital, Piazza Sant'Onofrio 4, 00165 Rome, Italy

Summary

The clinical features of childhood temporal lobe seizures are unhomogeneous and often hardly recognizable, especially in the very young age group, in contrast to the well defined seizures in the syndrome of temporal lobe epilepsy (TLE) in adults. We describe the electroclinical features of 29 children, 12 girls and 17 boys, who presented complex partial seizures of temporal lobe origin as their main or only seizure type, considering family history, antecedents of febrile convulsions, psychomotor development, seizure semiology, MRI and EEG features, responsiveness to antiepileptic drug treatment. We identified three aetiology-based subgroups of TLE: the first group included five children with temporal lobe tumours; the second group had 12 patients with temporal lesions, hippocampal sclerosis in nine and other non-progressive malformations in three patients; the third group included 12 children with cryptogenic TLE. An aetiology-based subdivision of patients with TLE permits identification of different clinical patterns regarding both seizure type and epilepsy evolution and can be useful in determining prognosis and outcome.

Introduction

Complex partial seizures are one of the most common seizure types encountered in children and adults (Holmes, 1986; Wyllie *et al.*, 1989). The structures involved in most cases are the limbic formation and areas of the neocortex, mostly located within the temporal lobe. The semiology of complex partial seizures in adults is homogeneous and well described, whereas the clinical features in children and infants are controversial and often hardly recognizable (Brockhaus & Elger, 1995; Bourgeois, 1998) due to difficulty in assessing impairment of consciousness, especially in the very young age group. Most clinical studies of temporal lobe epilepsy (TLE) derive from patients with refractory seizures and brain lesions undergoing surgical treatment. The syndrome of mesial temporal lobe epilepsy is a well described syndrome (Wieser *et al.*, 1993; Engel *et al.*, 1997); less information is available on cryptogenic TLE (Engel, 1996), which is still a clinical challenge and requires further research.

Our study is an approach to a classification of TLE in childhood based on aetiology and to the determination of prognostic features and outcome.

Patients and methods

We selected retrospectively 29 children, 12 girls and 17 boys, currently aged 2 years 10 months to 18 years 8 months, with a diagnosis of temporal lobe epilepsy, attending the Division of Neurology, Bambino Gesù Children's Hospital in Rome, Italy, between the years 1983 and 1999. These patients presented complex partial seizures of temporal lobe origin as their only or main seizure type, with onset between 6 months and 12 years 8 months. Complex partial seizures were defined as seizures in which the predominant symptomatology consisted of an alteration of consciousness defined as unresponsiveness or decreased responsiveness that is not caused by motor alterations, with or without automatisms. The temporal lobe involvement was defined by electroencephalographic findings, confirmed in the symptomatic cases by MR imaging.

The study considered the family history, antecedents of febrile convulsions, psychomotor development, seizure semiology, MRI features, responsiveness to AED treatment, interictal EEG. Ictal EEG was obtained in 12 children. Follow-up continued at least 3 years; one patient was lost after 8 years of follow-up.

We identified three groups according to aetiology. The first group included five children with temporal lobe tumours; in the second group, 12 patients had temporal lobe lesions, nine of them had hippocampal sclerosis, and the other three patients had different lesions such as cortical dysplasia, arachnoid cyst and a complex cortical lesion consisting of an association of dysembryoplastic neuroepithelial tumour (DNT), cortical malformation and harmartoma. The third and last group included 12 children who showed a normal MRI and were classified as cryptogenic TLE.

Results

First group: temporal lobe tumours

The group included five boys with temporal lobe tumours: one patient had grade I astrocytoma in the left temporal lobe; two had grade II astrocytoma, one in the left, the other in the right temporal lobe; one had grade III astrocytoma in the right and one ganglioma in the left temporal lobe. Two patients had family history of epilepsy or febrile seizures; nobody presented antecedent febrile convulsions and all children showed normal psychomotor development. Ages at seizure onset were between 2 months and 16 months. All had drug resistant, severe epilepsy; four patients had several seizures a day; one patient presented a monthly recurrence of seizures.

The brief stereotyped seizures consisted of motor arrest and staring as the main and often only manifestation, accompanied by autonomic symptoms, such as slight cyanosis of the lips in four cases, pallor in two and perspiring combined with shudder-like motor manifestations in one case. Oroalimentary automatisms, present in two patients at the beginning of epilepsy, were not very evident. In two other patients they occurred later in the course of the epilepsy, with a distance of at least 2 months from the first seizure. One patient presented unilateral blinking ipsilateral to the lesion. All children showed signs of reaction when called by persons present during the seizures.

Interictal EEG showed unilateral temporal or temporal-frontal epileptiform or slow abnormalities congruent to the lesion side in four patients, one patient had normal interictal EEG. Ictal EEG showed rapid activity, then theta and delta activity of increasing amplitude involving unilateral temporal-frontal region, congruent to the lesion side detected by MRI; the discharge became bilateral only in patients with a prolonged history of epilepsy before surgical treatment.

In three patients, MR imaging failed to detect the tumour at the first examination, performed at seizure onset. In these cases, a second examination after an interval of 4 months to 3 years permitted diagnosis.

Surgical treatment was performed after a course of 7 months to 3.3 years of epilepsy. All children clearly improved with surgery, but just one patient became seizure free, four continued to have sporadic or monthly seizures. (See Tables 1 and 2 for semiological and EEG features.)

Table 1. Semiological features

	Tumours $n = 5$	Lesional TLE $n = 12$	Cryptogenic TLE $n = 12$
Aura			
epigastric sensation	0	1	1
abdominal pain	0	5	6
olfactory symptoms	0	0	2
fear of strangeness	0	3	3
déjà-vu	0	0	1
visual symptoms	0	1	1
Semiological features	Psychomotor arrest, staring, impairment of consciousness with unresponsiveness or partial responsiveness		
oroalimentary automatisms	4	8	9
gestural automatisms	0	2	4
dysphasia	0	1	4
sudden fall	0	1	0
Autonomic signs and symptoms			
cyanosis	4	4	4
pallor and/or sweating	3	2	8
nausea and vomit	0	2	2
Contralateral motor manifestation	0	5	2
Ipsilateral eyelid blinking	1	1	0
Head and eye deviation	0	5	0
Frequent isolated auras	0	4	6
Duration < 1 min	4	6	8
> 1min	1	6	4
Postictal symptoms			
somnolence	3	4	7
sleep	2	2	3
headache	0	0	2
confusion	0	0	1
Secondary generalization			
sporadic or isolated	0	5	4
Status epilepticus (except febrile seizures)	0	3	0

Table 2. EEG features

	Tumours $n = 5$	Lesional TLE $n = 12$	Cryptogenic TLE $n = 12$
Interictal EEG			
unilateral involvement of temporal / temporal-frontal region			
– sharp waves and/or spikes	3	9	5
– slow waves	1	0	5
bilateral			1
– sharp waves and/or spikes	0	2	0
– slow waves	0	1	1
Normal	1	0	
Ictal EEG ($n = 12$)			
– recruiting then rhythmic theta-delta activity involving temporal/temporal-frontal region unilateral	5	1	2
– recruiting fast rhythm followed by hemispheric delta activity	0	2	1
– generalization	0	1	0

Second group: lesional temporal lobe epilepsy

We studied twelve patients with TLE due to a non progressive lesion, eight girls and four boys.

The most characteristic neuroradiological substrate was hippocampal sclerosis (HS), revealed in nine patients by repeated MR images, which showed unilateral hippocampal atrophy and/or an increase in hippocampal T2 signal intensity. In this subgroup, familial antecedents for epilepsy were present in two cases and for febrile convulsions also in two cases. Five of nine patients with hippocampal sclerosis had antecedent febrile convulsions; the febrile seizures consisted of unilateral convulsions in two cases and manifested as status epilepticus in three patients. The afebrile fits occurred after a mean interval of 3.2 years. Psychomotor development was normal in all children except one, who had learning difficulties. Age at epilepsy onset was 6 months to 12 years. Outcome was favourable in three patients, currently aged 17 years 10 months, 17 years 2 months and 11 years 6 months, who became seizure free after a mean epilepsy duration of 9.7 years. Follow-up after seizure disappearance was 6 years 7 months, 2 years 6 months and 6 years respectively. Two patients showed sporadic seizure recurrence. Four patients suffered from intractable severe and frequent seizures and were selected for neurosurgical treatment after a mean duration of epilepsy of 6.6 years.

Other pathologies in the lesional group of TLE included a complex cerebral lesion consisting of DNT, cortical malformation and harmartoma, as a histological finding after left temporal lesionectomy and corticectomy in a girl who is currently 9 years old. This patient, with seizure onset at 6 years 9 months, normal psychomotor development and severe intractable seizures with a frequency of several seizures a day, is now seizure-free after surgical treatment. Lastly, MR imaging revealed pathologies such as arachnoid cyst and dysplastic lesion: in the first case the patient benefited from AED treatment and became seizure free after a duration of epilepsy of 1 year 8 months, the latter patient with intractable frequent seizures was lost in the follow-up.

In this group with lesional temporal lobe epilepsy, seizures lasted less than 1 min in 50 per cent of cases. The other half of the patients showed a seizure duration of up to 3 min. In 75 per cent of the patients, seizures were preceded by auras, described as abdominal pain or undefined epigastric sensation, fear or feeling of strangeness. One patient had visual auras characterized by unformed luminous hallucinations in the visual hemicampus contralateral to the lesion; four patients had frequent and isolated auras lasting some seconds as an additional finding. Psychomotor arrest and vacant stare were accompanied by oroalimentary automatisms, such as swallowing and chewing or gestural automatisms. Sudden falling down occurred in one patient; dysphasia was reported in another. Autonomic symptoms such as cyanosis, pallor or nausea were frequent findings; ictal vomiting occurred in two patients. Tonic or dystonic posturing of the upper limb contralateral to the lesion side, present in five patients, was a reliable lateralizing sign. Head and eye deviation had no lateralizing significance. Sporadic or isolated secondary generalization occurred in five patients. Postictal symptoms consisted mostly of somnolence; deep sleep was an occasional finding.

Interictal EEG showed unilateral involvement of the temporal-frontal region congruent to the lesion side in 75 per cent of the patients, consisting of sharp waves and/or spikes; the other patients showed bilateral epileptiform or slow abnormalities. Ictal EEG in four patients was characterized by rhythmic theta-delta activity in the temporal-frontal region of the lesional side. (See Tables 1 and 2 for semiological and EEG features.)

Third group: cryptogenic temporal lobe epilepsy

This group, consisting of four girls and eight boys, showed familial antecedents for epilepsy in two cases, for epilepsy and febrile seizures in one and only for febrile seizures in another case. Two children had a single simple febrile seizure respectively 2 years 3 months and 7 years 3 months prior to the onset of afebrile fits. All children had normal psychomotor development, and normal cerebral MR images. One patient had a concomitant history of migraine, one boy had behavioural disturbances.

The patients showed two peaks concerning age at afebrile seizure onset: in nine patients age at onset was between 12 months and 4 years, and in three patients between 8 years 1 month and 10 years 5 months.

Ictal semiology consisted of psychomotor arrest, staring and impairment of consciousness, preceded by auras in 10 of 12 patients, characterized by abdominal discomfort, fear or strangeness, olfactory symptoms; visual symptoms referred as macropsia were present in one and experiential symptoms such as *déjà-vu* in another patient; frequent isolated auras were reported by six patients. Automatisms were oroalimentary or gestural; dysphasic symptoms were reported in four patients. Autonomic symptoms occurred frequently and were characterized mainly by pallor or perspiring. A tonic posturing of the arm as lateralizing sign contralateral to a constant epileptic focus was found in only two patients; secondary generalization as sporadic events occurred in four patients. Seizures lasted less than 1 min in most cases, postictal symptoms consisted of somnolence, more rarely sleep, headache or confusion.

Interictal EEG showed unilateral frontal-temporal epileptiform or slow abnormalities and rarely bilateral slow abnormalities. One patient showed a normal interictal EEG; in this case temporal lobe involvement was detected by an ictal EEG. Ictal EEG was obtained in only three patients and showed unilateral rhythmic theta-delta activity in the frontal-temporal region.

In the group with earlier onset, a more favourable outcome under antiepileptic drug therapy could be established: of these nine patients, four became seizure free after a mean duration of epilepsy of 2 years 7 months. Three of them already discontinued the AED treatment, the other one is in a phase of slow tapering (follow-up after seizure disappearance was at least 3 years and maximal 13 years). The remaining five patients in this group continue to present seizures, three of them show just sporadic, very brief seizures. In the three children with late onset of epilepsy, seizures persisted despite antiepileptic drugs with sporadic to monthly recurrence. (See Tables 1 and 2 for semiological and EEG features.)

Discussion

In our series epilepsy in temporal lobe tumours manifested within the first 16 months of life. This age group posed most difficulties in recognizing and determining the nature of the seizures. Seizures were characterized predominantly by behavioural arrest and autonomic symptoms and all patients showed signs of reaction during the brief seizures, confirming the absence of complete loss of consciousness. Automatisms were minimal and inconstant. This data has been reported also by other authors (Wyllie et al., 1993). Subtle seizure semiology can mislead and prevent the diagnosis of epileptic seizures. Great care must be used in interpreting an MRI that may be apparently normal; in three out of five tumour patients, the first imaging was referred as normal. In all these cases, when MRI was analysed keeping in mind clinical data and EEG localization, the tumour lesion was always very evident already at first examination.

Patients with temporal lobe lesions differed from the group with temporal tumours by later age at seizure onset. In children with hippocampal sclerosis we found an association with previous febrile seizures in 55 per cent, mostly complicated, in contrast to the group with temporal tumours where antecedent febrile seizures were not present, and to the cryptogenic group with these antecedents in only 16 per cent. Harvey found an association between significant antecedents of TLE, including complicated febrile seizures, meningitis and hypoxic-ischaemic encephalopathies, and HS in 29 per cent (Harvey et al., 1997). Murakami revealed prolonged convulsions as presumed causes of HS in 63.2 per cent of his cohort (Murakami et al., 1996). Furthermore the occurrence of status epilepticus during the course of epilepsy was found in our series only in patients with HS. According to Harvey (Harvey et al., 1997), the electroclinical and neuroradiological features of the group with HS most closely resemble the syndrome of mesial temporal lobe epilepsy described by Wieser and other authors (Wieser et al., 1993; Engel et al., 1997). In our series of nine patients with HS, outcome was favourable in three patients, who became seizure-free after a mean duration of epilepsy of 9.7 years. These data on possible favourable outcome in patients with HS contrast with most studies (Zix et al., 1999) and need to be confirmed by further prospective studies.

In the group with cryptogenic TLE, in which no aetiology could be detected by history or neuroradiological findings, familial antecedents for epilepsy and/or febrile seizures were present in 33 per cent of cases. Harvey observed familial antecedents in 16 per cent of patients with cryptogenic TLE (Harvey et al., 1997). We found two peaks concerning afebrile seizure onset age; the group with an earlier onset showed more favorable outcome under AED treatment, suggesting benign evolution. To date, an idiopathic form has not been detected. According to Engel (Engel, 1996), future clinical and laboratory investigations concerning this cryptogenic syndrome should be conducted to identify aetiology and outcome and determine a possibly benign course of TLE.

Our clinical study leads to the following concepts:

> (1) The syndrome of temporal lobe epilepsy does exist also in early infancy, with seizure onset in the first months of life;
>
> (2) An aetiology-based subdivision of patients affected by TLE into three groups permits

identification of different clinical patterns regarding both seizure type and epilepsy evolution;

(3) Automatisms considered as main features of the temporal ictal semiology are absent in very young children with TLE and tend to appear later in the seizure history, misleading at times the diagnosis of epilepsy at early onset;

(4) Early onset of partial epilepsy is usually connected with unfavourable evolution; a contrast to this common data is the finding of more favourable outcome in early onset cryptogenic TLE in our cohort.

References

Bourgeois, B.F. (1998): Temporal lobe epilepsy in infants and children. *Brain Dev.* **20**, 135–141.

Brockhaus, A. & Elger, C.H. (1995): Complex partial seizures of temporal lobe origin in children of different age groups. *Epilepsia* **36**, 1173–1181.

Engel, J., Jr. (1996): Introduction to temporal lobe epilepsy. *Epilepsy Res.* **26**, 141–150.

Engel, J., Jr., Williamson, P.D. & Wieser, H.G. (1997): Mesial temporal lobe epilepsy. In: *Epilepsy: a comprehensive textbook*, eds. J. Engel, Jr. & J. Pedley, vol. 3, chapter X, p. 231. New York: Lippincott-Raven.

Harvey, A.S., Berkovic, S.F., Wrennall, J.A. & Hopkins, I.J. (1997): Temporal lobe epilepsy in childhood: clinical, EEG and neuroimaging findings and syndrome classification in a cohort with new-onset seizures. *Neurology* **49**, 960–968.

Holmes, G.L. (1986): Partial seizures in children. *Pediatrics* **77**, 725–731.

Murakami, N., Ohno, S., Oka, E. & Tanaka, A. (1996): Mesial temporal lobe epilepsy in childhood. *Epilepsia* **37** (Suppl. 3), 52–56.

Wieser, H.G., Engel, J.Jr., Williamson, P.D., Babb, T.L. & Gloor, P. (1993): Surgically remediable temporal lobe syndromes. In: *Surgical treatment of the epilepsies*, 2nd edn., ed. J. Engel Jr., pp. 49–63. New York: Raven Press.

Wyllie, E., Rothner, A.D. & Lueders, H. (1989): Partial seizures in children: clinical features, medical treatment, and surgical considerations. *Pediatric. Clin. N. Am.* **36**, 343–364.

Wyllie, E., Chee, M., Granstrom, M.L., Del Giudice, E., Estes, M., Comair, Y., Pizzi, M., Kotagal, P., Bourgeois, B. & Lüders, H. (1993): Temporal lobe epilepsy in early childhood. *Epilepsia* **34**, 859–868

Zix, C., Billard, C. & Motte, J. (1999): Epilepsy due to mesiotemporal sclerosis in children: 10 cases. *Arch. Pediatr.* **6**, 398–405.

Chapter 16

Aetiological role of febrile convulsive attacks in limbic epilepsy

Andrea Van Lierde and Laura Mira*

Istituto di Pediatria e Neonatologia dell'Università di Milano, via Commenda 9, 20122 Milan, Italy;
*Fondazione Pierfranco e Luisa Mariani, viale Bianca Maria 28, 20129 Milan, Italy

Summary

Febrile convulsions (FC) occur in 2–4 per cent of all children; their relationship to epilepsy has been the subject of a long-standing debate, especially because they form a heterogenous group within this definition. The vast majority of true febrile convulsions are brief, non focal and benign events (so called simple febrile convulsions) and it is generally thought that they do not cause brain injury. However, it is now accepted that FC represent a risk factor for later development of epilepsy.

When epilepsy develops after simple FC, it is usually generalized and probably genetically determined. On the other hand, complex FC are followed by epilepsy more often than simple FC, but in these cases partial epilepsy is observed.

It is still controversial whether partial epilepsy, and particularly temporal lobe epilepsy, follows FC and, if any association exists, what is the role of FC in the pathogenesis of mesial temporal sclerosis (the most common cause of temporal lobe epilepsy, pathologically characterized by neuronal loss and gliosis of areas CA1, CA3, CA4 and dentate gyrus of hippocampal formation).

Although no conclusion has been reached so far, an aetiologic role FC in the genesis of temporal lobe epilepsy appears likely. The significance of this role, if any, remains to be determined. Currently, available evidence does not justify systemic preventive treatment of FC, but certainly supports aggressive efforts to promptly interrupt convulsive activity in convulsions lasting more than a few minutes.

Introduction

The Consensus Development Panel on febrile convulsions (FC) defined febrile seizures as 'an event in infancy or childhood, usually occurring between 3 months and 5 years of age, associated with fever but without evidence of intracranial infection or other definable cause. Seizures with fever in children who have suffered a previous nonfebrile seizure are excluded' (Consensus Development Panel, 1980).

Febrile convulsions occur in 2–4 per cent of all children, with higher rates in selected populations (Stanhope *et al.*, 1972). Their relationship to epilepsy has been the subject of a long-standing debate, especially because, within this definition, they constitute a heterogenous group. The vast majority of true febrile convulsions (i.e. convulsions only in response to fever) are brief, non focal and benign events (so called simple febrile convulsions, SFC) and it is generally thought that they do not cause brain injury. However, it is now accepted that FC represent a risk factor for later development of epilepsy, that affects children with FC two to 10 times more frequently than controls (Maher & McLachlan, 1995; Van den Berg & Yerushalmy, 1969; Nelson & Ellenberg, 1976; Annegers *et al.*, 1979; Lee *et al.*, 1981).

When epilepsy develops after SFC, it is usually generalized and probably genetically determined (Berkovic & Sheffer, 1998). On the other hand, complex febrile convulsions (CFC) – defined as FC lasting longer than 15 min and/or with evidence of focal or lateralized convulsive activity and/or recurring within 24 h – and febrile status epilepticus (FSE) – defined as a single CFC, or a series of CFC without recovery between seizures, with a total duration exceeding 30 min – are followed by epilepsy more often than SFC, but in this case it consists of partial epilepsy (Annegers *et al.*, 1987).

It is still controversial whether partial epilepsy, particularly temporal lobe epilepsy (TLE), follows FC and, if any association exists, what is the role of FC in the pathogenesis of mesial temporal sclerosis (MTS), the most common cause of TLE (identified in 50–60 per cent of lobectomies for TLE), pathologically characterized by neuronal loss and gliosis of areas CA1, CA3, CA4 and dentate gyrus of hippocampal formation.

Several retrospective studies have found a history of FC, often prolonged (30 min) and severe, in 20–38 per cent of patients with TLE. In a retrospective study, Ounsted *et al.* (1966) found that in 32 of their 100 patients childhood temporal lobe epilepsy had followed prolonged febrile convulsions in infancy. Rocca *et al.* (1987), in a population-based, case-controlled study of patients with CPS, reported that 20 per cent of 82 patients with TLE had a history of FC compared to 2 per cent of 150 controls. In contrast, prospective cohort studies have shown that the proportion of partial seizures was no higher in FC patients that in the general population and this may even apply to patients with febrile status epilepticus. These conflicting results may be explained by the fact that TLE frequency increases only in children with prolonged FC, which are infrequent, whereas the usual, brief FC are followed by generalized seizures. When focal seizures follow prolonged FC, there is an excellent correlation between the lateralization of the FC and that of the subsequent epileptic foci. It has been proposed that prolonged CFC produce mesial temporal injury, but it is still unsettled whether the injury to the highly susceptible hippocampus is due to the seizure itself or to secondary systemic factors such as hypoxia or hypotension. A similar process has been reported in many animal models of limbic status epilepticus. Wallace (1976) found that 10 out of 49 patients with prolonged and lateralized febrile convulsions, followed up for more than 3 years, developed partial complex seizures. However, since the average latency between FC and TLE onset is greater (8–9 years), a longer follow up is required to determine the risk of developing TLE (Mathern *et al.*, 1995; French *et al.*, 1993).

A number of features related to FC have been proposed as risk factors for the development of epilepsy: seizure duration, focality, recurrence, early age, seizures occurring with low-grade fever. To the exclusion of all others, focality and long duration of CFC have been found to be significant risk factors, but it is not yet clear whether they are independent risk factors (Annegers *et al.*, 1987; Berg & Shinnar, 1996a). Berg & Shinnar (1996a) found a high association between them. According to Annegers *et al.* (1987) the occurrence of FC longer than 30 min, focal seizures and seizures recurring within 24 h increases the probability of developing CPS by the age of 25 and their effect is additive: 50 per cent of children with all the three features had CPS by the age of 25. In other studies, with a shorter follow up, the risk factors did not prove to be additive (Berg & Shinnar, 1996b).

It has been suggested that MTS may precede and actually be the cause of both CFC and later TLE (Davies *et al.*, 1996; Annegers *et al.*, 1987; Cendes *et al.*, 1993). This is consistent with clinical studies demonstrating that severity of hippocampal atrophy does not correlate either with duration of TLE or frequency of seizures (Davies *et al.*, 1996; Cendes *et al.*, 1993; Tronerry *et al.*, 1993) or with the occurrence of MTS in children presenting initially with intractable TLE.

MTS could be acquired before CFC as the result of prenatal or perinatal injury, meningitis, encephalitis or head trauma and be the cause both of CFC and later TLE. If this were the case, we should find a high incidence of preceding cerebral insults in the clinical history of patients with CFC. In fact, there is no convincing evidence either to accept or reject this hypothesis. MRI of infants with a history of hypoxic-ischaemic perinatal damage may later show MTS (Rutherford *et al.*, 1995), but in the few reported cases MTS was accompanied by additional MRI signs of the preceding injury. It is still unknown whether birth trauma can cause isolated MTS without any other MRI abnormality.

The recent findings of a dual pathology consisting of hippocampal sclerosis and an additional pathology in the temporal lobe, usually a developmental lesion like microdysgenesis, cortical dysplasia or a dysontogenetic tumour, have led to the hypothesis that a pre-existing subtle brain abnormality could predispose to FC which in turn may cause an additional, acute seizure-induced injury, later evolving into MTS. (Raymond *et al.*, 1994; Ho *et al.*, 1998; Gunay & Aysun, 1996).

It is also well possible that MTS is the result of the combined effects of multiple pathogenic mechanisms. Recent studies suggested that fever and convulsions interact to cause MTS and then TLE through excitatory amino-acid neurotransmitters and their receptors (Olney *et al.*, 1972; Meldrum & Garthwaite, 1990; Meldrum, 1991).

Imaging studies

Imaging studies have shown that the atrophy of the hippocampus (AH), characterized by decreased T1 and increased T2 signal and loss of internal structure, is a common finding in TLE cases and correlates well with the presence of MTS at surgery and pathological examination. The increased signal on T2-weighted sequences is probably the consequence of gliosis, replacing in part the loss of neurons.

Mesial temporal sclerosis or hippocampal sclerosis is the term used to designate gliosis and neuronal loss that particularly affect the CA1 and CA3–4 or Sommer's sectors of the Ammon's horn. Aside from being detected by MRI studies, it is possible to make volume measurements of the hippocampus (Jack *et al.*, 1990, 1992). Measurements of the intensity of T2 signal may allow detection of unilateral or bilateral involvement in patients with apparently normal MRI scans obtained by routine techniques.

Normally, both hippocampi are of equal volume; asymmetry of more than a few per cent is considered abnormal (Jack *et al.*, 1990). The lesions may be limited to one part of the hippocampal formation (Bertram *et al.*, 1990). They sometimes extend in a homogeneous or patchy manner to other parts of the temporal cortex, often predominating in the anterior segment of the first temporal gyrus (Cavanagh & Meyer, 1956), although they may involve the other temporal gyri and even structures outside the temporal lobe (insula, fronto-basal and opercular cortex, a lesion termed pararhinal sclerosis) (Degen, 1978).

Results are conflicting, but further evidence may be gained by MRI. Using T2 signal changes and hippocampal volume measurements it may be possible to differentiate acute seizure-induced brain damage after CFCs from chronic pre-existing injury (Tronerry *et al.*, 1993; Lewis, 1999). Evidence from cohort studies points to a relationship between duration and focality of CFCs and later CPSs.

MTS is unilateral in 80 per cent of cases.

Twenty to 43 per cent of patients with atrophy of the hippocampus have a history of severe convulsions before the age of 4, while FC are rare in patients with other lesions such as hamartomas or developmental tumours. While this evidence is suggestive for a role of FC, it does not explain why the majority of AH cases occur in patients without a history of febrile seizures, therefore suggesting that other factors may be involved. The association of AH with other lesions in the temporal lobe or elsewhere (dual pathology) also confirms heterogeneity within the AH group. Febrile convulsions in patients with both MTS and focal cortical dysgenesis (FCD) may represent the early manifestation of the high epileptogenicity of FCD.

Fernandez *et al.* (1998) report two families with frequent FC and several family members affected by subtle hippocampal dysgenesis, with or without previous FC. These data seem to support the hypothesis that the disturbance of neuronal migration facilitates FC (though, in this case, they were mostly SFC).

Pathological findings

Pathological findings also point to an important role of FC. The association of prolonged FC with MTS has been repeatedly confirmed on patients with medically intractable TLE, even though the incidence varied in different series (Gloor, 1991; Abou-Khalil *et al.*, 1993). The results of these studies suggest that MTS is more closely related to a history of prolonged FC rather than to the frequency or severity of other seizure types (Cendes *et al.*, 1993; Kuks *et al.*, 1993). However, the interpretation of MTS is far from straightforward.

Recent work indicates that MTS predominantly unilateral and localized to the anterior hippocampus, selectively affecting the H1 sector and the dentate gyrus, is the typical lesion following prolonged seizures and differs from more diffuse and often bilateral lesions (Davies *et al.*, 1996). It also differs from the mostly bilateral AH found in meningitis and in encephalitis. However, a detailed histological study is rarely available and even typical. Moreover, AH may not be associated with a history of FC.

Experimental studies

Experimental evidence shows that prolonged convulsive activity does produce neuronal lesions similar to those of AH. It has been demonstrated that induction of status epilepticus (SE) by pilocarpine in adult rats causes later development of seizures in association with neuronal loss in the hippocampus. The extent of pathological changes was directly proportional to the duration of SE. This did not apply to younger animals. Kainic acid-induced SE in rat pups was not followed by later seizures or morphological changes in the brain, suggesting a protective mechanism in very young animals (Okada *et al.*, 1984). On the contrary, rat pups with dysgenesis have been shown to be more susceptible to hyperthermia-induced seizures and hyperthermia-induced neuronal dropout (Germano *et al.*, 1998).

Conclusions

These data represent conclusive evidence of an association between FC, MTS and TLE, still the nature of this association is not necessarily causal and several alternative hypotheses must be taken into account:

(1) MTS may indeed be the consequence of prolonged FC;

(2) MTS and TLE may be due to a common underlying factor responsible for both the FC and subsequent TLE;

(3) A previous abnormality (e.g. dysplasias) may cause the FC (or be a factor of localization and severity) which, in turn, results in MTS.

At present we do not have any definite answer. However, it might be possible to determine whether AH develops following prolonged FC by repeated MRI studies, to demonstrate the initial absence of AH and its later development. Preliminary results in one such study showed normal-sized hippocampi in a small group of patients with status including febrile status (Bertram *et al.*, 1990; Tronerry *et al.*, 1993). In these cases, high T2 signal was detected in one hippocampus, especially in cases of febrile status, but late MR results are not available yet.

Although no conclusion has been reached so far, an aetiologic role of FC in the genesis of TLE appears likely. The significance of this role, if any, remains to be determined. Currently, available evidence does not justify systemic preventive treatment of FC, but certainly supports aggressive efforts to promptly interrupt convulsive activity in convulsions lasting more than a few minutes.

References

Abou-Khalil, B., Andermann, E., Andermann, F., Olivier, A. & Quesney, L.F. (1993): Temporal lobe epilepsy after prolonged febrile convulsions: excellent outcome after surgical treatment. *Epilepsia* **34**, 878–883.

Annegers, J.F., Hauser, W.A., Elveback, L.R. & Kurland, L.T. (1979): The risk of epilepsy following febrile convulsions. *Neurology* **29**, 297–303.

Annegers, J.F., Hauser, W.A., Shine, S.B. & Kurland, L.T. (1987): Factors prognostic of unprovoked seizures after febrile convulsions. *N. Engl. J. Med.* **316**, 493–498.

Berg, A.T. & Shinnar, S. (1996a): Complex febrile seizures. *Epilepsia* **37**, 126–133.

Berg, A.T. & Shinnar, S. (1996b): Unprovoked seizures in children with febrile seizures: short term outcome. *Neurology* **47**, 562–568.

Berkovic, S.F. & Scheffer, J.E. (1998): Febrile seizures: genetics and relationship to other epilepsy syndromes. *Curr. Opinion Neurol.* **11**, 129–134.

Bertram, E.H., Lothman, E.W. & Lenn, N.J. (1990): The hippocampus in experimental chronic epilepsy: a morphometric analysis. *Ann. Neurol.* **271**, 43–48.

Cavanagh, J.B. & Meyer, A. (1956): Aetiological aspects of Ammon's horn sclerosis associated with temporal lobe epilepsy. *Br. Med. J.* **2**, 1403–1407.

Cendes, F., Andermann, F., Gloor, P., Lopes-Cendes, I., Andermann, E., Melanson, D. et al. (1993): Atrophy of mesial temporal structures in patients with temporal lobe epilepsy: cause or consequence of repeated seizures?. *Ann. Neurol.* **34**, 795–801.

Consensus Development Panel (1980): Febrile seizures: long term management of children with fever-associated seizures. *Pediatrics* **66**, 1009–1012.

Davies, K.G., Hermann, B.P., Dohan, F.C., Foley, K.T., Bush, A.J. & Wyler, A.R. (1996): Relationship of hippocampal sclerosis to duration and age of onset of epilepsy and childhood febrile seizures in temporal lobectomy patients. *Epilepsy Res.* **24**, 119–125.

Degen, R. (1978): Epilepsy in children. An etiological study based on their obstetrical record. *J. Neurol.* **217**, 145–158.

Fernandez, G., Effenberger, O., Vinz, B., Steinlein, O., Elger, C.E., Dohring, W. & Heinze, H.H. (1998): Hippocampal malformation as a cause of familial febrile convulsions and subsequent hippocampal sclerosis. *Neurology* **50**, 909–912.

French, J.A., Williamson, P.D., Thadani, V.M., Darcey, T.M., Mattson, R.H., Spencer, S.S. & Spencer, D.D. (1993): Characteristics of medial temporal lobe epilepsy: I. Results of history and physical examination. *Ann. Neurol.* **34**, 774–780.

Germano, I.M., Sperber, E.F., Ahuja, S. & Moshé, S.L. (1998): Evidence of enhanced kindling and hippocampal neuronal injury in immature rats with neuronal migration disorders. *Epilepsia* **39**, 1253–1260.

Gloor, P. (1991): Mesial temporal sclerosis: historical background and an overview from a modern perspective. In: *Epilepsy surgery*, ed. H.O. Lüders, pp. 689–703. New York: Raven Press.

Gunay, M. & Aysun, S. (1996): Neuronal migration disorders presenting with mild clinical symptoms. *Pediatr. Neurol.* **14**, 153–154.

Ho, S.S., Kuzniecky, R., Gilliam, F., Faught, E. & Morawetz, R.B. (1998): Temporal lobe developmental malformations and epilepsy. *Neurology* **50**, 909–912.

Jack, C.R., Sharbrough, F.W. & Twomey, C.K. (1990): Temporal lobe seizures: lateralization with MR volume measurements of the hippocampal formation. *Radiology* **175**, 423–429.

Jack, C.R., Sharbrough, F.W., Cascino, G.D., Hirschorn, K.A., O'Brien, P.C. & Marsh, R. (1992): Magnetic resonance image-based hippocampal volumetry: correlation with outcome after temporal lobectomy. *Ann. Neurol.* **31**, 138–146.

Kuks, J.B., Cook, M.J., Fish, D.R., Stevens, J.M. & Shorvon, S.D. (1993): Hippocampal sclerosis in epilepsy and childhood febrile seizures. *Lancet* **342**, 1391–1394.

Lee, K., Diaz, M. & Melchior, J.C. (1981): Temporal lobe epilepsy – not a consequence of childhood febrile convulsions. *Acta Neurol. Scand.* **63**, 231–236.

Lewis, D.V. (1999): Febrile convulsions and mesial temporal sclerosis. *Curr. Opinion Neurol.* **12**, 197–201.

Maher, J. & McLachlan, R.S. (1995): Febrile convulsions: is seizure duration the most important predictor of temporal lobe epilepsy? *Brain* **118**, 1521–1528.

Mathern, G.W., Babb, T.L., Vickrey, B.G., Melendez, M. & Pretorius, J. (1995): The clinical pathogenic mechanism of hippocampal neuron loss and surgical outcome in temporal lobe epilepsy. *Brain* **118**, 105–118.

Meldrum, B. (1991): Excitotoxicity and epileptic brain damage. *Epilepsy Res.* **10**, 55–61.

Meldrum, B. & Garthwaite, J. (1990): Excitatory aminoacid neurotoxicity and neurodegenerative disease. *Trends pharmacol. Sci.* **11**, 379–387.

Nelson, K.B. & Ellenberg, J.H. (1976): Predictors of epilepsy in children who have experienced febrile seizures. *N. Engl. J. Med.* **295**, 1029–1033.

Okada, R., Moshé, S.L. & Albala, B.J. (1984): Infantile status epilepticus and future seizure susceptibility in the rat. *Brain Res.* **317**, 177–183.

Olney, J.W., Sharpe, L.G. & Feigin, R.D. (1972): Glutamate-induced brain damage in infant primates. *J. Neuropathol. Exp. Neurol.* **31**, 464–488.

Ounsted, C., Lindsay, J. & Norman, R. (1966): *Biological factors in temporal lobe epilepsy. Clinics in Developmental Medicine*, no. 2. London: Spastic Society and Heinemann Medical.

Raymond, A.A., Fish, D.R., Stevene, J.M., Cook, M.J., Sisodiya, S.M. & Shorvon, S.D. (1994): Association of hippocampal sclerosis with cortical dysgenesis in patients with epilepsy. *Neurology* **44**, 1841–1843.

Rocca, W.A., Sharbrough, F.W., Hauser, W.A., Annegers, J.F. & Schoenberg, B.S. (1987): Risk factors for complex partial seizures: a population-based case-control study. *Ann. Neurol.* **21**, 22–31.

Rutherford, M.A., Pennock, J.M, Schwieso, J.E., Cowan, F.M. & Dubowitz, L.M.S. (1995): Hypoxic ischemic encephalopathy: early magnetic resonance imaging findings and their evolution. *Neuropediatrics* **26**, 183–191.

Stanhope, J.M., Brody, J.A., Brink, E. & Morris, C.E. (1972): Convulsions among the Chamorro people of Guam, Mariana islands. Part II. Febrile comvulsions. *Am. J. Epidemiol.* **95**, 299–304.

Tronerry, M.R., Jack, C.R., Jr, Sharbrough, F.W., Cascino, G.D., Hirschorn, K.A., Marsh, W.R. *et al.* (1993): Quantitative MRI hippocampal volume: association with onset and duration of epilepsy, and febrile convulsions in temporal lobectomy patients. *Epilepsy Res.* **15**, 247–252.

Van den Berg, B.J. & Yerushalmy, J. (1969): Studies on convulsive disorders in young children. I. Incidence of febrile and non febrile convulsions by age and other factors. *Pediatr. Res.* **3**, 298–304.

Wallace, S.J. (1976): Factors predisposing to a complicated initial febrile convulsion. *Arch. Dis. Childh.* **50**, 943–947.

Chapter 17

Memory disturbances in early hippocampal pathology

Daria Riva, Veronica Saletti, Sara Bulgheroni, Irene Bagnasco and Francesca Nichelli

*Divisione di Neurologia dello **Sviluppo**, Istituto Nazionale Neurologico 'C. Besta', via Celoria 11, 20133 Milan, Italy*

Summary

The role of the hippocampal and parahippocampal regions in the organization of long term declarative memorys are reviewed and confirmed also in developmental age. Parahippocampal regions, which are reciprocally interconnected with the cerebral neo-cortex, process memories which are semantically related. Vice versa hippocampal circuits, which are connected only with the parahippocampal circuits, process episodic memory, forming a sort of personal frame where memory constitutes a cognitive memory which belongs only to a given person. This means that lesions of these regions can produce a dissociation between semantic and episodic memory. If the lesion occurs very early in life, the impact on learning in general can be devastating; if the lesion occurs later in life, it results in anterograde amnesia of varying severity.

The hippocampus is particularly vulnerable to the effects of protracted hypoxia and global brain blood hypoperfusion. The reasons for this vulnerability are not yet fully understood. Using MRI techniques, this is now clear to be the case in humans regardless of the age at which the incident occurs.

Thus hypoxic–ischaemic episodes in infancy and later in life can result in bilateral hippocampal damage that can be severe and selective, while other cerebral areas seem to remain intact.

When these episodes occur neonatally or very early in life, the selective impairment of the hippocampal processes is not immediately evident. Later, however, between the ages about 5 and 8 years, the affected children begin to manifest a sort of global anterograde amnesia that is chronically disabling.

The syndrome is not the same as described in adults who, particularly in the cases with extensive, medial temporal damage, appear to be nearly totally unable to acquire new long term cognitive memory of any kind. On the contrary in the early lesioned children, the amnesia is comparatively limited either in extent or in severity or both.

However, the clinical picture also worsens in children when the hypoxic episodes do recur and are part of a more complex neurological disease in which the epilepsy originating from these structures is particularly severe and drug resistant. In these particular cases the impact is devastating.

The term 'temporo-mesial sclerosis' precisely defines a syndrome characterized by limbic epileptic seizures, a temporal focus, morphologically altered temporo-mesial structures and, in adults who are not operated, a neuropsychological pattern (Hermann et al., 1997) consisting of:

1. a deficit in the ability to learn and recall new information, depending on the side of the focus and the severity of the lesion;

2. a memory deficit that is more clearly apparent in relation to verbal tests;

3. a concomitant neurocognitive dysfunction that correlates with the type, frequency and duration of seizures, the antiepileptic therapy administered, and the duration of the disease.

Temporo-mesial sclerosis (TMS) during the developmental age is rarely observed (Murakami et al., 1996) and its aetiopathogenesis is not fully understood: in particular, it is not known whether it is the cause or effect of repeated (and especially long-lasting) seizures. It is certainly rare in children aged less than five years, although it has been encountered in children of 2–4 years and also in children who have experienced one long febrile seizure. It is much more frequent in adults but, in this case, the duration of epilepsy is usually more than 21 years and the frequency of seizures must be more than twice a year (Salmenpera et al., 1998).

TMS has only very recently been considered in research studies, most of which have mainly dealt with the neuropsychological and behavioural aspects of (particularly focal) paediatric neurological diseases. In fact it has only recently been generally accepted that the specialization of the brain areas processing specific functions occurs at an early stage of development and that therefore even the earliest of lesions may cause highly specific deficits (Riva, 1995). This means that also early hippocampal pathology can result in well defined deficits in memory processes.

A large number of experimental and clinical studies have demonstrated that temporo-mesial structures play a fundamental role in the organization of memory.

The clinical studies have been based on descriptions of patients affected by amnesic syndrome after surgery for bilateral temporo-mesial lesions or patients with more selective partial verbal and non-verbal memory deficits due to either left or right unilateral surgical lesions (Frisk & Milner, 1990; Jones-Gotman, 1986;. Jones-Gotman et al., 1997; Press et al., 1989; Rausch & Babb, 1993).

The enormous flow of studies in this field began in 1957 with Scoville and Milner's original description of what has now become the historical case of 'H.M.', because it has since been the subject of further studies by Milner and other authors (Scoville & Miller, 1957; Corkin, 1984; Milner et al., 1968; Gabrieli et al., 1988).

H.M. underwent bilateral ablation of the temporo-mesial structures because of intractable epilepsy. The intervention caused severe anterograde amnesia. The organization of memory showed clear signs of dissociation among its various components, fundamentally represented by an important deficit in the acquisition of new long-term episodic memories, preserved procedural memory, good short-term memory function, and good cognitive and sensory functioning.

The evidence provided by H.M., and many others after him, made it possible to arrive at the definition of a memory system organized into short- and long-term components. Long-term memory is sub-divided into implicit (or procedural) and explicit (or declarative) memory (Tulving, 1972, 1983).

Procedural memory is at most only partially conscious and consists of a collection of different skills; it is expressed by means of 'activities', does not respond to the criterion of true/false, progressively increases with experience, and generally represents a predisposition to behave in a particular way on the basis of previous memories. On the contrary, declarative memory is conscious and expressed by means of words, concepts and propositions; it is also expressed by means of images and the recall of previously encountered facts and events.

Declarative memory is further sub-divided into semantic and episodic memory. Semantic memory represents our knowledge of the world beyond any context or temporal parameters, is automatically expressed and lives in the present; episodic memory is based on facts/events occurring in a precise temporal and spatial context in which the fundamental reference point is the person remembering.

Amnesia appears related to long-term declarative memory (Baddeley, 1984).

Given the existence of different types of memory, it follows that they are processed by different brain areas and based on different neuronal circuits (Gabrieli et al., 1997).

Short-term memory is probably processed by the inferior parietal lobe (although not everybody agrees on this point); declarative long-term memory is processed by the temporo-mesial structures, in particular, the hippocampus and parahippocampal regions, whereas procedural memory seems to be processed by the striatum and the cerebellum.

Given that different brain areas process different components of the memory system, it follows that these components may be independently deficient depending on the damaged area.

Short-term memory deficits can therefore exist in the presence of a perfectly functioning long-term memory, and vice versa; a deficient declaratory memory in the presence of an intact procedural memory, and vice versa; and (not for all authors) a deficient episodic memory in the presence of an integral semantic memory (Baddeley, 1984; Ellis & Young, 1988).

In Mishkin et al. (1997) and Elchenbaum et al.'s (1997) model of the anatomy of the temporo-mesial structures, the memory is seen as being very flexible and based on representations stored in the neocortex in a highly precise and sophisticated manner.

The representations are grouped into semantic associations in the parahippocampal region, whose memories are faithfully coded in such a way that they can be re-evoked particularly when they are contiguous (i.e. if they belong to similar semantic categories), whereas the hippocampus is the anatomical site to which the personal context is attached. The memory is positioned in time and place, and it or some of its parts can be manipulated and associated with other parts of other memories in order to create an infinity of rearranged complex memories (Mishkin et al., 1998).

The hippocampus is an extraordinary structure because, guided by a sort of metacognitive and decision-making capacity, it is capable of extracting items or parts of episodes, processing them by means of associations, and rearranging them in such a wide variety of ways as to allow inferences to be drawn. It is thus capable of combining our memories in order to form the cognitive map of personal experiences that each of us carry with us.

Systematic studies of animal temporo-mesial structures have made it possible to validate the model in an irrefutable manner (Mishkin et al., 1997; Suzuki & Amaral, 1994a, b).

Within the context of clinical neurology, the syndrome of anterograde amnesia defines a total incapacity to learn and recall recent events: it may be semantic, episodic or affect both components.

The large number of studies involving patients who have undergone surgical ablation of the temporo-mesial structures have revealed differences in the severity of memory deficit depending on whether the surgery was mono- or bilateral: bilateral ablation leads to a very severe form of amnesia, whereas unilateral ablation causes a memory deficit relating to the type of information typical of the hemisphere involved (Frisk & Milner, 1990; Jones-Gotman, 1986).

In particular, it has been noted (Jones-Gotman et al., 1997) that ablation of the anterior portion of the temporal lobe + amygdala + part of the hippocampus or excision of the temporal cortex/neocortex (excluding the amygdala and hippocampus), or selective ablation of the amygdala and hippocampus, cause similar learning and delayed recall deficits respectively relating to verbal or non-verbal stimuli (the latter being generally less severe). The underlying pathogenic mechanism has been interpreted as a disconnection of the cortex from the hippocampus: although the neocortex is still capable of storing the memories, it cannot pass them to the hippocampus and the parahippocampal structures, and so they cannot be recalled as such or rearranged.

Furthermore, although it is true that early lesions can sometimes be easily compensated for, it must also be said that some localizations cannot be substituted and that these include structures such as the basal nuclei and the hippocampus.

De Long & Heinz (1997) described four children who had been affected by a severe form of West's syndrome during their first months of life, and who showed a bilateral reduction in hippocampal volume and bilateral anterior lobe hypometabolism at PET in two cases. Despite adequate motor and sensory functions, all four presented extremely severe developmental impairment, with a total absence of verbal communication with autistic-like social behaviour, peculiar social skills and purposive or adaptive activity, even after epilepsy was controlled.

Chugani et al. (1996) described 14 post-West children in whom PET revealed bilateral hippocampal atrophy. All suffered from severely reduced language and severely delayed psychomotor development, but the most important element was that ten of them were autistic. In the children with only unilateral temporo-mesial lesions, the impairment was generally less severe and, although badly organized and retarded, language was not completely absent.

These dramatic cases can perhaps be interpreted in the light of the fact that language organization (especially the components involved in spontaneous creative production and not just rigid repetition) is the first example of a flexible expression of memory with a high degree of rearranging ability. Early hippocampal atrophy from the time of the beginning of the natural organization of language, and the consequent persistent deficit in memory, also underlies isolated social behaviour because affected children are incapable of personalizing their memories by inserting them in a specific context defined by spatio-temporal parameters, and therefore cannot construct a cognitive map of their experiences. It follows that early hippocampal lesions impede the normal development of the network of language, and personal and communication memories that forms the basis of more complex human social behaviours.

If the onset of hippocampal lesions is later, the deficits are more selective and impinge upon a cognitive, linguistic and social development that is already under way; the picture is therefore more similar to that observed in adults. Wood's case of a nine-year-old child with amnesia post herpetic encephalitis (Wood et al., 1989), as well as Ostergaard's (1987) and Ostergaard &

Squire's (1990) case of a 10-year-old with the same disease, presented dissociation between a preserved procedural memory and a deficient declarative memory with, perhaps, episodic memory more impaired than the semantic one.

In 1997, Vargha-Khadem *et al.* described three subjects with bilateral hippocampal atrophy whose intelligence was within normal limits, semantic memory preserved and school performance slow but satisfactory. On the other hand, their everyday memory was deficient and there was a deficit in multimodal mnemonic associations (e.g. they had difficulty in associating a voice with a particular face, or an object with the place in which it is located).

In order to detect memory consequences of early unilateral pathology, and to investigate the different components of the memory system, we also studied a sample of five children with temporal lobe epilepsy (three with a left and two with a right focus), and unilateral hippocampal pathology according to the EEG focus site. We compared them with five control subjects selected according to the age, sex, school level and socio-cultural background. All, either patients or controls, underwent the same radiological and neuropsychological examinations.

The pathologies underlying the limbic seizures in the patients with a left focus were TMS (two cases) and hippocampal dysplasia (one); both of the patients with a right focus were affected by hippocampal atrophy. All of the subjects underwent the following neuroradiological protocol:

1. NMR (Press *et al.*, 1989) with evaluations of:

    - hippocampal hypotrophy;
    - the internal morphology of the hippocampus;
    - alterations in T1 (hypointensity) and T2-weighted images (hyperintensity);
    - the volume of the hippocampal structures.

2. Spectroscopy (Gadian *et al.*, 1996; Cendes *et al.*, 1994) to evaluate the reduction in N-acetyl aspartate acid at the sites of the NMR alterations, which correspond to the neuronal loss.

The results of these examinations provided radiological confirmation that the hippocampal lesions were homolateral to the site of the focus.

The patients had a bilateral reduction in hippocampal volume (Lencz *et al.*, 1992) that was more marked on the side of the NMR alterations; spectroscopy revealed a reduction in N-acetyl aspartate acid that was also more marked on the side of the focus.

The neuropsychological examinations evaluated general intelligence; short-term spatial and verbal memory; long-term episodic memory, tested by means of a story, verbally uncodifiable abstract drawings, and a daily memory questionnaire; long-term semantic memory; and verbal and non-verbal learning.

The results were:

- Intelligence in patients was normal or low average;
- Performance or non-verbal intelligence was particularly defective in subjects compared to controls;
- Verbal and spatial short-term memory were relatively preserved;
- All patients, despite the unilateral pathology, performed worse than controls, either in verbal or non-verbal learning and long term-recall;
- Left-affected patients were more impaired than right ones in all tasks, particularly in verbal memory tests;

- Semantic components were mildly impaired in all subjects;
- The difference in everyday memory between patients and controls was highly significant.

The patient with a tumour involving the hippocampus, parahippocampus and amygdala regions had the same deficits as those of the other patients with left lesions, but also a marked reduction in semantic memory and a bizarre communication characterized by social isolation and echolalia.

General conclusions

The results reported here demonstrate the fact that the temporo-mesial structures process long-term declarative memory at developmental age. This not only means that the architecture of the anatomical structures is established very early in life, but also that an early lesion affecting these structures cannot be compensated for by the establishment of alternative pathways and, furthermore, that the degree of impairment is age-related (i.e. it is greater in patients who are affected at a younger age). Very early lesions of the hippocampus irreversibly compromise the possibility of acquiring complex modalities of verbal and social communication, as well as the possibility of organizing an absolutely personal cognitive map.

Later lesions only cause amnesia of various degrees of severity, with a more severe impairment of episodic than semantic memory if localized in the hippocampus, or with impairment of both memory components in the case that they involve both the hippocampus and parahippocampus.

Finally, it is very interesting to note that these results not only confirm that dissociations in the memory system components are also possible at a very early developmental age, but also confirm the structure of the circuit.

The cortex/neocortex faithfully stores the information. The parahippocampal regions codify the information belonging to the same categories in a contiguous manner, and are also capable of re-evoking simple connections with the cortex/neocortex under the impulse of simple stimuli, particularly if they are contiguous and monomodal. The hippocampus analyses different elements of various experiences and stimuli, acquired in different spatio-temporal contexts and via a wide range of modalities (sight, touch, smell, sound, emotion, etc.), and is capable of relating them to each other in a myriad of different combinations and in a totally flexible and inexhaustible manner.

Studies of the temporo-mesial structures therefore not only highlight specific neuropsychological deficits, but also provide an extremely interesting insight into the pathologies typical of childhood development, such as infantile autism.

Further studies of this type of pathology are necessary not only in order to better define the disease affecting a given child with a temporal focus and limbic seizures, but also in order to overcome the rigid scheme of thought and interpretation characterizing many of the most serious pathologies affecting children of developmental age.

References

Baddeley, A. (1984): *La memoria umana*. Bologna: Il Mulino.

Cendes, F., Andermann, F., Preul, M.C. & Arnold, D.L. (1994): Lateralization of temporal lobe epilepsy based on regional metabolic abnormalities in proton magnetic resonance spetroscopic images. *Ann. Neurol.* **35**, 211–216.

Chugani, H.T., Silva, E.D. & Chugani, D.C. (1996): Infantile spasm: III. Prognostic implications of bitemporal hypometabolism on positron emission tomography. *Ann. Neurol.* **39**, 643–649.

Corkin, S. (1984): Lasting consequences of bilateral medial temporal lobectomy: clinical course and experimental findings in H.M. *Sem. Neurology* **4**, 252–262.

De Long, R. & Heinz, E.R. (1997): The clinical syndrome of early-life bilateral hippocampal sclerosis. *Ann. Neurol.* **42**, 11–17.

Eichenbaum, H. (1997): How does the brain organize memory? *Science* **277**, 330–332.

Ellis, W.A. & Young A.W. (1988): Memory. In: *Human cognitive neuropsychology*. Hove, London & Hillsdale: Lawrence Erlbaum.

Frisk, V. & Milner, B. (1990): The role of the left hippocampal region in the acquisition and retention of story content. *Neuropsychologia* **28**, 349–359.

Gabrieli, J.D.E., Cohen, N.J. & Corkin, S. (1988): The impaired learning of semantic knowledge following medial temporal lobe resection. *Brain Cognition* **7**, 157–177.

Gabrieli, J.D.E., Brewer, J.B., Desmond, J.E. & Glover, G.H. (1997): Separate neural bases of two fundamental memory processes in the human medial temporal lobe. *Science* **276**, 264–266.

Gadian, D.G., Isaacs, E.B., Cross, H.J., Connelly, A., Jackson, G.D., King, M.D., Neville, B.G. & Vargha-Khadem, F. (1996): Lateralization of brain function in childhood revealed by magnetic resonance spectroscopy. *Neurology* **46**, 974–977.

Hermann, B.P., Seidenberg, M. *et al.* (1997): Neuropsychological characteristics of the Syndrome of mesial temporal lobe epilepsy. *Arch. Neurol.* **54**, 369–376.

Jones-Gotman, M. (1986): Right hippocampal excision impair learning and recall of a list of abstract design. *Neuropsychologia* **24**, 659–670.

Jones-Gotman, M., Zatorre, R.J., Olivier, A., Andermann, F., Cendes, F., Stauton, H., McMackin, D., Siegel, A.M. & Wieser, H.G. (1997): Learning and retention of words and designs following excision from medial or lateral temporal-lobe structures. *Neuropsychologia* **35**, 963–973.

Lencz, T., McCarthy, G., Bronen, R.A. *et al.* (1992): Quantitative magnetic resonance imaging in temporal lobe epilepsy: relationship to neuropathology and neuropsychological function. *Ann. Neurol.* **31**, 629–637.

Milner, B., Corkin, S. & Teuber, H.L. (1968): Further analysis of the hippocampal amnesic syndrome: 14 years follow-up study of H.M. *Neuropsychologia* **6**, 215–234.

Mishkin, M., Suzuki, W., Gadian, D.G. & Vargha-Khadem, F. (1997): Hierarchical organization of cognitive memory. *Phil. Trans. R. Soc. London* (B) **352**, 1461–1467.

Mishkin, M., Vargha-Khadem, F. & Gadian, D.G. (1998): Amnesia and the organization of the hippocampal system. *Hippocampus* **8**, 212–216.

Murakami, N., Shigeru, O., Oka, E. & Tanaka, A. (1996): Mesial temporal lobe epilepsy in childhood. *Epilepsia* **37** (Suppl. 3), 52–56.

Ostergaard, A. (1987): Episodic, semantic and procedural memory in a case of amnesia at an early age. *Neuropsychologia* **25**, 341–357.

Ostergaard, A. & Squire, L.R. (1990): Childhood amnesia and distinctions between forms of memory: a comment on Wood, Brown, and Felton. *Brain Cognition* **14**, 127–133.

Press, A.G., Amaral, D.G. & Squire L.R. (1989): Hippocampal abnormalities in amnesic patients revealed by high resolution magnetic resonance imaging. *Nature* **341**, 54–57.

Rausch, R. & Babb, T.L. (1993): Hippocampal neuron loss and memory scores before and after temporal lobe surgery for epilepsy. *Arch. Neurol.* **50,** 812–817.

Riva, D. (1995): Le lesioni cerebrali focali. In: *Manuale di neuropsicologia dell'età evolutiva*. A cura di G. Sabbadini. Bologna: Zanichelli.

Salmenpera, T., Kalviainen, R., Partanen, K. & Pitkanen, A. (1998): Hippocampal damage caused by seizures in temporal lobe epilepsy. *Lancet* **351,** 35.

Scoville, W.B. & Milner, B. (1957): Loss of recent memory after bilateral hippocampal lesions. *J. Neurol. Neurosurg. Psych.* **25**, 251–255.

Suzuki, W.A. & Amaral, D.G. (1994a): Perirhinal and parahippocampal cortices of the macaque monkey: cortical afferents. *J. Comp. Neurol.* **350**, 497–533.

Suzuki, W.A. & Amaral, D.G. (1994b): Topographic organization of the reciprocal connections between monkey entorhinal cortex and the perirhinal and parahippocampal cortices. *J. Neurosci.* **14**, 1856–1877.

Tulving, E. (1972): Episodic and semantic memory. In: *Organization of memory*, eds. E. Tulving & W. Donaldson. New York: Academic Press.

Tulving, E. (1983): In: *Elements of episodic memory*. Oxford: Oxford University Press.

Vargha-Khadem, F., Gadian, D.G., Watkins, K.E., Connely, A., Van Paeschen, W. & Mishkin, M. (1997): Differential effects of early hippocampal pathology on episodic and semantic memory. *Science* **277**, 376–380.

Wood, F.B., Brown, I.S. & Felton, R.H. (1989): Long term follow-up of a childhood amnesic syndrome. *Brain Cognition* **10,** 76–86.

Chapter 18

Psychic alterations in temporal lobe seizures in children

Charlotte Dravet and Michelle Bureau

Centre Saint-Paul, 300 Boulevard de Sainte Marguerite, 13009 Marseille, France

'Often the seizure disorder is only the most pressing
but not the only or even the worst dysfunction.'
D.C. Taylor, 1996

Summary

In the literature it is assumed that psychic alterations are frequent in children with epilepsy, particularly when it is a temporal lobe epilepsy (TLE). We reviewed the studies published in the last 30 years and came across many contradictory findings. Hyperkineticism, aggressiveness, catastrophic rages, antisocial conducts, formal thought disorders, communication deficits, affective disorders, and psychosis were the common features mentioned and analysed. Their relationships with different factors were studied: age at seizure onset, poor control of seizures, lateralization of the EEG focus, type of lesion, cognitive performance, family structure and pathology. Some studies compared the data obtained in patients with TLE to those either in patients with generalized epilepsy, or in patients with other chronic non-neurological diseases. Other prospective studies reported the long-term outcome of these children and showed it was rather favourable. Some authors considered the outcome after epilepsy surgery, often without valuable quantitative measures. The recruitment and the methodology used in these reports were very heterogeneous and made drawing firm conclusions difficult. Moreover, in the oldest studies many patients were not submitted to modern neuroimaging and in the absence of surgery the diagnosis of TLE was not always well-established. However it seems probable that in some children there is an association of TLE with aggressiveness, hyperkineticism, more rarely psychosis, leading to poor school achievement and anti-social conducts. These disorders are related to poor neuropsychological performances. They can be improved by surgery when it is successful and makes the seizures disappear.

The literature about relationships between epilepsy and psychiatric disturbances is extremely rich, but also confusing. Most of the studies concern adult patients, particularly for temporal lobe epilepsy (TLE). In 1970, Rutter *et al.*, by carrying out an epidemiological study on children aged 5 to 14 in the Isle of Wight, demonstrated a very high prevalence of psychiatric disorders in epilepsy relative either to the general population, or to non-neurological diseases (Table 1). After exclusion of children with a low IQ, this prevalence was lower in uncomplicated epilepsy (28.65 per cent) than in epilepsy associated to a neurological disease (58.3 per cent). But the quality of the disorders was the same in epileptic and non-epileptic patients.

Table 1. Psychiatric disorders in children in the Isle of Wight (Rutter et al., 1970)

Children from 5 to 14 years:	11,865	Psychiatric disorders	Percentage
Children with epilepsy:	86 (7.2 per 1000)	No.	
2,189	without any disease	144	6.6%
138	not neurological disease	16	11.6%
64	not complicated epilepsy	18	28.6%
24	neurological disease without epilepsy	9	27.5%
22	neurological disease with epilepsy	7	58.3%

In the literature it is assumed that psychic alterations are frequent in children with TLE and have some particular characteristics: hyperactivity, antisocial behaviour, aggressiveness, catastrophic rages, as well as formal thought disorders, communication deficits and even psychosis. Some authors admit that epilepsies with complex partial seizures are specifically related to psychotic disorders. Affective disorders and cognitive impairments are often associated and reciprocally interact. Their relationships with different factors were studied: age at seizure onset, poor control of seizures, lateralization of the focus, type of lesion, cognitive performance, family structure and pathology. Some authors also considered long-term evolution and outcome after surgery. Others compared either TLE and different other types of epilepsy, or epilepsy and other chronic pathology such as asthma. But the different studies are heterogeneous and provide often contradictory data. The role of antiepileptic drugs in behavioural and learning disorders was taken into consideration, mainly for barbiturates, phenytoin and carbamazepine, but no studies with comparison of different plasma levels were conducted in children.

In this paper we make a review of the most important studies, without pretending to be exhaustive, which would be nearly impossible.

Type of disturbances and related factors

The only large prospective study on the psychological aspects of TLE in childhood is that by Ounsted et al. (1987). They collected 100 successive cases of patients with TLE from 1948 to 1954 and have followed them up to 1977. The two criteria used to include children in the TLE group were: clinical diagnosis of seizures conforming to temporal lobe attacks, and presence in the EEG of a focal discharge in one or both temporal regions. They coded the data in 1964 and reanalysed them in 1977. No patient has been lost to follow-up. Only 15 per cent of the patients did not have any behavioural disturbance at any time. Three main types of disorders were observed: *mental defect*, *hyperkinetic syndrome* and *cataclysmic rage outbursts*. Unstable home contexts, schooling difficulties unrelated to intelligence, and antisocial conducts were also noticed.

Mental defect with a verbal IQ of less than 70 was present in nearly a quarter of the sample population, and implied a bad prognosis: recovery was not a factor, early death was common and total care was needed for survivors. Moreover, 32 children required special schooling, largely dependent of behaviour more than on cognitive defects. The objective fact of exclusion clearly has a negative prognosis, only one child of this group being fully recovered.

The true *hyperkinetic syndrome* (as defined by Hutt & Hutt, 1970) affected 26 children and carried a bad prognosis in adult life: only two patients belonged to the group of patients completely recovered, four died, and the other 20 were uncontrolled. It was more frequent in boys, often associated to brain damage (88 per cent of cases), to an early onset of seizures (81 per cent before 2 years 4 months), and to a low IQ (median IQ of 70 *vs.* 100 for the whole group). This syndrome, probably due to a number of factors, amongst which antiepileptic drugs such as phenobarbitone and primidone, is now rare.

Catastrophic rages were a major problem for 36 of these children. They were similar to the cataclysmic rages of infants and also carried a poor prognosis in adulthood: only five patients belonged to the group of patients completely recovered, three died before 15 years, and the other 28 were uncontrolled. Sixteen were in the group of adults with psychiatric disorders. There was no significant difference in the incidence between the sexes. Boys and girls differed only in the age of onset at the first seizure, lower in the girls (9 months vs. 16 months). They could be associated to brain damage (47 per cent), and to epileptic status (33 per cent).

The problem of aggressiveness in epileptic children has been underlined by many authors for decades, as well documented by Bagley (1971). Among the oldest we cite only Lennox & Lennox (1960) who found 25 per cent of 1270 patients 'irritable, quick-tempered, highly strung'. Few studies have tried to correlate aggressiveness with the seizure types. Nuffield (1961) studied 332 epileptic children and showed that the 40 children with TLE were significantly more aggressive that the remainder of the children. Surprisingly he did not find an influence of the environmental factors, but his concept of environment was not well defined (Bagley, 1971). However this study is probably biased by the type of recruitment. Patients were referred to the Maudsley Hospital which is known to treat a highly selected psychiatric population, and the children studied were not representative of children with TLE in general. Whitman *et al.* (1982) compared 35 children with TLE and 48 children with primary generalized epilepsies on standardized measures of social competence, aggression and overall behaviour disorder via analyses of covariance. The presence of TLE *per se* bore no relationship to aggression, social competence or overall behavioural disorder. However, some specific subject- and seizure-related variables were found to be associated with increased aggression and behavioural dysfunction in children with TLE.

Other features have been described in children with TLE: inattentiveness, maladjustment at school, stubbornness, emotional dependence (Stores, 1978; Camfield *et al.*, 1984; Elger *et al.*, 1998), as well as formal thought disorder, communication deficits (Caplan *et al.*, 1992, 1994), affective disorders and even psychosis (Caplan *et al.*, 1991; Taylor, 1996). The factors causing these psychological impairments are complex and not easy to establish. Every author has his own methodology and the data are often contradictory.

Stores (1978) performed four studies in epileptic children (average age of 10 to 11 years) attending ordinary school, in order to identify those at greatest risk of behavioural complications. The results suggest that boys are more vulnerable than girls and that a persistent left temporal spike discharge is associated with reading retardation, inattentiveness, emotional dependency, overactivity, social isolation. Affective, personality and cognitive disorders are not easy to separate. The possibility is raised that phenytoin can adversely affect cognitive functions. The association between a left temporal focus and psychosis has been pointed out by

Sherwin *et al.* (1982) in adult patients. However, Pritchard *et al.* (1980) did not find significant differences between left and right focus lateralization in 56 adolescents and adults with TLE onset in childhood (mean 6.1 years). Twenty had obvious psychopathology: character disorders, confrontations with school authorities, psychosis, suicide attempt, emerging during adolescence. In the same way, Camfield *et al.* (1984) carried out a study with 27 children (6–17 years), with a normal or quite normal IQ, 14 with right and 13 with left TLE. Cognitive abilities, personality profile, school success were considered. Ten were 'maladjusted' with psychological problems not related to the focus lateralization, but related to greater cognitive deficits. Only one had rage attacks and none was hyperkinetic. Recently, Elger *et al.* (1998) carried out two studies in children selected for TLE surgery. The first study analysed cognitive functions and compared the results with findings in adults. The data indicated a particular risk of cognitive impairments in children suffering from an epilepsy of the dominant temporal lobe but only for the language, in agreement with Adams *et al.* (1990), but in disagreement with other studies which gave the same results as in adults (Fedio & Mirsky, 1969; Cohen, 1992; Jambaqué *et al.*, 1993). The second study attended to the occurrence and determinants of behavioural disorders and their development after surgery. In the latter, 32 per cent of 37 children demonstrated behavioural disorders, the most frequent being rage outbursts, aggressiveness and maladjustment. No differences were found concerning anticonvulsive medication, frequency of febrile convulsions, gender, seizure type, side of the focus, age at onset, age at surgery, average seizure frequency. However, multiple regression analysis demonstrated a focus with a high spike frequency in the EEG (9/12, $P < 0.01$) and a neoplastic lesion in the MRI (10/12, $P < 0.05$) significantly more frequent in the group of children with impaired behaviour. After surgery, seven of the 12 children showed an impressive improvement of behaviour, none of the included variables being predictive for the postoperative outcome in this small sample.

Williams *et al.* (1998) also studied cognition and behaviour after temporal lobectomy in children. Patients were nine children 8–15 years of age, five girls, four boys, all right handed. They were evaluated before and at one year (8–17 months) after surgery. Antiepileptics were not reduced at the time of the initial evaluation and all patients continued taking their medication at the time of follow-up evaluations, although dosages had been reduced in some patients. The tests used for neuropsychological assessment measured overall intellectual function, verbal and visual memory, reading recognition, spelling, maths, reading comprehension, executive function, fine motor speed. Behavioural status was assessed by the Child Behavior Checklist, anxiety by the Revised Children's Manifest Anxiety Scale, depression by the Children's Depression Inventory. Repeated measures analysis of variance did not indicate differences in performance on the basis of laterality of surgery (five left and four right resections). Paired comparison *t* tests did not suggest marked changes in cognitive functioning after surgery, although decreases in delayed verbal memory were evident. Positive effects on quality of life during the first year after surgical intervention were suggested by reduced internalizing symptoms and increased social interaction. However, before surgery these children were not rated as having significant behavioural difficulties, except mild elevations in scores for social problems, thought and attention problems. That could be explained by the absence of gross brain pathology: only one case of tuberous sclerosis, the others having mesial temporal sclerosis (five), cortical temporal gliosis (two), normal cortex (one). Surgery consisted of tailored lobectomies usually without extension to other tissues. Seizure outcome was class 1 in the Engel classification in six patients, class 2 in two, class 3 in one. Thus, this small number of children seems to have a true TLE, which is rare in the other series where quantitative psychological evaluations were performed. These results require confirmation by other prospective studies of the same type, but they provide arguments against the existence of a link between behavioural disorders and TLE.

The report by Hermann (1982) is of particular interest. This author specifically investigated the interrelationship between the adequacy of neuropsychological functioning and psychopathology in children with epilepsy. He studied 50 children, aged 8–12, attending regular school classes, classified into two groups on the basis of their performance on a standardized battery of neuropsychological measures (the Luria-Nebraska Neuropsychological Test Battery – Children's Version). Twenty-five children with good neuropsychological function were compared to a closely matched group of 25 children with poor neuropsychological function on measures of aggression, overall behavioural pathology, and overall social competence, which were derived from a standardized behavioural assessment inventory (interview with the child's parents utilizing the Child Behaviour Checklist). Overall, poor neuropsychological functioning was associated with significantly elevated aggression and overall behavioural dysfunction scores and significantly lower social competence indices. The children with TLE were equally distributed in the two groups. These results are in agreement with the observation by Rutter *et al.* (1970) that psychiatric disturbances were very common in 'neuro-epileptic' children with a low IQ, the rate being 50 per cent.

Psychosis

The concept of psychosis in children is different from that in adults which makes the study of this symptom difficult in epileptic children. In the literature, we find data concerning psychotic disorders and childhood epilepsy, but few are specifically orientated towards TLE. Taylor (1996) indicates that the closest associations with autism or autistic behavioural features are through infantile spasms and the Lennox–Gastaut syndrome. The epilepsy most frequently arises in the first year of life and the autistic syndrome appears to be a sequel. Caplan & Gillberg (1997) underline the difficulty of differentiating epileptic seizures and autistic behaviours in children affected by the two disorders. Many bizarre behaviours are similar to clinical seizure activity (staring gaze, complex gestures and postures, tic-like movements, excitation bursts etc.). The EEG and video-monitoring are very helpful in differential diagnosis, but often extremely difficult to perform in these children. The cases reported by Deonna *et al.* (1993) are particularly important because they show that autistic behaviour can appear simultaneously with epilepsy from temporal lobe origin. Of two children with tuberous sclerosis, the first boy considerably improved after remission of the seizures and removal of the lesion (subependymal glial nodule). In the second boy, lesions, situated in the two temporal lobes, could not be removed and the outcome was less favourable. However, in this latter case we wonder whether the diagnosis of tuberous sclerosis is actually acceptable.

Taylor (1996) assumes that schizophrenia is rare in childhood and is less commonly associated with epilepsy than autistic disorders but often appears during adolescence or early adulthood. With Marsh (Taylor & Marsh, 1977) he showed that some types of lesions, notably gangliomas, bear a higher risk of association with later psychosis. We have already quoted the study by Ounsted *et al.* (1987). In their cohort only 26 adult patients among 87 presented with psychiatric disorders. Three categories were identified at follow-up: nine patients (10.3 per cent) have developed psychosis, both diagnosed and treated for schizophrenic signs and symptoms; twelve (13.8 per cent) have exhibited antisocial personality disorders (delinquents); only five have been treated for neurotic symptoms. The nine patients who developed overt psychosis in adulthood were eight males and one female. Seven had a left-sided focus and two had bilateral discharges. All had severe epilepsy and were on anticonvulsants when psychotic. This small number of psychotic adult patients contrasted with the large number of children showing disorders of personality (85 per cent) in this cohort. The authors believe there are powerful restorative forces and strong inhibitory mechanisms acting during development. In the same way, major family troubles, as experienced by 27 of their patients, were not predictive of any form of adult social or psychiatric disorder. This favourable outcome of behavioural disturbances in adulthood has been also underlined by Lindsay et al. (1979).

The link between left-sided temporal focus and occurrence of psychosis has been also emphasized by Taylor (1975) and Flor-Henry (1969) in adults, and by Falconer (1973) and Caplan et al. (1993) in patients submitted to epilepsy surgery. For Caplan et al. (1991) the schizophrenia-like psychosis appears to be associated with poor seizure control, hallucinations, delusions, and illogical thinking but no loose associations or negative signs of schizophrenia. Beside the well defined autism and psychosis there are other types of behavioural disturbances which could be diagnosed as 'pervasive developmental disorders'. They are described in childhood epilepsy without reference to TLE by Caplan & Gillberg (1997). They are also described by Soulayrol (1999) in his study of the mental structures of epileptic children. This author does not treat this problem according to the epilepsy type. He reports his experience of one epileptologist being also a psychoanalyst, and he tries to understand the psychopathology of epileptic children from a psychodynamic point of view, taking the history and the psychic functioning of the child and of his family into account, with all the implications of seizures at the different levels of the personality structuration. This original approach allows us to understand why the same epilepsy cannot have the same consequences in different subjects who do not have the same 'background', the same internal conflicts, the same way of appropriation of their seizures, the same relationship with their mother, the same place among their siblings, etc.

TLE and other epilepsies or chronic diseases

Hermann et al. (1980) compared 47 patients with TLE and 28 with generalized epilepsy according to the age at seizure onset in order to evaluate the effects of age at onset of different epilepsy types on psychological dysfunction in patients. They used the MMPI clinical scales. Previous studies with this method resulted in contradictory findings (Guerrant et al., 1962; Lachar et al., 1979) and failed to clearly demonstrate overall differences between seizure groups. Hermann's study revealed that the group with adolescent-onset TLE was at higher risk of developing psychological dysfunctions than the others (childhood and adult onset TLE and generalized epilepsy whatever the onset age). They assume that it is obviously not simply a reaction to the adolescent onset of a chronic disorder, since the group with generalized epilepsy of adolescent onset had lower scores on the scale used (MMPI scale 4, which measures impulsivity, anger, non-conformity and rebelliousness). Later on, the same author (Hermann et al., 1988), with another methodology, showed that the presence of complex partial seizures (CPS) was not correlated with any of the dependent measures, nor was it a significant predictor in any of the regression analyses. For them, CPS of temporal origin are the most often hypothesized and empirically investigated risk factor. Nonetheless, empirical evidence remains equivocal.

Kaminer et al. (1988) made a study of 26 adolescents, aged 13–18, suffering from TLE, using a structured psychiatric interview (kiddie SADS Epidemiological Version) with patients and parents. In addition to categorical diagnoses, symptom cluster scores were determined in a similar manner to those determined by Spitzer & Endicott for adults. A control group of 26 adolescents suffering from asthma and matched for intelligence, age at onset, rough estimate of disease severity and for other demographic variables, was also examined. Applying strict DSM-III criteria, only one patient, an epileptic subject, met the conditions for a psychiatric diagnosis. The analysis of the symptom cluster scores exposed a high incidence of depressive features, conduct disorders and aggression in both subjects and controls, although only one epileptic patient fulfilled the criteria for an affective disorder. Patients receiving carbamazepine had lower conduct disorder and aggression scores than those taking hydantoin, but preponderance of broken homes was associated to hydantoin treatment. Thus, TLE may not be a specific cause of psychopathology in adolescence and the depression might result from the suffering involved in chronic illness. This conclusion is in agreement with the conclusions of Guerrant *et al.* (1962) in adults but it must be tempered by the small number of subjects.

Perini *et al.* (1996) conducted a controlled study of psychiatric disorders in different forms of epileptic and non-epileptic chronic conditions. They compared two groups of epileptic patients, 20 with TLE and 18 with juvenile myoclonic epilepsy (JME) between them and with 20 matched diabetic patients and 20 matched normal controls. They assessed them by structured interviews (SADS), self-rating scales (Beck depression inventory), the state and trait anxiety scales. Sixteen patients with TLE (80 per cent) fulfilled the criteria for a psychiatric diagnosis versus 22 per cent of those with JME and 10 per cent of those with diabetes ($P < 0.0001$). The most frequent disorder in TLE was a mood disorder: depression in 11 TLE patients (55 per cent) vs. three with JME and two diabetic ($P < 0.001$). Eight TLE patients also had a co-morbid personality or anxiety disorder. These results are in complete opposition to those in the previous study, perhaps because the conditions compared are not the same. The authors conclude that these psychiatric disorders are not an adjustment reaction to a chronic disease but rather reflect a limbic dysfunction.

Discussion

All these data do not allow us to have a clear idea of the psychological alterations in childhood TLE. The data in adults are also heterogeneous and have been accurately criticized by Stevens (1975, 1980). This author has extensively reviewed the literature and did not find any proof that TLE was specifically associated with behavioural disorders, particularly with psychosis. She showed that most of the studies were biased either by the methodology or by the recruitment or by the lack of precise information concerning the epilepsy type. For example, she remarked that the cohort reported by Ounsted *et al.* (1966) includes patients with a wide variety of cerebral pathologies. The selection was made on the basis of a 'discharging focus' over one or both temporal lobes, which is not enough to define TLE even if associated with complex partial seizures. Nearly half of the subjects were mentally retarded and had aetiologies or neurological signs attesting to coexistent widespread cerebral pathology. 'As the authors note', she said, 'among the small group of 12 children in this series who had temporal lobe epilepsy but no other kind of seizure disorders, not a single child manifested catastrophic rage'. She conducted different studies, with different methodologies, in order to discern whether there were significant psychological differences between the patients with TLE and generalized epilepsies (Mirsky *et al.*, 1960; Small *et al.*, 1962; Stevens, 1966). The results were negative in all the three studies. Then she discussed anatomical lesions in patients, and experimental data concerning the role of hippocampus and amygdala in aggressive behaviours, as well as the effects of drugs and temporal lobectomy in the treatment of interictal behaviour disturbances. She concluded that 'patients with major and psychomotor epilepsy are subject to an increased risk of psychiatric disturbance but that, except for the immediate postictal psychotic state, the risk appears to reflect the site and extent of brain damage and the individual's psychosocial history and opportunities more than a diagnosis of epilepsy. This suggests that epileptic seizures themselves are not often the cause of the interictal disorders when they are present, but that the psychological disturbance relates to interactions between environmental causes and the neurological disorder underlying epilepsy.' These conclusions are similar to those drawn by Bagley (1971) in children. Moreover, this author did not find any influence of the temporal localization of the EEG focus, but he did not define a group of children with TLE.

Bruton et al. (1994) examined the relationship between epilepsy and psychosis. They compared clinical, EEG, and neuropathological data from a group of subjects who suffered from both epilepsy and psychosis and from another group of patients who had epilepsy but no evidence of psychotic illness. There were 10 patients diagnosed with epilepsy plus schizophrenia-like psychosis, nine subjects with epilepsy plus 'epileptic psychosis', and 36 individuals with epilepsy without history of psychosis. They examined gross and microscopic material from whole-brain specimens. Three neuropathological features emerged which separated the psychotic from non-psychotic groups: enlarged ventricules, periventricular gliosis and an excess of acquired brain damage (focal cystic softenings, calcification in the basal ganglia, plaques of demyelination in the white matter). Two additional findings also emerged: significant increase of widespread small-vessel disease in the cerebral white matter in the group of the schizophrenia-like patients, when compared to the two other groups; no difference in frequency, degree and type of temporal lobe damage between the schizophrenic and other psychotic patients and the non-psychotic epilepsy group. Thus, epileptic patients with psychosis have more severe and widespread brain damage than do epileptic patients with no evidence of psychotic illness. From the clinical point of view it is noted that the age of onset of seizures was more often around puberty and that the frequency of generalized tonic–clonic seizures was higher in the groups with psychosis compared with the others. However, it is important to remark that this study was retrospective for the clinical data, which were collected over 40 years (1950–1990). The diagnosis of seizures was made only on the 'case note history' of the patients. EEGs were recorded on 4-, 5- or 8 channels and the authors had only factual reports written at the time of recording, the originals not being available for examination. In such conditions it is probable that the diagnosis of TLE is not well established in all patients. On the other hand, this study was made in the department of neuropathology of a large institution for the mentally ill. Even if this department received the brains of many patients coming from other places, because of its reputation, the majority of the patients deceased in this institution (75) or in long-stay epileptic colonies (21), only 15 being deceased in the community. Therefore they represent a group of very severely affected patients.

Conclusion

At the end of this review, it seems that in some children there is an association of TLE with aggressiveness, hyperkineticism, more rarely psychosis, leading to poor school achievement and anti-social conducts. For some authors these disorders are related to poor neuropsychological performance. They can be improved by surgery when it is successful and causes the seizures to disappear. But no study, before the era of paediatric epilepsy surgery, has taken both the seizure types and the exact topography of the epileptogenic zone into consideration. Often the diagnosis of TLE is based only upon the association of complex partial seizures and the presence of a temporal focus in the EEG. Now, we know how difficult it is to differentiate temporal lobe from frontal lobe epilepsy and that in many children we deal with a fronto-temporal epilepsy, sometimes a more complex situation (Battaglia et al., 1998). For patients not submitted to surgery and not investigated by MRI, as in the oldest studies, the pathological substratum of the epilepsy remains unknown and lesions could have been more responsible for psychological disorders than the epilepsy by itself. In most of the reports on results of paediatric epilepsy surgery the outcome in terms of behavioural disorders and quality of life is not considered or is considered without valid methodology (Gilliam, 1997; Munari et al., 1998). At present, accurate psychological and neuropsychological assessments can be performed by the paediatric epilepsy surgery teams in various centres. We may hope to have a better knowledge of these problems in order to help our patients and their families. Moreover, the effect of antiepileptic drugs, not considered in this paper, plays a role which is difficult to estimate. Perhaps the use of new molecules can allow us to improve the benefit/risk ratio in the patients recently affected. We would like also not to forget the interest of one psychoanalytic approach, when possible, which lightens the deep resonance of epilepsy on a fragile personality, on the way of its structuration, and the upsets caused by its sudden occurrence in the child–mother relationship, different from one child to another.

References

Adams, C.B.T., Beardsworth, E.D., Oxbury, S.M., Oxbury, J.M. & Fenwick, P.B.C. (1990): Temporal lobectomy in 44 children: outcome and neuropsychological follow-up. *J. Epilepsy* **3** (Suppl.), 157–168.

Bagley, C. (1971): *The social psychology of the child with epilepsy*. London and Prescot: Routledge and Kegan Paul.

Battaglia, D., Dravet, C., Gelisse, P., Pinto, P., Bureau, M. & Genton P. (1998): Pronostic des épilepsies partielles non idiopathiques chez l'enfant de moins de six ans. In: *Epilepsies partielles graves pharmaco-résistantes de l'enfant*, eds. M. Bureau, P. Kahane & C. Munari, pp. 55–66. Montrouge: John Libbey Eurotext.

Bruton, C.J., Stevens, J.R. & Frith, C.D. (1994): Epilepsy, psychosis, and schizophrenia: clinical and neuropathologic correlations. *Neurology* **44**, 34–42.

Camfield, P.R., Gates, R., Ronen, G., Camfield, C., Ferguson, A. & MacDonald, G.W. (1984): Comparison of cognitive ability, personality profile, and school success in epileptic children with pure right versus left temporal lobe EEG foci. *Ann. Neurol.* **15**, 122–126.

Caplan, R., Shields, W.D., Morin, L. & Yudovin, S. (1991): Middle childhood onset of interictal psychosis: case studies. *J. Child Adolesc. Psychiatry* **30**, 893–896.

Caplan, R., Guthrie, D., Shields, W.D. & Mori, L. (1992): Formal thought disorder in pediatric complex partial seizure disorder. *J. Child. Psychiatr. Psychol.* **33**, 1399–1412.

Caplan, R., Guthrie, D., Shields, W.D. et al. (1993): Communication deficits in children undergoing temporal lobectomy. *J. Am. Acad. Child Adolesc. Psychiatry* **32**, 604–611.

Caplan, R., Guthrie, D., Shields, W.D. & Yudovin, S. (1994): Communication deficits in pediatric complex partial seizure disorder and schizophrenia. *Dev. Psychopathol.* **6**, 499–517.

Caplan, R. & Gillberg, C. (1997): Child psychiatric disorders. In: *Epilepsy. A comprehensive textbook*, eds. J. Engel, Jr & T.A. Pedley, pp. 2125–2139. Philadelphia, New York: Lippincott-Raven.

Cohen, M. (1992): Auditory/verbal and visual/spatial memory in children with complex partial epilepsy of temporal lobe origin. *Brain Cogn.* **20**, 315–326.

Deonna, T., Ziegler, A.L., Moura-Serra, J. & Innocenti, G. (1993): Autistic regression in relation to limbic pathology and epilepsy: report of two cases. *Dev. Med. Child Neurol.* **35**, 166–176.

Elger, C.E., Lendt, M., Helmstaedter, C. & Kowalik, A. (1998): Pre- and postoperative neuropsychological assessment of children with pharmaco-resistant epilepsies. In: *Epilepsies partielles graves pharmaco-résistantes de l'enfant*, eds. M. Bureau, P. Kahane & C. Munari, pp. 173–180. Montrouge: John Libbey Eurotext.

Falconer, M.A. (1973): Reversibility by temporal-lobe resection of the behavioral abnormalities of temporal lobe epilepsy. *N. Engl. J. Med.* **289**, 451–455.

Fedio, P. & Mirsky, A.F. (1969): Selective intellectual deficits in children with temporal lobe or centrencephalic epilepsy. *Neuropsychologia* **7**, 287–300.

Flor-Henry, P. (1969): Psychosis and temporal lobe epilepsy. *Epilepsia* **10**, 363–395.

Gilliam, F. (1997): Measuring the effect of paediatric epilepsy surgery on quality of life. In: *Paediatric epilepsy syndromes and their surgical treatment*, eds. I. Tuxhorn, H. Holthausen & H. Boegnik, pp. 85–90. London: John Libbey.

Guerrant, J., Anderson, W., Fischer, A., Weinstein, M. & Jaros, R.M. (1962): *Personality in epilepsy*. Springfield, IL: Charles C. Thomas.

Hermann, B.P. (1982): Neuropsychological functioning and psychopathology in children with epilepsy. *Epilepsia* **23**, 545–554.

Hermann, B.P., Schwartz, M.S., Karnes, W.E. & Vahdat, P. (1980): Psychopathology in epilepsy: relationship of seizure type to age at onset. *Epilepsia* **21**, 15–23.

Hermann, B.P., Whitman, S., Hugues, J.R., Melyn, M.M. & Dell, J. (1988): Multietiological determinants of psychopathology and social competence in children with epilepsy. *Epilepsy Res.* **2**, 51–60.

Hutt, S.J. & Hutt, C. (1970): Direct observation and the measurement of behaviour. Springfield IL: Charles .C. Thomas.

Jambaqué, I., Dellatolas, G., Dulac, O., Ponsot, G. & Signoret, J.L. (1993): Verbal and visual memory impairment in children with epilepsy. *Neuropsychologia* **31**, 1321–1337.

Kaminer, Y., Apter, A., Lerman, P. & Tyano, S. (1988): Psychopathology and temporal lobe epilepsy in adolescents. *Acta Psychiatr. Scand.* **77**, 640–644.

Lachar, D., Lewis, R. & Kupke, T. (1979): MMPI in differentiation of temporal lobe and non temporal lobe epilepsy: investigation of three levels of test performance. *J. Clin. Consult. Psychol.* **47**, 186–188.

Lennox, W. & Lennox, M.A. (1960): *Epilepsy and related disorders*. London: Churchill.

Lindsay, J., Ounsted, C. & Richards, P. (1979): Long-term outcome in children with temporal lobe seizures: social outcome and childhood factors. *Dev. Med. Child Neurol.* **21**, 285–298.

Mirsky, A.F., Primac, D.W., Marsan, C.A., Rosvold, H.E. & Stevens, J.R. (1960): A comparison of the psychological test performances of patients with focal and non-focal epilepsy. *Exp. Neurol.* **2**, 75–89.

Munari, C., Lo Russo, G., Minotti, L., Tassi, L., Francione, S., Hoffmann, D., Kahane, P., Pasquier, B., Baudain, D. & Benabid, A.L. (1998): Traitement chirurgical des épilepsies partielles graves de l'enfant: ce que la littérature peut nous apprendre. In: *Epilepsies partielles graves, pharmaco-résistantes de l'enfant: stratégies diagnostiques et traitements chirurgicaux*, eds. M. Bureau, P. Kahane & C. Munari, pp. 195–208. Montrouge: John Libbey Eurotext.

Nuffield, E. (1961): Neuro-physiology and behaviour disorders in epileptic children. *J. Ment. Sci.* **107**, 348–358.

Ounsted, C., Lindsay, J. & Norman, R. (1966): Biological factors in temporal lobe epilepsy. *Clinics in Developmental Medicine*, no. 22. Lavenham, Suffolk: The Lavenham Press Ltd.

Ounsted, C., Lindsay, J. & Richards, P. (1987): Temporal lobe epilepsy: a biographical study 1948–1986. Blackwell, Oxford: MacKeith Press.

Perini, G.I., Tosin, C., Carraro, C. *et al.* (1996): Interictal mood and personality disorder in temporal lobe epilepsy and juvenile myoclonic epilepsy. *J. Neurol. Neurosurg. Psychiatry* **61,** 601–605.

Pritchard, P.B., Lombroso, C.T. & McIntyre, M. (1980): Psychological complications of temporal lobe epilepsy. *Neurology* **30,** 227–232.

Rutter, M., Graham, P. & Yule, W. (1970): A neuropsychiatric study in childhood. *Clinics in Developmental Medicine*, Nos. 35–36. London: S.I.M.P. with Heinemann Medical.

Sherwin, I., Peron-Magnan, P., Bancaud, J., Bonis, A. & Talairach, J. (1982): Prevalence of psychosis in epilepsy as a function of the laterality of the epileptogenic lesion. *Arch. Neurol.* **39,** 621–625.

Small, J., Milstein, V. & Stevens, J.R. (1962): Are psychomotor epileptics different? *Arch. Neurol.* **7,** 330–338.

Soulayrol, R. (1999): *L'enfant foudroyé*. Paris: Odile Jacob.

Stevens, J.R. (1966): Psychiatric implications of psychomotor epilepsy. *Arch. Gen. Psychiat.* **14,** 461–471.

Stevens, J.R. (1975): Interictal clinical manifestations of complex partial seizures. In: *Advances in Neurology*, vol. 11, eds. J.K. Penry and D.D. Daly, pp. 85–112. New York: Raven Press.

Stevens, J.R. (1980): Biologic background of psychosis in epilepsy. In: *Advances in epileptology*, eds. R. Canger, F. Angeleri & J.K. Penry, pp. 167–172. New York: Raven Press.

Stores, G. (1978): School children with epilepsy at risk for learning and behavioral problems. *Dev. Med. Child Neurol.* **20,** 502–508.

Taylor, D.C. (1975): Factors influencing the occurrence of schizophrenia-like psychosis in patients with temporal lobe epilepsy. *Psychol. Med.* **5,** 249–254.

Taylor, D.C. (1996): Psychiatric aspects. In: *Epilepsy in children*, ed. S. Wallace, pp. 601–616. London: Chapman & Hall Medical.

Taylor, D.C. & Marsh, S.M. (1977): Neuropathology and social pathology: the effects of small lesions in the temporal lobe. In: *Tegretol in epilepsy: proceedings of an international meeting*. Macclesfield: Geigy.

Whitman, S., Hermann, B.P., Black, R.B. & Chhabria, S. (1982): Psychopathology and seizure type in children with epilepsy. *Psychol. Med.* **12,** 843–853.

Williams, J., Griebel, M.L., Sharp, G.B. & Boop, F.A. (1998): Cognition and behavior after temporal lobectomy in pediatric patients with intractable epilepsy. *Pediatr. Neurol.* **19,** 189–194.

Chapter 19

Perceptual and intellectual disturbances

Heinz Gregor Wieser

Department of Neurology, University Hospital, Frauenklinikstrasse 26, 8091 Zürich, Switzerland

Summary

Epileptic seizures may interfere with a normal life in several ways. Whereas in adults psychosocial restrictions, such as problems with the professional career and driving licence, often prevail, children present with different problems. These are due to substantial biologic differences in types of epilepsy seen in children, plasticity of the developing brain, different developmental stages during childhood, and psychosocial issues, including embarrassment, ridicule by their peers, and discrimination, as well as stress on the family. Children with intractable epilepsy may be unable to attend regular educational programmes or participate in normal recreational and social activities for their age. Normal development is often severely handicapped by recurrent seizures and high-dose antiepileptic drug treatment. Limbic seizures in children are often drug-resistant, might be associated with certain neurobehavioural peculiarities and might have a different aetiology compared to adults. In general, cortical dysgenesis is frequently encountered in childhood epilepsy. We list the various forms of migration disorders and report our experience with epilepsy surgery in children, concentrating on the Zürich amygdalohippocampectomy series. In particular we report histological findings of resected hippocampi showing granule cell dispersion of the dentate fascia. In agreement with most paediatric epilepsy surgery programmes we conclude that early surgery should be contemplated if a child with intractable epilepsy fulfills the criteria for epilepsy surgery.

Neurobehavioural, neuropsychological and psychiatric aspects of temporal lobe epilepsy

There is a long-standing interest in the psychiatric aspects of the epilepsies in general, and of temporal lobe epilepsy (TLE) in particular (Morel, 1860; Falret, 1860; Jackson, 1875, 1931–32; Glaus, 1931; Gibbs, 1951; Hill, 1953; Slater & Beard, 1963; Tellenbach, 1965; Ferguson & Rayport, 1984; Blumer, 1984; Smith *et al.*, 1991). Complex partial seizures themselves have been viewed as short-lived psychoses and the psychomotor status epilepticus (temporal lobe (TL) status epilepticus) is certainly a unique possibility to bridge the gap between neurology and psychiatry, as are other peri-ictal psychoses and mood changes (Wieser, 1980, 1992; Wieser *et al.*, 1985). For most doctors, seizures are the prime target of diagnostic and therapeutic efforts. A considerable number of patients and their relatives, however, suffer quite a lot in the interictal state and seek help because of the consequences of having seizures, or of having a brain disease which produces both seizures and neurobehavioural as well as psychiatric signs and symptoms.

Several general factors are associated with psychiatric morbidity, such as brain damage, difficulties with schooling and employment, interpersonal relationships, medication, and the stigma of epilepsy. In addition, more 'specific' personality and behavioural features associated with TLE have been described. The prevalence of psychiatric morbidity in the epilepsies is estimated by some psychiatrists as high as one third to one half (Fenwick et al., 1993). Although it remains controversial whether patients with TLE, compared to other types of the epilepsies, have an increased risk of psychopathology (Stevens, 1991), many authors have presented data which point in this direction (Gudmundson, 1966; Pond & Bidwell, 1960; Rodin et al., 1976; Trimble & Perez, 1980). The modern debate about the psychiatric disorders associated with epilepsy centres on personality and behaviour changes including irritability, on psychoses, and on mood disorders.

For many centuries epilepsy patients were forced into patterns of abnormal behaviour. 'Epileptic personality' traits have been discussed at length by psychiatrists (Freud, 1961; Szondi, 1963) and neurologists (Alajouanine, 1963; Geschwind, 1984). Formal studies of epileptic behavioural disturbances and personality aberrations performed since the advent of modern antiepileptic therapy, however, failed to demonstrate either an excess of psychiatric disorders in the epilepsy patients or a specific epileptic personality. Therefore, the term 'epileptic personality disorder', which suggests that behavioural problems exist in many epilepsy patients, is no longer acceptable.

The Geschwind Syndrome

Despite this, Geschwind described a set of behavioural abnormalities that he had observed in patients with TL seizure disorders. According to him the main characteristics of this syndrome are (i) increased concern with philosophical, moral, or religious issues; (ii) hypergraphia; (iii) hyposexuality; and (iv) irritability (Waxman & Geschwind, 1974, 1975; Geschwind, 1979). Blumer (1984) has described the following main features: (a) sexual changes, (b) impulsive/irritable behaviour, (c) good naturedness/religiosity, (d) deepening of emotional response (viscosity), and (e) alternating moods and epileptic psychoses. Benson (1991) then, in agreement with Geschwind and Blumer, Bear (1979) summarized the syndrome by listing three major areas of abnormalities: (i) **circumstantiality**, i.e. a tendency to be overinclusive, involving excessive and detailed verbal output, excessive writing (hypergraphia), and a clinging, tenacious attitude (viscosity); (ii) **altered sexuality**, i.e. almost always in the direction of hyposexuality, although rare instances of homosexuality, transvestitism, fetishism, etc., have been reported; and (iii) **intensification of cognitive and emotional behaviour**, i.e. tendency to develop a strong and deep interests in philosophic, religious, and emotional aspects of life. Geschwind and others have stressed the fact that this syndrome is specific for TLE, i.e. does not occur in extratemporal epilepsies and not in patients with TL damage without seizures. Consequently they hypothesized that the presence of an 'active epileptic focus' is necessary for the development of this syndrome, in the sense that the interictal discharges alter the synaptic reagibility. This kind of 'kindling' would then lead to a kind of 'sensory-limbic hyperconnection'.

Psychoses and **mood disorders** in epilepsy have often been regarded as a model for understanding psychiatric illness, in particular schizophrenia, since epilepsy opens a way of investigating organic mechanisms for episodic abnormal behaviour (Bruens, 1980). One of the essential questions is that of the causal relationships of epilepsy and psychosis, when both occur together. It is most obvious in ictal and postictal psychosis, such as psychomotor status and postictal delirious states. It is less obvious in the so-called alternating psychosis (Tellenbach, 1965). The observation of 'forced normalization' brought Landolt (1955, 1958, 1960) to the hypothesis that the psychosis would be a kind of physiologic reaction to the epileptic disturbance in the sense of an antithetical concept (Wieser, 1998). A similar reasoning led to the convulsive therapy of Meduna (1935).

A severe drawback of much of the work in this field is that 'psychosis' has been used without satisfactory definition by many authors. With regard to the schizophrenia-like psychosis and epilepsy, only the more recent work used the concepts of Kurt Schneider for the diagnosis of schizophrenia-like illness, relying in particular on the presence of first-rank symptomatology. In doing so, Perez & Trimble (1985) have stressed the fact that the syndrome profile of patients with schizophrenia-like symptoms and epilepsy, when compared to that of patients with schizophrenia without epilepsy, shows few but significant differences. These are the preservation of affective warmth and failure of personality deterioration in the majority of patients with schizophrenia-like psychosis and epilepsy, as described by Slater & Beard (1963) and Slater *et al.* (1965). The problem of laterality has been discussed ever since (Flor-Henry, 1969, 1972; Sherwin, 1981). There is some evidence that schizophreniform features are associated with left-sided temporal lobe lesions, but Flor-Henry's suggestion that right-sided abnormality is linked with a manic-depressive picture is less well supported from available data (Trimble, 1991).

Limbic seizures in children

Whereas in adults psychosocial restrictions, such as problems with the professional career and driving license, often prevail, children with epilepsy present with different problems. These relate to substantial biologic differences in types of epilepsy seen in children, plasticity of the developing brain, different developmental stages during childhood, and psychosocial issues, including embarrassment, ridicule by their peers, and discrimination, as well as stress on the family. Children with intractable epilepsy may be unable to attend regular educational programmes or participate in normal recreational and social activities for their age. Schooling and normal development is often severely handicapped by recurrent seizures and high-dose antiepileptic drug treatment.

In the literature on limbic seizures in children, differing opinions can be found regarding the question of whether the clinical, electrical and behavioural manifestations are similar in children and adults. Moshé *et al.* (1995) found a remarkable similarity, whereas other authors, such as Wyllie *et al.* (1993), reported major differences. For example Wyllie and collaborators found that the majority of children with TL tumours associated with seizures had much more 'complex' EEG findings with prominent extratemporal interictal spikes and sharp-waves and poorly defined seizure onset or false lateralization of EEG seizure patterns. Wide-spread and poorly localized sharp-waves were also noted by Glaser & Golub (1955). Furthermore, the pathological substrate of TLE in young children differs significantly from adults in that developmental rather than acquired or neoplastic lesions predominate. Cortical dysplasia is a common pathological substrate in paediatric TL-ectomy series.

Seizure onset in the 1st decade of life, especially infancy, is often associated with arrested development or frank regression. Neurobehavioural problems are frequently encountered in children with intractable epilepsy, in particular TLE, including specific learning deficits, mental retardation, attention problems, hyperactivity, rage attacks and aggression. Psychiatric disturbances, such as psychosis, depression, anxiety, and personality disorders may also be present, but are more often seen in older children and adolescents.

Benefits of early TL epilepsy surgery, and in particular mesial-limbic TL surgery in paediatric patients, include (a) cure of seizures, (b) improved personal and family quality of life, (c) and prevention of the long-term detrimental effects of intractable seizures in the developing years (Lindsay *et al.*, 1979a, b, c). The Bonn group, when analysing their paediatric epilepsy series with a view towards predictive factors for the development of behavioural disorders in children, came to the conclusion that density of focal spike activity and a neoplastic lesion were significantly associated with behavioural disorders, whereas the factors 'age of onset of epilepsy', 'age at surgery' as well as 'average seizure frequency' did not reach statistical significance (Elger *et al.*, 1997).

In larger surveys epilepsy surgery in children below age 15 years accounts for 20–25 per cent of surgical series (Table 1).

Table 1. Epilepsy surgery in children (less than 15 years)

ILAE survey (Silfvenius & Wieser, 1997)	428/1997	21.4%
Maudsley Hospital series (Polkey, 1996)	598/2340	24.6%

The Zürich amygdalohippocampectomy series

In Zürich TLE surgery was initiated in 1949 by the neurosurgeon H. Krayenbühl (Krayenbühl *et al.*, 1954). At that time, the patients admitted for surgical intervention and suffering from TLE received a 'classical', anterior two-third temporal, resection. A refinement of the presurgical evaluation was achieved by the introduction of the stereoelectroencephalography (SEEG) in 1969 with the aim of improving surgical results. The analysis of these SEEG findings resulted in the development of a microsurgical selective operation, the selective amygdalohippocampectomy (AHE; Wieser & Yasargil, 1982; Wieser, 1991), for the main subtype of the TLE, the syndrome of mesial temporal lobe epilepsy (MTLE; Wieser *et al.*, 1993; Wieser, 1997).

AHE is performed with a 'curative' (causal) or a 'palliative' intention. AHE is a rather standardized type of epilepsy surgery, although to a certain extent it is always individually tailored according to the preoperative and intraoperative findings.

Criteria for 'curative' AHE consist of (a) unequivocal unilateral mesial temporal focal seizure onset associated with typical clinical symptoms; (b) intact contralateral hippocampal functions, as determined by neuropsychological testing for learning and memory performance, including the selective memory amobarbital tests; (c) convergent results of non-invasive evaluation, such as MRI, PET, SPECT, ^{1}H-MRS, and electrophysiological findings.

A 'palliative' operation of this type might be indicated in patients in whom the primary epileptogenic zone is located in eloquent cortex (language-dominant posterior temporal neocortex) and cannot be removed without intolerable functional deficits. A palliative AHE, however, is only indicated when the ipsilateral hippocampal formation is rapidly involved by the ictal discharges and acts as a 'secondary pacemaker', i.e. a seizure sustaining substrate.

Table 2. Selective amygdalohippocampectomy series Zürich with type of lesions in children (grouped into < 3, 3–12, and 12–16 years) and postoperative seizure outcome

Age at op. (years)	n %	Neuropathology	Seizure Outcome Class*				
			I	II	III	IV	n.a.
0.2–2.9	4 0.7%	Hamartoma 1; Cort. Dysgenesis 1; Astrocyt. 2	2 50%	–	1 25%	1 25%	–
3–11.9	22 5.4%	Ganglioglioma 4; DNET 1; other Tumours 12; AVM 1, Tub. scl. 1	19 86%	–	–	1 4%	2 9%
12–16	24 5.9%	Ganglioglioma 5, Tub.scl. 2; Hamartoma 1; AVM 3	14 58%	3 12%	3 12%	2 8%	2 8%
0.2–16	50 12.1%		35 70%	3 6%	4 8%	4 8%	4 8%
Total series	406 100%		67%	8%	8%	12%	13%

n.a., not available; * Seizure outcome classification according to Engel et al. (1993) into classes I-IV is as follows:

Class I: Free of disabling seizures[a]

A. Completely seizure-free since surgery
B. Nondisabling simple partial seizures only since surgery
C. Some disabling seizures after surgery, but free of disabling seizures for at least 2 years
D. Generalized convulsions with antiepileptic drug withdrawal only

Class II: Rare disabling seizures ('almost seizure-free')

A. Initially free of disabling seizures but has rare seizures now
B. Rare disabling seizures since surgery
C. More than rare disabling seizures since surgery, but rare seizures for the last 2 years
D. Nocturnal seizures only

Class III: Worthwhile improvement[b]

A. Worthwhile seizure reduction
B. Prolonged seizure-free intervals amounting to greater than half the followed-up period, but not less than 2 years.

Class IV: No worthwhile improvement[b]

A. Significant seizure reduction
B. No appreciable change
C. Seizures worse

[a] Excludes early postoperative seizures (first few weeks).

[b] Determination of 'worthwhile improvement' will require quantitative analysis of additional data such as percentage seizure reduction, cognitive function, and quality of life.

However, the postsurgical epileptological and behavioural outcome depends, of course, on the underlying lesion. Cortical dysplasia was a common pathological substrate in the paediatric TL-ectomy series at Miami Children's Hospital (Duchowny et al., 1997): 53/61 paediatric patients showed cortical dysplasia (ectopic white matter neurons 52; cortical dyslamination 25; large and/or dysplastic neurons, nine), and 25/61 had tumours/hamartomas (glial-neuronal hamartoma 12, DNET 10, gangioglioma three, oligoastrocytoma one). In the Maudsley children series 21 per cent of resected specimens in children below 15 years had cortical dysplasia (Table 3).

Table 3. Pathology in resected specimens in children (Maudsley series; from Polkey, 1996)

	0–5 years	6–10 years	11–15 years	All	%
MTS	0	1	6	7	9%
Tumour	5	6	10	21	28%
Rasmussen's Disease	5	7	4	16	21%
Cortical dysplasia	4	5	7	16	21%
Other	1	4	8	13	18%
Non-specific	0	0	2	2	3%
All	15	23	37	75	
%	20%	31%	49%		100%

In our own experience the results of epilepsy surgery in children with well circumscribed lesions are better the earlier the operation and the shorter the time with persisting seizures. Fifty patients (12.1 per cent) of the Zürich amygdalohippocampectomy series were operated below age 16, and had a good seizure outcome (70 per cent seizure-free). This compares well with the seizure outcome of the entire AHE series (67 per cent seizure-free) (see Table 2).

It is obvious that patients with more widespread migration disorders usually show less good results in both epileptological and behavioural outcome measures. Therefore the frequency and types of neurodevelopmental abnormalities in a rather homogeneous series of 400 patients who underwent AHE in Zürich since 1975 because of drug-resistant MTLE was recently re-evaluated. In this retrospective study we described the histopathological abnormalities, classifying them into the classification scheme for cortical dysgenesis presenting with epilepsy (Raymond et al., 1995, 1996). The aetiology of cortical dysgenesis comprises defective genes and chromosomes, as well as extraneous factors affecting neuroblasts, guiding glial cells, or both. It might be acute or chronic. Cortical dysgenesis can be grouped as follows:

- **Abnormalities of gyration** comprise:
  - Lissencephaly ('smooth brain')
  - Type I & II [agyria-pachygyria]
  - Diffuse polymicrogyria
  - Focal macrogyria
  - Focal macrogyria/polymicrogyria associated with a cleft

- **Heterotopias** comprise of
  - Subependymal grey-matter heterotopias (nodular or diffuse)
  - Subcortical laminar grey matter heterotopias
  - Subcortical nodular grey matter heterotopias
  - Subarachnoid glioneuronal heterotopias

- **Cortical dysgenesis associated with neoplasia** comprise of
  - Dysembryoplastic neuroepithelial tumour (DNET)
  - CD with ganglioglioma
  - CD with low grade astrocytoma

- Within the **Schizencephaly group** one can list
  - Type I 'closed lip' schizencephaly
  - Type II 'open lip' schizencephaly

- Congenital bilateral perisylvian syndrome
  (= bilateral opercular polymicrogyria with widened Sylvian fissures; Kuzniecky et al., 1993)

In our epilepsy surgery series, besides minor gyral abnormalities, we found heterotopias, focal cortical dysplasia/microdysgenesis, and cortical dysgenesis associated with dysembryoblastic neuroepithelial tumour (DNET), with ganglioglioma, and with low-grade astrocytoma, as well as tuberous sclerosis-like abnormalities and duplication/dispersion of the dentate fascia.

Of particular interest is the disorganization of the granule cell layers of the dentate gyrus, and above all its duplication (Houser, 1990; Houser et al., 1992). This abnormality was viewed by some authors as dysgenesis of the archicortex (Raymond et al.,1996), although others discuss it as a consequence of and in association with hippocampal sclerosis.

Neuropathological – clinical correlations in patients with hippocampal sclerosis

From the Zürich AHE series of presently 426 patients we recently re-evaluated the available histopathological specimens of 75 patients with the diagnosis of hippocampal sclerosis. This histopathological re-evaluation comprised of the following hippocampal abnormalities including a ranking (not present, mild, marked, severe) of the degree of the following pathology: (1) gliosis, (2) neuronal loss, and (3) granule cell dispersion of the dentate fascia. Alteration of the hippocampal CA regions were carefully studied in order to classify the hippocampal sclerosis as typical (versus atypical) for MTLE. The typical ('classical') hippocampal sclerosis consists of marked gliosis and neuronal loss in CA1, CA3 and CA4, with CA2 spared.

Marked and severe gliosis were found in 97 per cent, marked and severe neuronal loss in 70 per cent and granular cell dispersion in 60 per cent of the 75 patients.

Patients with marked and severe hippocampal pathology differed significantly from those with normal or less severe hippocampal pathology with regard to outcome and age at surgery. Seizure onset was at younger age, duration of illness was longer, and the age at surgery was significantly higher in the group of patients with hippocampal pathology. The seizure outcome following AHE was significantly better in the presence of hippocampal pathology. Patients with hippocampal pathology had more often febrile convulsions. Patients with febrile convulsions had a trend for more severe granule cell dispersion.

Table 4. Correlation between some clinical data of all re-evaluated AHE patients and the types of hippocampal pathology

Correlation Coefficient	Gliosis	Neuronal loss	CA-regions	GC-dispersion	Age and seizure onset	Duration of illness	Age at surgery	Febrile convulsions
Neuronal loss	0.78***							
CA-regions	0.51***	0.25***						
GC-dispersion	0.66***	0.88***	0.21**					
Age and seizure onset	0.14	–0.15	0.22**	–0.06				
Duration of illness	0.09	0.20**	–0.02	0.16*	–0.45***			
Age at surgery	0.21*	0.02	0.20**	0.10	0.46***	0.55***		
Febrile convulsions	0.10	0.20**	0.01	0.26***	–0.14	–0.06	–0.15	
Outcome	0.33***	0.43**	0.11	0.34***	–0.14	0.11	–0.02	0.18*

CA-regions, alteration of the architecture of CA-regions; GC-dispersion, granule cells dispersion of the dentate fascia; *$P < 0.10$; **$P < 0.05$; ***$P < 0.01$

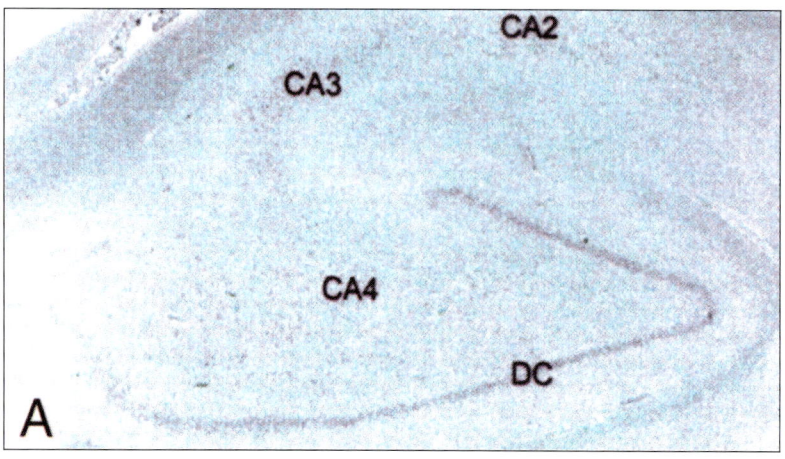
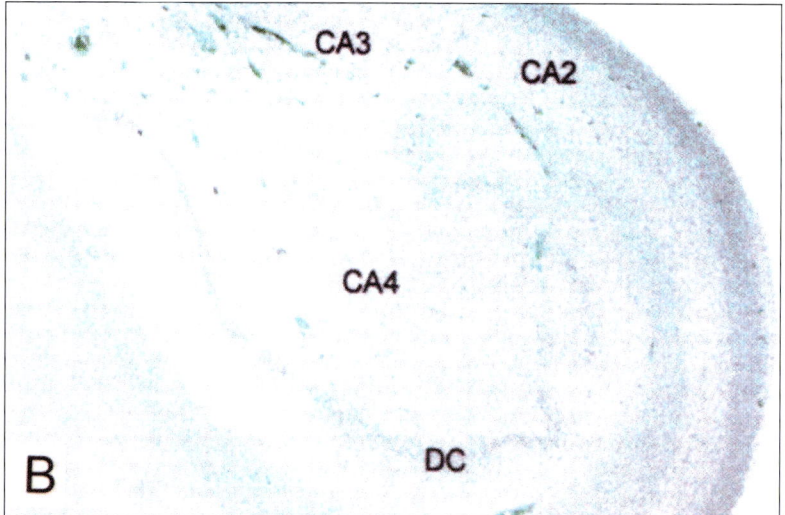
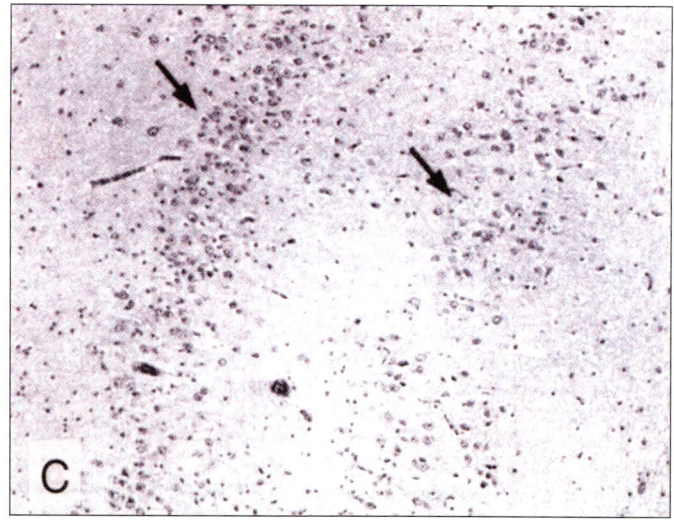

Fig. 1. Representative histopathological examples of human hippocampus.

A: H&E staining of a normal autopsy control. Regions CA4, CA3, CA2 and dendritic cell layer (DC).
B: Hippocampal sclerosis. H & E staining. Note the dispersed granule cell layer (DC), severe damage and neuronal loss of CA4 and CA3. In CA2 there are some neurons left.
C: Dispersed granule cells that form a bilaminar pattern (arrows) with a relatively neuron-free zone between the two layers (x 25).

Thus, from the analysis of our own surgical series we advocate early surgery in refractory epileptic children provided that there are reasonably good chances that a limited resection can significantly ameliorate the seizure tendency. If a tumour or a hamartoma is found, the chances that surgical removal of the lesion and its vicinity will render the patient seizure-free are high. The same holds true for the syndrome of MTLE in children.

Children with TLE have a higher risk of deficits in cognitive functioning. Many different factors contribute to cognitive impairment (Kastelejin-Nolst Trenité, 1996) and most of them are interrelated. The most important are: underlying brain pathology, seizures and so-called 'sub-clinical' brain epileptiform EEG discharges, antiepileptic drugs, and psychosocial factors, such as 'family support' (Crandall *et al.*, 1987). Behavioural syndromes of limbic TL, such as the 'impulse-dyscontrol syndrome' in the sense of a 'sensory-limbic hyperconnection' with hyperactivity and aggressive outbursts may play an important role in MTLE of children (Wieser, 1997).

Without surgery the prognosis of medically refractory patients with MTLE is relatively poor. Both severity and frequency of seizures may increase, and memory may decline, which may result in severe psychosocial disturbances. Early surgical intervention, i.e. relief of disabling seizures before the negative consequences of MTLE interfere critically with vocational and social development, results in best psychosocial outcome (Khan & Wieser, 1992) and should be envisaged in this prototype of a surgically remediable epileptic syndrome. Several groups have reported good surgical results in children with TLE (Meyer *et al.*, 1986; Drake *et al.*, 1987; Wieser, 1988; Fish *et al.*, 1991; Munari, 1995). Today the diagnosis of MTLE can be often made without resorting to invasive methods. If lateralization is a problem, 'semi-invasive' foramen ovale electrodes may be very helpful (Wieser & Moser, 1988; Wieser & Morris, 1996) and have been used to good effect in children by the Zürich group.

Pre- and postoperative antiepileptic drug treatment in the Zürich AHE series

It is reasonable to assume that for the development of a child the types and amounts of drug intake are of considerable importance. Therefore seizure outcome measures alone, without quality-of-life and AED measurement, are not very useful. With this in mind we have studied the amount and type of AED treatment before and after AHE in relation to seizure outcome on a year-to-year basis.

Pre-operatively all non-tumoural patients were by definition drug-resistant. They had taken all first-line AEDs, and most of the patients had taken more than two 'new AEDs'. At time of surgery the majority of patients took three AEDs. One year postoperatively 65 per cent of the entire AHE patients were seizure-free, but only 24 per cent of the seizure-free patients had discontinued AED treatment. Considering all patients of this series (including so-called 'lesional' cases, i.e. tumours and other gross lesions), 1 year postoperatively 16 per cent had no AED, 46 per cent had one AED, 24 per cent had two AEDs, and 14 per cent had more than two AEDs. Considering only so-called 'non-tumoural' cases, 1 year postoperatively 1 per cent, 2 years postoperatively 11 per cent, 5 years postoperatively 35 per cent, and 10 years postoperatively 65 per cent of the seizure-free patients were off AEDs.

Concluding remarks

Among the localization-related epilepsies TLE is the most common when the medically refractory patients are considered. It has also been known for many years that cortical dysgenesis is common in children. The most common pathologic substrate of TLE is hippocampal sclerosis. Data accumulated from surgical series strongly suggest that TLE associated with hippocampal sclerosis represents a distinctive epileptic syndrome, the so-called 'Mesial temporal lobe epilepsy' (MTLE). Early diagnosis of the situation is important because disabling seizures and their consequences can be prevented by surgical intervention, either by limited anterior temporal lobectomy or selective amygdalohippocampectomy in 70–90 per cent of patients (Engel & Pedley, 1997; Tuxhorn et al., 1997; Wallace, 1996; Roger et al., 1992).

MTLE is remediable by surgery when it is correctly identified and differentiated from other TLE types. The diagnosis is based on aetiology, seizure history, clinical presentation, progressive nature, intractability, and special features in electrophysiological, neuropsychological, structural and functional imaging, and histopathological examinations. For the correct diagnosis and treatment the entire clinical and paraclinical set of findings has to be taken into consideration, not only one parameter. With the availability of special high-resolution MRI techniques, including volumetry and densimetry, the preoperative diagnosis and recognition of MTLE with hippocampal sclerosis undoubtedly became much easier and, most importantly, less invasive. In many previously published surgical series patient data was mainly evaluated according to the type and localization of gross pathological findings, but without considering in detail whether the key features of a MTLE syndrome were present or not. With this in mind we re-evaluated the available histological specimens of those patients who had the initial diagnosis of hippocampal sclerosis and correlated some clinical data with the various hippocampal pathology categories. In doing so highly significant correlations were seen between seizure outcome and gliosis, neuronal loss, and granule cell dispersion of the dentate fascia. Patients with hippocampal pathology had significantly better seizure outcome. Patients with febrile convulsions had a trend for better seizure outcome, and a severe granule cell dispersion.

With a progressive epilepsy with the seizure focus in the limbic cortex it is well understandable that children with intractable epilepsy may be unable to attend regular educational programmes or participate in normal recreational and social activities for their age. All this may prevent a normal development and may lead to neurobehavioural peculiarities.

References

Alajouanine, T. (1963): Dostojevski's epilepsy. *Brain* **86**, 209–218.

Bear, D.M. (1979): Temporal lobe epilepsy. A syndrome of sensory-limbic hyperconnection. *Cortex* **15**, 357–384.

Benson, D.F. (1991): The Geschwind syndrome. In: *Neurobehavioural problems in epilepsy,* eds. D. Smith, D. Treiman & M. Trimble, *Advances in Neurology,* vol. 55, pp. 411–421. New York: Raven Press.

Blumer, D. (1984): *Psychiatric aspects of epilepsy.* Washington, DC: American Psychiatric Press.

Bruens, J.H. (1980): Psychosis in epilepsy: historic concepts and new developments. In: *Advances in epileptology,* eds. R. Canger, F. Angeleri & J.K. Penry, XIth Epilepsy International Symposium, pp. 161–166. New York: Raven Press.

Crandall, P.H., Rausch, R. & Engel, J., Jr. (1987): Preoperative indicators for optimal surgical outcome for temporal lobe epilepsy. In: *Presurgical evaluation of epileptics,* eds. H.G. Wieser & C.E. Elger, pp. 325–334. Berlin: Springer.

Drake, J., Hoffmann, H.J., Kobayashi, J., Hwang, P. & Becker, L.E. (1987): Surgical management of children with temporal lobe epilepsy and mass lesions. *Neurosurgery* **21**, 792–797.

Duchowny, M., Harvey, A.S., Jayakar, P., Resnick, T., Alvarez, L., Gilman, J. & Dean, P. (1997): The preoperative evaluation of pediatric temporal lobe epilepsy. In: *Paediatric epilepsy syndromes and their surgical treatment*, eds. I. Tuxhorn, H. Holthausen & H. Boenigk, pp. 261–273. London: John Libbey.

Elger, C.E., Brockhaus, A., Lendt, M., Kowalik, A. & Steidele, S. (1997): Behaviour and cognition in children with temporal lobe epilepsy. In: *Paediatric epilepsy syndromes and their surgical treatment*, eds. I. Tuxhorn, H. Holthausen & H. Boenigk, pp. 311–325. London: John Libbey.

Engel, J. Jr. & Pedley, T.A. (eds.) (1997): *Epilepsy. A comprehensive textbook*. Volumes I–III. Philadelphia: Lippincott-Raven.

Engel, J. Jr, Van Ness, P.C., Rasmussen, T. & Ojemann, L.M. (1993): Outcome with respect to epileptic seizures. In: *Surgical treatment of the epilepsies*, ed. J. Engel, Jr., pp. 609–621. New York: Raven Press.

Falret, J. (1860): De l'état mental des épileptiques. *Arch. Gen. Med.* **16,** 661–679.

Fenwick, P.B.C., Blumer, D., Caplan, R., Ferguson, S.M., Sarard, G. & Victoroff, J.I. (1993): Presurgical psychiatric assessment. In: *Surgical treatment of the epilepsies*, 2nd edn., ed. J. Engel, Jr., pp. 273–290. New York: Raven Press.

Ferguson, S.M. & Rayport, M. (1984): Psychosis and epilepsy. In: *Psychiatric aspects of epilepsy*, ed. D. Blumer, pp. 229–270. Washington, DC: American Psychiatric Press.

Fish, D.R., S.J. Smith, F., Quesney, F., Andermann, F. & Rasmussen, T. (1991): Surgical treatment of children with medically intractable frontal or temporal lobe epilepsy: results and highlights of 40 years experience. *Epilepsia* **34,** 244–247.

Flor-Henry, P. (1969): Psychosis and temporal lobe epilepsy. *Epilepsia* **10,** 363–395.

Flor-Henry, P. (1972): Ictal and interictal psychiatric manifestations of epilepsy. Specific or non-specific? *Epilepsia* **13,** 773–783.

Freud, S. (1961): Dostojevsky and parricade. In: *The Standard Edition of the Complete Works of Sigmund Freud*, ed. J. Strachey, vol. 21, pp. 177–196. London: Hogarth Press.

Geschwind, N. (1979): Behavioural changes in temporal lobe epilepsy. *Psychol. Med.* **9,** 217–219.

Geschwind, N. (1984): Dostojevski's epilepsy. In: *Psychiatric aspects of epilepsy*, ed. D. Blumer, pp. 325–334. Washington, DC: American Psychiatric Press.

Gibbs, F.A. (1951): Ictal and nonictal psychiatric disorders in temporal lobe epilepsy. *J. Ment. Dis.* **133,** 522–528.

Glaser, G.H. & Golub, L.M. (1955): The electroencephalogram of psychomotor seizures in childhood. *Electroencephalogr. Clin. Neurophysiol.* **7,** 329–340.

Glaus, A. (1931): Ueber Combination von Schizophrenie und Epilepsie. *Zbl. Neurol. Psychiatr.* **135,** 450–550.

Gudmundson, G. (1966): Epilepsy in Iceland: a clinical and epidemiological investigation. *Acta Neurol. Scand.* **23** (Suppl. 25), 100–114.

Hill, D. (1953): Psychiatric disorders of epilepsy. *Med. Press* **229,** 473–475.

Houser, C.R. (1990): Granule cell dispersion in the dentate gyrus of humans with temporal lobe epilepsy. *Brain Res.* **535,** 195–204.

Houser, C.R., Swartz, B.E., Walsh, G.O. & Delgado-Escueta, A.V. (1992): Granule cell disorganisation in the dentate gyrus: possible alterations of neuronal migration in human temporal lobe epilepsy. In: *Molecular neurobiology of epilepsy*, eds. J. Engel Jr., C. Wasterlain, E.A. Calvalheiro, U. Heinemann & G. Avanzini, pp. 41–49. Amsterdam: Elsevier.

Jackson, J.H. (1875): On temporary mental disorders after epileptic paroxysms. In: *Selected Writings of John Hughlings Jackson*, ed. J. Taylor, vol. 1, pp. 119–134. London: Staples Press.

Jackson, J.H. (1931–1932): *Selected writings of John Hughlings Jackson* (2 vols). London: Hodder & Stoughton.

Kasteleijn-Nolst Trenité, D. (1996): Cognitive aspects. In: *Epilepsy in children,* ed. S. Wallace, pp. 581–599. London: Chapman & Hall Medical.

Khan, N. & Wieser, H.G. (1992): Psychosocial outcome of patients with amygdalohippocampectomy. *J. Epilepsy* **5**, 128–134.

Krayenbühl, H., Hess, R. & Weber, G. (1954): Elektroenzephalographische und therapeutische Ergebnisse in der Behandlung von 21 Fällen mit sogenannter Temporallappenepilepsie. *Zentralbl. Neurochir.* **14** (4/5), 205–211.

Kuzniecky, R., Andermann, F. & Guerrini, R. (1993) The CBPS Multicenter Collaborative Study. *Lancet* **341**, 608–612.

Landolt, H. (1955): Ueber Verstimmungen, Dämmerzustände und schizophrene Zustandsbilder bei Epilepsie. *Schweiz. Arch. Neurol. Psychiatr.* **76**, 313–321.

Landolt, H. (1958): Serial electroencephalographic investigations during psychotic episodes in epileptic patients and during schizophrenia attacks. In: *Lectures on Epilepsy,* ed. A. Lorentz de Haas, pp. 91–133. Amsterdam: Elsevier.

Landolt, H. (1960): *Die Temporallappenepilepsie und ihre Psychopathologie. Ein Beitrag zur Kenntnis psychophysischer Korrelationen bei Epilepsie und Hirnläsionen.* Basel, New York: Karger.

Lindsay, J., Ounsted, C. & Richards, P. (1979a): Long-term outcome in children with temporal lobe seizures. I: Social outcome and childhood factors. *Dev. Med. Child Neurol.* **21**, 285–298.

Lindsay, J., Ounsted, C. & Richards, P. (1979b): Long-term outcome in children with temporal lobe seizures. II: Marriage, parenthood and sexual indifference. *Dev. Med. Child Neurol.* **21**, 433–440.

Lindsay, J., Ounsted, C. & Richards, P. (1979c): Long-term outcome in children with temporal lobe seizures. III: Psychiatric aspects in childhood and adult life. *Dev. Med. Child Neurol.* **21**, 630–636.

Meduna, L. Von (1935): Versuche über die biologische Beeinflussung des Ablaufs der Schizophrenie. I. Campher- und Cardiazolkrämpfe. *Z. Gesamte Neurol.Psychiatr.* **152**, 235–262.

Meyer, F.B., Marsh, R.W., Laws, E.R. & Sharbrough, F.W. (1986): Temporal lobectomy in children with epilepsy. *J. Neurosurg.* **64**, 371–376.

Morel, B.A. (1860): D'une forme de délire, suite d'une surexcitation nerveuse se rattachant à une variété non encore décrite d'épilepsie (épilepsie larvée). *Gaz. Hebd. Med. Chir.* **7**, 773–775, 819–821, 836–841.

Moshé, S.L., Shinnar, S. & Swann, J.W. (1995): Partial (focal) seizures in developing brain. In: *Brain development and epilepsy,* eds. P.A. Schwartzkroin, S.L. Moshé, J.L. Noebels & J.W. Swann, pp. 34–65. New York: Oxford University Press.

Munari, C. (1995): Methodologies, results and limits of epilepsy surgery in children. *Gaslini* **27** (Suppl. I al N 2), 48–53.

Perez, M. & Trimble, M.R. (1985): Epileptic psychosis – a diagnostic comparison with process schizophrenia. *Br. J. Psychiatry* **146**, 155–163.

Polkey, C.E. (1996): Surgical treatment of epilepsy in children. In: *Epilepsy in children,* ed. S. Wallace, pp. 561–579. London: Chapman & Hall Medical.

Pond, D. & Bidwell, B. (1960): A survey of epilepsy in 14 general practices. II: social and psychosocial aspects. *Epilepsia* **1**, 285–299.

Raymond, A.A., Fish, D.R., Sisodiya, S.M., Alsanjari, N., Stevens, J.M. & Shorvon, S.D. (1995): Abnormalities of gyration, heterotopias, tuberous sclerosis, focal cortical dysplasia, microdysgenesis, dysembryoplastic neuroepithelial tumour and dysgenesis of the archicortex in epilepsy. Clinical, EEG and neuroimaging features in 100 adult patients. *Brain* **118**, 629–660.

Raymond, A.A., Fish, D.R., Sisodoya, S.M. & Shorvon, S.D. (1996): The developmental basis of epilepsy. In: *The treatment of epilepsy,* eds. S. Shorvon, F. Dreifuss, D. Fish & D. Thomas, pp. 20–54. Oxford: Blackwell Science.

Rodin, E., Katz, M. & Lennox, D. (1976): Differences between patients with temporal lobe seizures and those with other forms of epileptic attacks. *Epilepsia* **17**, 313–320.

Roger, J., Bureau, M., Dravet, Ch., Dreifuss, F.E., Perret, A. & Wolf, P. (eds.) (1992): *Epileptic syndromes in infancy, childhood and adolescence,* 2nd edn. London: John Libbey.

Sherwin, I. (1981): Psychosis associated with epilepsy: significance of laterality of the epileptogenic lesion. *J. Neurol. Neurosurg. Psychiatry* **44**, 83–85.

Silfvenius, H. & Wieser H.G. (1997): ILAE Commission Report: A global survey on epilepsy surgery, 1980–1990: a report by the Commission on Neurosurgery of Epilepsy, The International League against Epilepsy. *Epilepsia* **38**, 249–255.

Slater, E. & Beard, A.W. (1963): The schizophrenia-like psychoses of epilepsy. *Br. J. Psychiatry* **109**, 95–150.

Slater, E., Beard, A.W. & Glithero E. (1965): Schizophrenia-like psychosis of epilepsy. *Int. J. Psychiatry* **1**, 6–8.

Smith, D., Treiman, D. & Trimble, M.R. (eds.) (1991): *Neurobehavioral problems in epilepsy. Advances in neurology*, vol. 55, pp. 411–421. New York: Raven Press.

Stevens, J.R. (1991): Psychosis and the temporal lobe. In: *Neurobehavioral problems in epilepsy. Advances in Neurology*, vol. 55, eds. D. Smith, D. Treiman & M.R. Trimble, pp. 79–96. New York: Raven Press.

Szondi, L. (1963): *Schicksalsanalytische Therapie*. Bern: Huber.

Tellenbach, H. (1965): Epilepsie als Anfallsleiden und als Psychose. Ueber alternative Psychosen paranoider Prägung bei 'forcierter Normalisierung' (Landolt) des Elektroencephalogramms Epileptischer. *Nervenarzt* **36**, 190–202.

Trimble, M.R. (1991): Interictal psychoses of epilepsy. In: *Neurobehavioral problems in epilepsy. Advances in Neurology*, vol. 55, eds. D. Smith, D. Treiman & M.R. Trimble, pp. 143–152.

Trimble, M.R. & Perez, P. (1980): The phenomenology of the chronic psychosis of epilepsy. *Adv. Biol. Psychiatry* **8**, 98–105.

Tuxhorn, I., Holthausen, H. & Boenigk, H. (eds.) (1977): *Paediatric epilepsy syndromes and their surgical treatment*. London: John Libbey.

Wallace, S. (ed.) (1996): *Epilepsy in children*. London: Chapman & Hall Medical.

Waxman, S.G. & Geschwind, N. (1974): Hypergraphia in temporal lobe epilepsy. *Neurology* **24**, 629–638.

Waxman, S.G. & Geschwind, N. (1975): The interictal behavioral syndrome of temporal lobe epilepsy. *Ann. Gen. Psychiatry* **32**, 1580–1586.

Wieser, H.G. (1988): Presurgical evaluation and surgical therapy of children suffering from drug-resistant partial epilepsies. *Electroenceph. Clin. Neurophysiol.* **70**, 16.

Wieser, H.G. (1991): Selective amygdalohippocampectomy: indications, investigative technique and results. In: *Advances and technical standards in neurosurgery*, eds. L. Symon *et al.*, vol. 13, pp. 39–133. Vienna: Springer.

Wieser, H.G. (1992): Behavioural consequences of temporal lobe resections. In: *The temporal lobes and the limbic system*, eds. M.R. Trimble & T.G. Bolwig, pp. 169–188. Petersfield, UK: Wrightson Biomedical Publishing.

Wieser, H.G. (1997): The syndrome of mesial temporal lobe epilepsy. In: *Paediatric epilepsy syndromes and their surgical treatment*, eds. I. Tuxhorn, H. Holthausen & H. Boenigk, pp. 242–250. London: John Libbey.

Wieser, H.G. (1998): Electrophysiological aspects of forced normalization. In: *Forced normalization and alternative psychoses of epilepsy*, eds. M.R. Trimble & Bettina Schmitz, pp. 95–119. Petersfield, UK: Wrightson Biomedical Publishing.

Wieser, H.G. & Morris, H. (1996): Foramen ovale and peg electrodes. In: *Epilepsy: a comprehensive textbook*, eds. J. Engel Jr. & T.A. Pedley. New York: Raven Press.

Wieser, H.G. & Moser, S. (1988): Improved multipolar foramen ovale electrode monitoring. *J. Epilepsy* **1**, 13–22.

Wieser, H.G. & Yasargil, M.G. (1982): Selective amygdalohippocampectomy as a surgical treatment of mesiobasal limbic epilepsy. *Surg. Neurol.* **17**, 445–457.

Wieser, H.G. (1980): Temporal lobe or psychomotor status epilepticus. A case report. *Electroenceph. Clin. Neurophysiol.* **48**, 558–572.

Wieser, H.G., Hailemariam, S., Regard, M. & Landis, T. (1985): Unilateral limbic epileptic status activity: Stereo-EEG, behavioural, and cognitive data. *Epilepsia* **26,** 19–29.

Wieser, H.G., Engel, J. Jr., Williamson, P.D., Babb, T.L. & Gloor, P. (1993): Surgically remediable temporal lobe syndromes. In: *Surgical treatment of epilepsies*, ed. J. Engel Jr., pp. 49–63. New York: Raven Press.

Wyllie, E., Chee, M., Granström, M.L., Del Giudice, E., Estes, M., Comair, Y., Pizzi, M., Kotagal, P., Bourgeois, B. & Lüders, H. (1993): Temporal lobe epilepsy in early childhood. *Epilepsia* **34,** 859–868.

Chapter 20

Ictal EEG during limbic seizures in children

Laura Tassi, Giorgio Lo Russo and Claudio Munari

Centro Regionale Chirurgia dell'Epilessia 'Claudio Munari', Ospedale Niguarda Ca' Granda, Piazza Ospedale Maggiore 3, 20162 Milan, Italy

Summary

Clinical data, ictal event observation, MRI and EEG data, possible morphologies of the first electrical changes, as well as the occurrence of some types of well-localized ictal discharges, together allow the formulation of some localizing hypotheses.

Several uncertainties as to the adult semiology of limbic seizures are even more marked in childhood population. Children are usually suffering from symptomatic epilepsy and sometimes their young age prevents identification of ictal subjective manifestations. We selected a sample of children for whom surgical treatment of drug-resistant partial epilepsy had been recommended, where temporal origin of seizures was unquestionable and surface or depth video recordings had been performed.

Localizing diagnosis was again based on anatomo-electroclinical correlations. Interictal EEG is inadequate to this aim, since it mostly localizes abnormalities in a much larger area than the temporal; whereas the recording of ictal events, and especially well localized low voltage fast activities, is much more relevant when carefully correlated to clinical events.

Among the different possible localizations, those originating in the temporal lobe are undoubtedly the most frequent. However, this defines the temporal lobe as a mere appendix to limbic structures, which are not necessarily related to an ictal discharge.

Further studies are needed, applying invasive procedures to record from mesial and lateral structures simultaneously, in order to define the true role of the limbic lobe in triggering temporal seizures, especially in children. Clearly, electrophysiological data must be related to clinical data gathered by careful clinical observation and by accurate ictal questioning.

Introduction

Among presurgical diagnostic procedures, EEG monitoring associated with video allows not only the identification of the very first electrical changes, but also to compare and relate them to clinical manifestations.

In order to define anatomo-electroclinical correlations, a few requirements must be met:

- a comprehensive clinical history, carefully gathered from the patient himself/herself and his/her relatives or any witness to the ictal event;
- adequate questioning in the course of the ictal event during video-EEG recording;
- neuroimaging studies focused on the area supposedly responsible for ictal discharges;
- analysis of interictal and especially ictal EEG findings, in the attempt to identify the first and possibly well localized EEG change related to the first clinical manifestation (whether subjective, reported by the patient, or objective, detected by the observer), keeping in mind that in most cases the ictal discharge precedes the clinical signs (Broglin et al., 1991; Bancaud et al., 1985).

On the basis of these data and the knowledge of the possible morphologies of the first electrical changes, the occurrence of some types of well localized ictal discharges (low voltage fast activity and flattening) allows some localizing hypotheses.

As far as the 'limbic' localization of children epilepsies is concerned, many questions are still unanswered:

- what are the boundaries of the limbic system;
- whether these epilepsies can be related to epilepsies originating in the temporal lobe, which nevertheless includes several extra limbic cortical structures;
- whether children and adult populations differ in any way.

All the uncertainties above are greater in the childhood population, about whom, for different reasons, even less is known (Aicardi, 1994; Marchini et al., 1988; Munari, 1995). Children are usually suffering from symptomatic epilepsy and sometimes their young age prevents identification of ictal subjective manifestations, even when present. We therefore selected a sample of children for whom surgical treatment of drug-resistant partial epilepsy had been recommended, temporal origin of seizures was unquestionable and surface or depth video recordings had been performed.

Material and methods

From 1990 to 1998, 13 children underwent surgery for drug-resistant partial epilepsy at the Grenoble and Milan Centres for Epilepsy Surgery (Fig. 1): the following were the criteria to enter the study:

- patients were studied by video-EEG and/or video-stereo-EEG, as part of presurgical evaluation, with recording of spontaneously occurring ictal events;
- seizures should originate from the temporal lobe;
- surgical resection did not extend beyond the anatomical boundaries of the temporal lobe;
- patients had been seizure-free since surgery.

Among others, the general features of the selected sample (Fig. 2) included a mean age of 12 years, a very early onset (mean age: 2 years) and a very long duration of disease (about 10 years). Seizure frequency was about 16 seizures in a month, i.e. at least four weekly seizures.

1990-1998
CHU Grenoble - Ospedale Niguarda Milano
13 children operated on for a partial drug-resistant epilepsy and:
temporal lobe origin
only temporal resection
seizure-free since surgery
Video-EEG and/or Stereo-EEG recorded seizures

Fig. 1.

GENERAL CHARACTERISTICS

13 children:	6 girls - 7 boys	
Age:	12,3 y	(5-16)
Onset:	2,2 y	(5m-8y)
Duration:	10,0 y	(1-15)
Seiz. Frequency:	16/m	(4-60)

ATCD:
 none: 8
 FC: 5
Symptomatic: 9 pts
Cryptogenetic: 4 pts (3MTS)

Fig. 2.

As for the previous history, it was silent in eight out of 13 children, while febrile convulsions had been present in five. Histological examination at surgery disclosed an anatomical lesion in nine out of 13 patients; in four children no specific lesions were found, except mesial temporal sclerosis in three cases. As part of the presurgical evaluation, 11 children underwent video-EEG monitoring and seven were studied by intracerebral implanted electrodes (Fig. 3). Stereotactic procedures were not necessary in two patients only. Surgical treatment consisted of cortectomy in four patients (with cryptogenic epilepsy) and lesionectomy with cortectomy in nine patients. All patients have been seizure-free since surgery (after a follow-up of more than 12 months in all cases).

Results

Video-EEG recordings

Video-EEG monitoring provide two different kinds of information: the distribution of interictal abnormalities and the electrical patterns during seizures.

GENERAL CHARACTERISTICS

Video-EEG:		11
Stereo-EEG		7
Video-EEG & Stereo-EEG		5
Video-EEG only		6
Stereo-EEG only		2
A+V:		8
A+V+Biopsies:		3
No stereotactic procedures:		2
Surgery	C:	4 pts
	C+L:	9 pts

Fig. 3.

INTERICTAL EEG

Background activity
 - symmetric: 5 pts
 - asymmetric: 8 pts

Slow-waves
 - lobar, well localized: 3 pts
 - lobar: 1
 - bilobar: 6
 - bilateral: 1
 - none: 2

Spikes
 - lobar, well localized: 6 pts
 - lobar: 0
 - bilobar: 2
 - multilobar: 1
 - none: 4
 - synchronous bilateral: 4

Fig. 4.

```
ICTAL Video-EEG

57 spontaneous seizures recorded:

- low voltage fast activity:    12/4 pts
- flattening:                   34/9 pts
- rhythmic spikes:               2/1 pt
- rhythmic slow waves:           1/1 pt
- not interpretable:             8/2 pts
```

Fig. 5.

```
Video-EEG: 57 spontaneous seizures recorded:

29/57: initial discharge well localized into
the temporal lobe.

  8 low voltage fast activity    18 flattening
  1 rhythmic slow waves           2 rhythmic spikes

  ─────────────────────────────────────

  6 without subjective manifestations
  7 isolated subjective manifestations
 16 with subjective and objectivable signs
```

Fig. 6.

Interictal abnormalities

In eight children background rhythm was asymmetric at the expense of the hemisphere where ictal discharges started. As often occurs in drug-resistant patients, interictal abnormalities could be well localized in few patients (in three cases for slow waves and in six cases for spike abnormalities), while they could involve two adjacent lobes in six patients with slow waves and in two patients with spikes. Four children showed interictal bilateral and synchronous spike-waves (Fig. 4).

Ictal activity

Fifty-seven seizures were recorded in 11 patients (Fig. 5). Twelve of them were characterized by a well localized low voltage fast activity and 34 by a similarly well localized flattening. Instances of rhythmic spikes or rhythmic slow wave discharges, once considered typical of temporal seizures, were only three out of 57.

Among these 57 spontaneous seizures, 29 were characterized by an early discharge well localized in the temporal lobe (Fig. 6). The clinical features of these 29 seizures consisted of isolated subjective disturbances in six cases, objective manifestations in seven and both in 16. The

```
Video-EEG
7 isolated subjective manifestations/2 pts

   7 epigastric feeling/2 pts

6 without subjective manifestations/3 pts

   arms elevation      1/1 pt
   polypnoea           3/1 pt
   smiling             1/1 pt
   lachrymation        1/1 pt
   staring             1/1 pt
   chewing             2/2 pts
```

Fig. 7.

```
Video-EEG
16 with subjective and objectivable signs/7 pts

   Subjective manifestations

      epigastric          9/4 pts
      cephalic            4/1 pt
      fear                3/1 pt
      gustatory hall.     1/1 pt
      olfactory hall.     1/1 pt
      auditory ill.       1/1 pt
      psych. manifest.    1/1 pt
      shiver              1/1 pt
```

Fig. 8.

isolated subjective disturbances recorded in two patients consisted of epigastric feeling. Among objective manifestations without subjective prodromic symptoms polypnea and chewing automatisms were the most frequent (Fig. 7).

In seizures in which subjective disturbances were followed by objective signs, the most frequent subjective symptoms were epigastric (nine cases) or cephalic sensations (four cases) and fear (three cases) (Fig. 8). Among objective signs (Fig. 9), staring (eight cases), fear expression (five cases) and gestural automatisms (four cases).

Video-stereo-EEG monitoring

Seven patients were studied by intracerebral implanted electrodes (stereo-EEG), unilaterally in all cases, with 67 electrodes (mean 9.5 in each patient) (Fig. 10) (Munari et al., 1994).

Only one patient did not present spontaneous attacks but only seizures induced by intracerebral electrical stimulation. Nineteen spontaneous seizures were recorded in the remaining six patients. Out of these 19 seizures (Fig. 11), six were characterized by early involvement of limbic structures; in one case the discharge was limited to the amygdala, without concomitant clinical symptomatology. In the other seizures the temporal neocortex was involved simultaneously. In the six seizures in which clinical manifestations accompanied a discharge limited to mesial temporal structures (Fig. 12), objective abnormalities were observed in one case only (staring, chewing and loss of contact), with an early discharge in the amygdala and hippocampus. In two cases the discharge induced epigastric feeling (in one case associated with fear, in the other ascending) and both the amygdala and the hippocampus were involved by the discharge. In three other cases the discharge involved the amygdala and the hippocampus (two cases) and only the amygdala (one case), accompanied by a cephalic sensation and subjective tachycardia.

Discussion

As to the procedures to define the syndromic features of epilepsy or merely to ascertain its presence, evidence from the literature suggests the need to perform video-EEG recordings in children with epilepsy, both to determine the extension of the epileptogenic zone in view of surgery and, at least preliminarily, to make diagnostic and therapeutic decisions.

Moreover, this diagnostic procedure is considered absolutely necessary in the children population also in order to limit invasive diagnostic investigations (Holmes, 1989; Mizrahi et al., 1990; Hopkins & Klug, 1991; Davies & Weeks, 1995; Blume et al., 1997). However, despite a generic agreement about the fact that video-EEG should be performed, even if expensive (Wyllie, 1991; Mitchell et al., 1991; Swick et al., 1996), in fact most groups utilize only interictal EEG recordings (Davidson & Falconer, 1975; Linsday et al., 1984; Goldring, 1987; Chugani et al., 1988; Lüders et al., 1989; Adler et al., 1991; Ribaric et al., 1991; Cascino & Herkes, 1993; Guldvog et al., 1994), often associated with so called 'non invasive' procedures such as anterior temporal, sphenoidal, nasopharyngeal and foramen ovale electrodes (Falconer et al., 1955; Davidson & Falconer, 1975; Duchowny, 1987; Wyllie et al., 1990; Lüders et al., 1989; Adler et al., 1991; Erba et al., 1992; Ventureya & Higgins, 1993).

From the clinical viewpoint, on the other hand, there is no agreement about a univocal definition of ictal clinical semiology, a problem still greater than in the adult population: unfortunately, from an analysis of studies which took the issue into account, the description of the seizures is often incomplete and children are not tested or questioned during the ictal events, and in any

Video-EEG	
16 with subjective and objectivable signs/7 pts	
Objectivable signs	
staring	8/5 pts
frightened look	5/2 pts
gestural autom.	4/3 pts
arms elevation	3/2 pts
face jerks	3/1 pts
pallor	2/2 pts
verbal autom.	2/2 pts
smiling	1/1 pt
blushing	1/1 pt
chewing	1/1 pt
contralateral jerks	1/1 pt

Fig. 9.

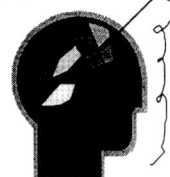

Stereo-EEG

7 pts: 67 depth electrodes (9,5/pt), unilateral

43 temporal lobe;
11 frontal lobe;
10 opercular region;
3 parietal.

19 spontaneous seizures recorded in 6 pts.
One pt only elicited seizures.

Fig. 10.

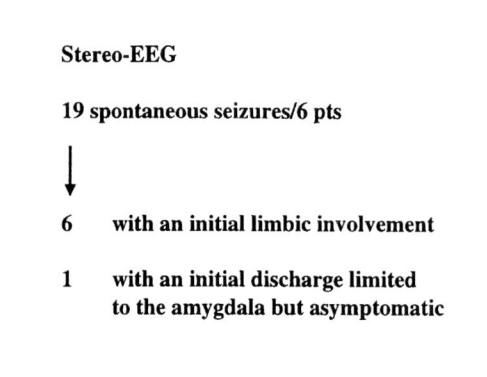

Fig. 11.

case they are judged to be unable to cooperate (Wyllie et al., 1993; Brokhaus & Elger, 1995; Acharaya et al., 1997).

An attempt has been made to arbitrarily separate the children into two groups, with more or less of 2 years or 6 years of age (Yamamoto et al., 1987; Brokhaus & Elger, 1995; Acharaya et al., 1997).

Unfortunately, it is still very difficult to outline the features of temporal lobe epilepsies in children. In our sample, localizing diagnosis was based as always on anatomo-electroclinical correlations. As already pointed out in the Results, interictal EEG alone is inadequate to this aim, since it localizes abnormalities in a much larger area than the temporal lobe itself in most patients. On the contrary, the recording of ictal events, and especially of well localized low voltage fast activities, is much more relevant, when carefully correlated to ictal clinical events (Allen et al., 1992).

The analysis of video-EEG data allows two types of approaches:

- the exact mapping of the epileptogenic zone and the direct feasibility to perform surgery;
- the opportunity to identify which structures may be involved early by ictal discharges and therefore, when possible, to plan stereo-EEG investigation.

In our population, seven children underwent exploration by intracerebral electrodes, with at least five electrodes implanted in the temporal lobe; spontaneous seizures could not be recorded in one patient only. In the 19 spontaneous seizures recorded in the remaining patients, in six cases (31.5 per cent) there was evidence of early involvement of limbic structures and in one case (5 per cent) it was limited to the amygdala, but without concomitant clinical correlates. This means that in 64.5 per cent of cases (12 seizures out of 19) ictal discharges in the temporal

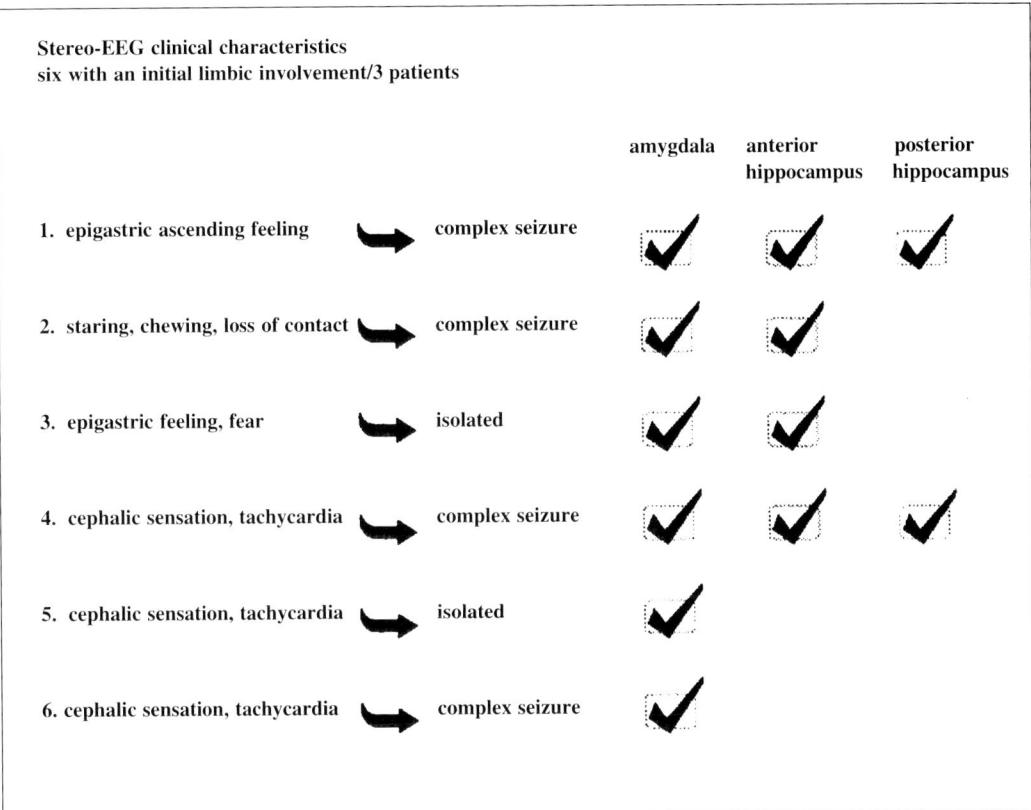

Fig. 12.

lobe originate from the neocortex or simultaneously involve the neocortex and the limbic structures. In the six cases in which the ictal discharge was confined to the limbic lobe, in five instances it was associated with a merely subjective sensation (epigastric in two cases, cephalic with tachycardia in three) and in one case it started with loss of contact and chewing automatisms.

At first sight it appears that the role of limbic structures has probably been overestimated to such a point that a temporal seizure is habitually considered of mesial origin. On the contrary, our data suggest just the opposite, since they show that only 31.5 per cent of seizures originate from the limbic structures. Especially in the US and Canada, there is a general tendency to ascribe the locus of origin of ictal discharges in temporal lobe seizures to the mesial temporal structures and particularly to the hippocampus. Two observations lead us to think otherwise:

- contrary to this theory, surgical resection involves both mesial temporal structures and neocortex (it should be noted that in cases of selective hippocampectomy rate of seizure-free patients does not exceed 30 per cent) (Engel, 1993).

- as for of invasive procedures, only a few centres can rely on adequate electrophysiological data to evaluate changes both in the mesial structures and the neocortex simultaneously. Usually only the mesial portion of the temporal lobe is explored.

Among the different possible localizations of epilepsies, those originating in the temporal lobe are undoubtedly the most frequent. This explains why temporal lobe epilepsies are the best known and studied. Moreover, in the case of a surgical approach their prognosis is certainly better than that of extratemporal epilepsies. However, this does not entitle us to consider the temporal lobe as a mere appendix to limbic structures which, though very important, are not essential to generate an ictal discharge.

Further studies are needed, applying invasive procedures to record from mesial and lateral structures simultaneously, to define the true role of the limbic structures in triggering temporal seizures, especially in children. Clearly, electrophysiological data must be related to clinical data gathered by careful clinical observation and by accurate ictal questioning.

References

Acharya, J.N., Wyllie, E., Lüders, H.O. et al. (1997): Seizure symptomatology in infants with localization-related epilepsy. *Neurology* **48**, 189–196.

Adler, J., Erba. G., Winston, K.R. et al. (1991): Results of surgery for extratemporal partial epilepsy that began in childhood. *Arch. Neurol.* **48**, 133–140.

Aicardi, J. (1994): *Epilepsy in Children*, pp. 1–555. New York: Raven Press.

Allen, P.J., Fisch, D.R. & Smith, S.J.M. (1992): Very high-frequency rhythmic activity during SEEG suppression in frontal lobe epilepsy. *Electroenceph. Clin. Neurophysiol.* **82**, 155–159.

Bancaud, J., Chodkiewicz, J.P., Munari, C. et al. (1985): Place de la chirurgie dans le traitement des épilepsies infantiles. *Les Epilepsies de l'Enfant*, Bordeaux, pp. 143–148. Paris: Labaz.

Blume, W.T., Girvin, J.P., McLachlan, R.S. & Gilmore, B.E. (1997): Effective temporal lobectomy in childhood without invasive EEG. *Epilepsia* **38**, 164–167.

Brockhaus, A. & Elger, C.E. (1995): Complex partial seizures of temporal lobe origin in children of different age groups. *Epilepsia* **36**, 1173–1181.

Broglin, D., Landré, E., Chauvel, P., Munari, C., Trottier, S., Chodkiewicz, J.P., Bancaud, J. & Talairach, J. (1991): Epilepsy surgery in adolescent and children: stereotactic preoperative evaluation and results. *Epilepsia* **32** (Suppl. 1), 21.

Cascino, G.D. & Herkes, G.K. (1993): Interpretation of interictal EEG. In: *The treatment of epilepsy: principles and practices*, ed. E. Wyllie, pp. 249–260. Philadelphia, MD: Lea & Febiger.

Chugani, H.T., Shewon, D.A., Peacock, W.J. et al. (1988): Surgical treatment of intractable neonatal-onset seizures. *Neurology* **38**, 1178–1188.

Davidson, S. & Falconer, M.A. (1975): Outcome of surgery in 40 children with temporal lobe epilepsy. *Lancet* **1**, 1260–1263.

Davies, K.G. & Weeks, D.R. (1995): Results of cortical resection for intractable epilepsy during epilepsy using intra-operative corticography without chronic intracranial recording. *Br. J. Neurosurg.* **9**, 7–12.

Duchowny, M. (1987): Complex partial seizures of infancy. *Arch. Neurol.* **44**, 911–914.

Engel, J., Jr. (1993): Update on surgical treatment of the epilepsies. Summary of the second Palm Desert Conference on the surgical treatment of the epilepsies. *Neurology* **43**, 1612–1617.

Erba, G., Winston, K.R., Adler, J.R., Welch. K., Ziegler, R. & Hornig, G.W. (1992): Temporal lobectomy for complex partial seizures that began in childhood. *Surg. Neurol.* **38**, 424–432.

Falconer, M.A., Hill, D., Meyer et al. (1995): Treatment of temporal lobe epilepsy by temporal lobectomy. *Lancet* **23**, 827–833.

Goldring, S. (1987): Pediatric epilepsy surgery. *Epilepsia* **28** (Suppl. 1), S82–S102.

Guldvog, B., Loyning, Y., Hauglie-Hanssen, H. et al. (1994): Surgical treatment for partial epilepsy among Norwegian children and adolescents. *Epilepsia* **35**, 554–565.

Holmes, G.L. (1989): Electroencephalographic and neuroradiological evaluation of children with epilepsy. *The Pediatric Clinics of North America* **26**(N2), 395–420.

Hopkins, L.J. & Klug, G.L. (1991): Temporal lobe surgery for the treatment of the intractable complex partial seizures of temporal lobe origin in early childhood. *Dev. Med. Child Neurol.* **33**, 26–31.

Linsday, J., Glaser, G., Richards, P. & Ounsted, C. (1984): Developmental aspects of focal epilepsies of childhood treated by neurosurgery. *Dev. Med. Child Neurol.* **26**, 574–587.

Lüders, H., Dinner, D.S., Morris, III H.H. *et al.* (1989): EEG evaluation for epilepsy surgery in children. *Clev. Clin. J. Med.* **56** (Suppl. 1), S53–S61.

Marchini, M., Munari, C. & Bancaud, J. (1988): Epilessie temporali gravi ad insorgenza infantile. *Boll. Lega It. Epil.* **64**, 197–198.

Mitchell, W.G., Chen, L.S. & Horton, E.J. (1991): Clinical utility of VEEG in seizure, epilepsy, or other paroxysmal events in infant and children. *Child Neurol. Soc.* **32**, 433.

Mizrahi, E.M., Kellaway, P., Grossman, R.G. Rutecki, P.A., Armstrong, D., Rettig, G. & Loewen, S. (1990): Anterior temporal lobectomy and medically refractory temporal lobe epilepsy of childhood. *Epilepsia* **31**, 302–312.

Munari, C. (1995): Methodologies, results and limits of epilepsy surgery in children. *Gaslini* **27** (Suppl. 1), 48–53.

Munari, C., Hoffmann, D., Francione, S., Kahane, P., Tassi, L., Lo Russo, G. & Benabid, A.L. (1994): Stereo-electroencephalography methodology: advantages and limits. *Acta Neurol. Scand.* **S152**, 56–67.

Ribaric, I.I., Nagulic, M. & Djurovic, B. (1991): Surgical treatment of epilepsy: our experiences with 34 children. *Child's Nerv. Syst.* **7**, 402–404.

Swick, C.T., Bouthillier, A. & Spencer, S.S. (1996): Seizures occuring during long-term monitoring. *Epilepsia* **37**, 927–930.

Ventureya, E.C.G. & Higgins, M.J. (1993): Complications of epilepsy surgery in children and adolescents. *Pediatr. Neurosurg.* **19**, 40–56.

Yamamoto, N., Watanabe, K., Negoro, T. *et al.* (1987): Complex partial seizures in children. *Neurology* **37**, 1379–1382.

Wyllie, E. (1991): Candidacy for epilepsy surgery: special considerations in children. In: *Epilepsy surgery*, ed. H. Lüders, pp. 127–130. New York: Raven Press.

Wyllie, E., Wyllie, R., Kotagal, P. *et al.* (1990): Comfortable insertion of sphenoidal electrodes in children. *Epilepsia* **31**, 521–523.

Wyllie, E., Chee, M., Granstrom, M.L. *et al.* (1993): Temporal lobe epilepsy in early childhood. *Epilepsia* **34**, 859–868.

Chapter 21

Focal seizures in infancy. Do ictal and interictal features suggest limbic involvement?

Silvana Franceschetti, Tiziana Granata, Simona Binelli, Laura Canafoglia, Marina Casazza, Elena Freri, Annalisa Pozzi and Giuliano Avanzini

Divisione di Neurofisiologia, Istituto Neurologico 'C. Besta', via Celoria 11, 20133 Milan, Italy

Summary

We report the video-EEG findings in 38 infants aged less than three years presenting with definitely focal seizures; the mean age at seizure onset was 2.3 ± 2.0 months; both cryptogenic and symptomatic epilepsies were included. The aim of the study was to characterize focal ictal events in infancy, especially those thought to arise from the temporal regions. In 15 cases (39 per cent), the ictal EEG discharges involved the temporal regions from the onset (13 cases) or later during the course of the seizure (two cases). In 10/13 cases whose ictal discharges involved the temporal regions from the onset, the seizures were characterized by autonomic signs or complex behavioural phenomena compatible with a limbic origin. Interictal epileptic activity was consistently confined to the temporal regions in only four cases, whereas multifocal interictal abnormalities were present in nine infants.

In our cases, the ictal clinical and EEG findings suggested that the limbic region and its circuitry can sustain seizures in infancy, even though temporal lobe involvement at this age may lead to fragmentary clinical phenomena. On the other hand, the partial seizures could not be considered an expression of 'temporal lobe epilepsy' in most patients, because a number of clinical and radiological findings and the presence of interictal EEG multifocal abnormalities suggested diffuse cortical hyperexcitability.

Introduction

Partial seizures are common manifestations of epilepsy in infancy and early childhood and may be symptoms of congenital or perinatal brain damage, or of a genetically determined progressive disorder. At this age, focal or multifocal brain damage may lead to apparently generalized epilepsies, such as West or Lennox–Gastaut syndromes (Vinters *et al.*, 1993; Jellinger, 1987; Commission on Classification, 1989); in these conditions the focal origin of the seizures is often suggested by focal EEG changes, although it is generally difficult to define the precise localization of ictal discharges. Conversely, in infants, definitely focal seizures are often associated with clearly recognizable and long-lasting ictal and interictal EEG discharges that are similar to those observed in older children or adult patients; in such cases, the discharges can be attributed to a definite cortical region as far as recognisable surface recordings. Nevertheless, the ictal events in infancy and early childhood are often difficult to define: subjective events cannot be reported by very young patients and the subjective content of mimicry and behavioural changes cannot be understood because we do not know what kind of information the associative brain structure really contains. Complex symptoms (e.g. alimentary or simple gestural automatisms), changes in mimicry or behavioural arrest can often be detected during focal seizures, but can hardly be attributed to a specific cortical region although the temporal onset of ictal EEG events has been reported (Yamamoto et al., 1987; Duchowny et al., 1992; Luna et al., 1989). The aim of the present study was to clarify and characterize focal ictal events in infancy, especially those thought to arise from the temporal regions. We here report the electroclinical characteristics of 38 infants with definitely focal seizures recorded using video-EEG.

Methods

Thirty-eight cases presenting with definitely focal seizures were selected among 127 children aged less than three years, of whom one or more ictal video-EEG recordings were obtained between 1993 and 1998. Infants with cryptogenic or symptomatic epilepsies were included, but not those with asymmetric spasms or series of subtle seizures, or those with multifocal myoclonic jerks fitting the definition of infantile epilepsia partialis continua.

All of the selected cases underwent repeated interictal and ictal EEG-polygraphic recordings associated with video monitoring; sleep recordings were also obtained in all cases. Scalp recordings were made using surface Ag–AgCl electrodes positioned according to the International 10–20 System, and the EEG and polygraphic signals were acquired using a Micromed computerized EEG system (sampling frequency 256 Hz; band pass filters 1.6–120 Hz for the EEG signals).

All of the patients underwent at least one brain MR examination. An extensive diagnostic protocol aimed at detecting genetically determined metabolic and/or degenerative disorders primarily involving the central nervous system was adopted whenever the aetiological factor of epilepsy could not be recognized. Thirty-five of the infants were followed for a mean period of 28 months.

Results

The series included 17 males and 21 females, whose age at seizure onset ranged from one day to ten months (mean 2.3 ± 2.0 months); the time interval between the onset of seizures and our first video-EEG recording ranged from a few days to 25 months (mean 7.2 ± 6.0 months). In 14 patients (45 per cent), the epilepsy was symptomatic of non-progressive encephalopathy (brain malformation in 10, foetal or perinatal brain damage in two, previous encephalitis in two). Three patients had tuberous sclerosis. In three cases (8 per cent), the epilepsy was due to a recognizable metabolic disorder (mitochondrial encephalopathy in two, leukodystrophy in one). The causative factor could not be identified in 18 patients, although a primary progressive disorder of unknown nature was suspected on the basis of clinical or radiological findings in 11 children, three of whom had a sibling with a similar clinical picture.

Ictal and interictal epileptic activity

In 13 cases (34.2 per cent), the ictal discharges involved the temporal regions from their onset: the earliest detectable location of an ictal EEG event was strictly temporal in five (13 per cent), fronto-temporal in five, and temporo-parieto-occipital in three. In two other infants, the ictal discharge apparently originated in other areas but involved the temporal region later during the course of the seizure. Figure 1 shows the distribution of the identifiable origin of the seizures in the population as a whole.

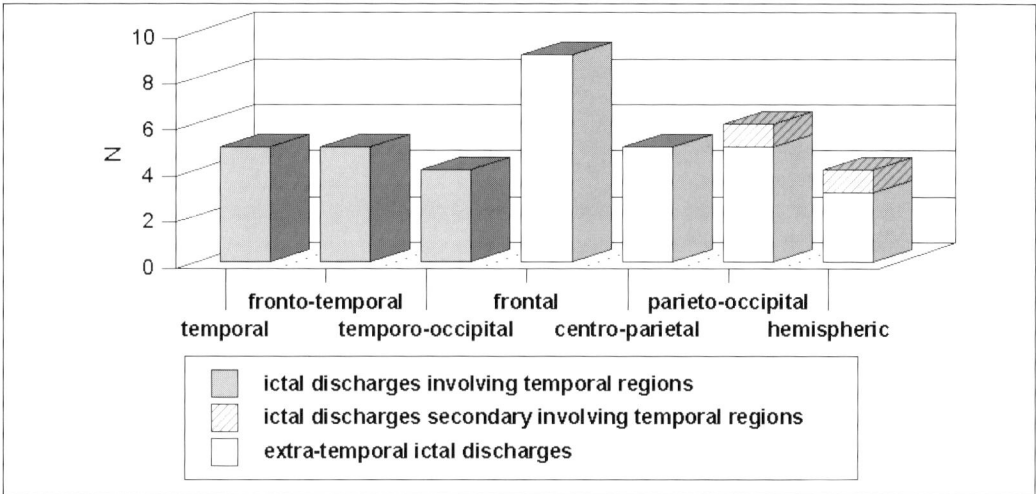

Fig. 1. Ictal discharge location in 38 infants with symptomatic or cryptogenic partial seizures.

The morphological characteristics of the ictal EEG events in the 13 patients whose seizures originated primarily in the temporal region did not differ significantly from those observed in patients with an extra-temporal onset. However, they had slightly more theta-delta rhythmic activity (46.1 per cent in the 'temporal' group vs. 30.7 per cent in the 'extratemporal' group), and signal attenuation was less frequent (15.3 per cent vs. 42.3 per cent). The duration of the discharges was similar in both groups of patients.

Interictal epileptic activity was focal in 16 patients, with a location consistent with that of the ictal EEG discharges; 18 had interictal EEG pictures characterized by multifocal epileptic abnormalities; four showed no interictal epileptic abnormalities. The multifocal interictal discharges were more often recorded in infants with temporal ictal EEG events (69 per cent) than in those with extra-temporal discharges (36 per cent) (Fig. 2).

Seizure semiology

With the aim of detecting a possible relationship between the location of the ictal EEG discharge and the characteristics of ictal behaviour, the observed clinical phenomena were classified as follows: motor fits (all motor phenomena including postural changes, head version, and focal clonic or myoclonic jerks); autonomic changes (e.g. early changes in breath rhythm, flushing); automatic behaviour (including alimentary or gestural automatisms associated or not with changes in mimicry); and staring episodes (including motionless episodes not associated with atonia). Staring episodes were observed in eleven cases, changes in mimicry in three,

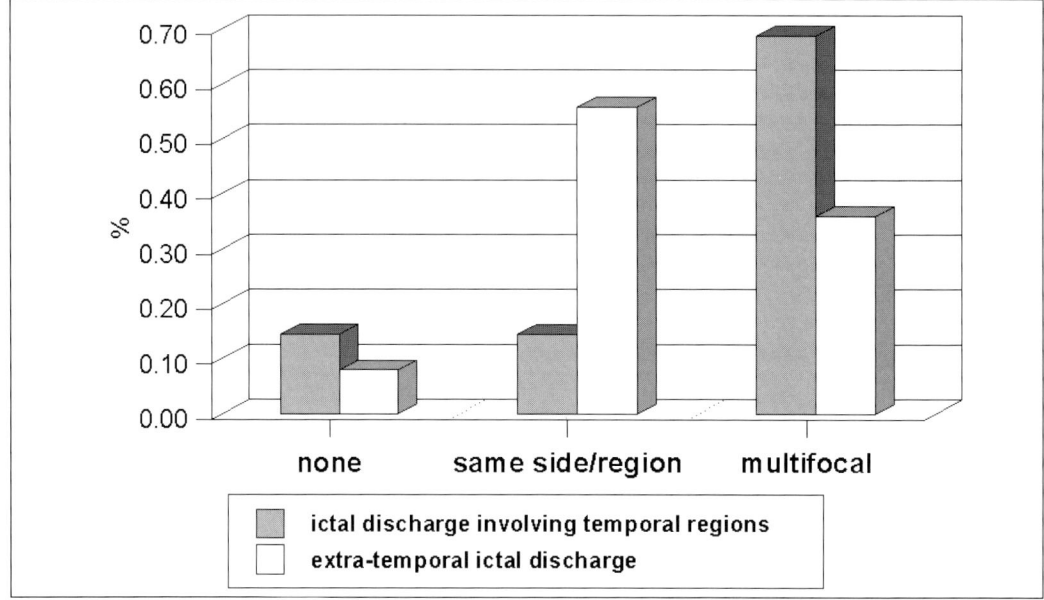

Fig. 2. Interictal epileptiform activity in patients with temporal versus extra-temporal ictal discharge.

simple gestural automatisms in three, alimentary automatisms in four, changes in respiratory frequency in four, and flushing in one.

Autonomic signs and/or complex behavioural phenomena were observed in 10 (78 per cent) of the thirteen patients whose ictal EEG discharges involved the temporal regions from their onset; they occurred as the earliest sign in six patients (staring in five cases, gestural automatisms in one), and appeared later during the seizure in the remaining four cases (changes in mimicry in two, oral or gestural automatisms associated with autonomic changes in two). Complex behavioural phenomena or autonomic symptoms were detected in 13 of the 25 infants with extra-temporal ictal discharges (52 per cent). Figure 3 shows the distribution of ictal clinical events in relation with the location of the EEG ictal discharge.

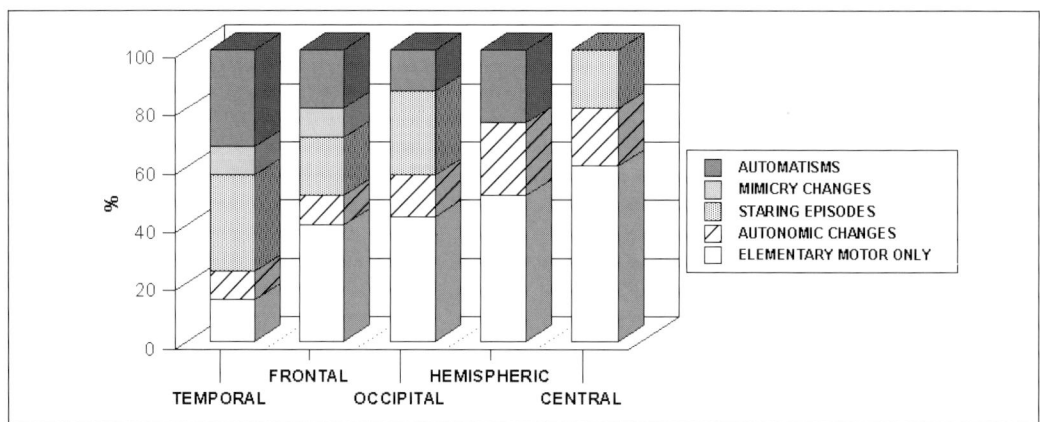

Fig. 3. Ictal symptoms in 38 infants with symptomatic or cryptogenic partial seizures.

Clinical background

Most of the infants experienced a very early onset of seizures, with no differences between those with temporal (mean age at onset = 2.0 ± 1.5 months) and those with extra-temporal ictal EEG discharges (mean age at onset = 2.5 ± 2.3 months). Moreover, there was no difference in age at the time of the EEG recordings in the two subgroups (8.5 ± 5.7 months vs. 11.8 ± 9.0 months).

The percentage of infants with non-progressive brain damage of unknown aetiology was especially high among those whose ictal discharges arose from the temporal regions (33 per cent); no difference was found in the distribution of the other causative factors.

Neuroradiological examination was unrevealing in six cases, but MRI revealed diffuse or multifocal brain damage in 23 (eight of the 13 cases with temporal and 15 of the 25 with extra-temporal ictal discharges); focal or lateralized brain damage consistent with the site of the ictal epileptic discharges was found in only eight cases (three with temporal and five with extra-temporal discharges). Abnormalities of the hippocampal structures (which appeared to be incompletely everted) were found in three patients, one of whom had temporal ictal discharges.

Thirty-one children were followed for at least one year (mean follow-up 28 months). The seizures were refractory to antiepileptic treatment in 27 cases: nine in the 'temporal' and 18 in the 'extra-temporal' group. In eight of these patients (one of whom continued to have temporal ictal discharges), the recordings made during follow-up consistently indicated that the seizures originated in the same cortical region. In the remaining 19 patients, the ictal discharges originated in different cortical regions and sometimes moved from one area to another during the same or consecutive seizures, thus showing their multifocal nature.

Discussion

Video-EEG recordings of 38 patients aged less than three years showed that 39 per cent had focal ictal discharges involving the temporal region from the time of onset (13 cases: 34 per cent), or which spread there from other areas (two cases: 5 per cent). This percentage is similar to that reported in comparable case series (Yamamoto et al., 1987; Duchowny et al., 1987; Blume, 1989).

However, the localization of the ictal discharges in our patients must be considered cautiously because most of the partial seizures were due to a severe and diffuse encephalopathy that often had a worsening (apparently progressive) course; furthermore, focal damage consistent with the location of ictal discharges could be identified in only a few cases. This was especially true in the case of those with temporal ictal discharges, whose partial seizures could not be considered an expression of 'temporal lobe epilepsy' because a number of clinical and EEG findings suggested diffuse cortical hyperexcitability. Multifocal interictal activity was detectable at the time of the first video-EEG recordings and, during the follow-up, most of the patients developed ictal discharges originating in another cortical region.

Despite these limitations relating to the localization of a stable epileptic focus, the ictal discharges involving the temporal regions were often associated with behavioural phenomena compatible with a limbic origin. Oral or gestural automatisms, autonomic changes and staring episodes appeared to be especially common during temporal discharges although they were not exclusively related to them.

A considerable amount of evidence derived from epilepsy models indicates that the limbic regions (especially the hippocampal structures) are highly epileptogenic in immature animals (Moshé, 1993), and some published data suggest the limbic origin of seizures in young children with apparently generalized or extratemporal ictal discharges (Brockhaus & Elger, 1995). Our findings suggest that the limbic region and its circuitry can sustain seizures in infancy, even though temporal lobe involvement at this age may lead to fragmentary clinical phenomena that are more subtle and less specific than in older patients. Moreover, the limited opportunity of interacting with the patients and interpreting their behavioural changes makes it extremely difficult (and potentially misleading) to try and attribute the observed clinical ictal findings to a specific cortical area.

References

Blume, W.T. (1989): Clinical profile of partial seizures beginning at less than four years of age. *Epilepsia* **30**, 813–819.

Brockaus, A. & Elger, C.E. (1995): Complex partial seizures of temporal origin in children of different age groups. *Epilepsia* **36**, 1173–1181.

Commission on Classification and Terminology of the International League Against Epilepsy (1989): Proposal for revised classification of epilepsy and epileptic syndromes. *Epilepsia* **30**, 389–399.

Duchowny, M. (1992): The syndrome of partial seizures in infancy. *J. Child Neurol.* **7**, 66–69.

Luna, D., Dulac, O. & Plouin, P. (1989): Ictal characteristics of cryptogenic partial epilepsies in infancy. *Epilepsia* **30**, 827–832.

Jellinger, K. (1987): Neuropathological aspects of infantile spasms. *Brain Dev.* **9**, 349–357.

Moshé, S.L. (1993): Seizures in developing brain. *Neurology* **43**(S5), S3–S7.

Vinters, H.V., De Rosa, M.J. & Farrel M.A. (1993): Neuropathologic study of resected cerebral tissue from patients with infantile spasms. *Epilepsia* **34**, 772–779.

Yamamoto, N., Watanabe, K., Negoro, T., Takaesu, E., Aso, K., Furune, S. & Takahashi, I. (1987): Complex partial seizures in children: ictal manifestations and their relation to clinical course. *Neurology* **37**, 1379–1382.

Chapter 22

Ictal SPECT in temporal lobe seizures in children

Catherine Chiron[*†], Pierre Véra[*‡], Andreas Hollo[*], Anna Kaminska[*†], Cécile Cieuta[*†], Dorothé Ville[*], Jean Louis Stiévenart[§], Isabelle Gardin[§], Perrine Plouin[†], Martine Fohlen[°], Olivier Delalande[°], Claude Jalin[°] and Olivier Dulac[†]

[*]CEA, Service Hospitalier Frederic Joliot, DSV/DRM, Orsay, France; [†]Department of Neuropediatrics, Saint Vincent de Paul Hospital, Paris, France and INSERM U29, Marseille, France; [‡]Department of Nuclear Medicine, Rouen University Hospital and Henri Becquerel Center, Rouen, France; [§]Department of Nuclear Medicine, Beaujon University Hospital, Clichy, France; [°]Rothschild Foundation, Paris, France

Summary

Ictal SPECT studies are increasingly used to localize seizure foci in patients with refractory temporal lobe epilepsy, but in children the experience is still limited. In our personal experience over 18 months, 10 children with temporal epilepsy and aged from 1.5 to 16 years underwent ictal ECD-SPECT (20 mCi/1.73m^2) combined with video-EEG and interictal ECD-SPECT plus 3D-MRI two days later. Ictal-interictal subtraction images were computed by registering and normalizing the ictal to the interictal SPECT scans for each child. The ictal, interictal SPECT and subtraction images were then superimposed to MRI.

Seizure onset was clearly temporal on ictal semiology in three children and confirmed by a temporal subtraction image in two (one ictal hyperperfusion, one postictal hypoperfusion, one without abnormality having been injected during aura). The temporal origin of the seizures was only suspected on clinical and/or EEG in five more children and there was a temporal image of hyperperfusion in four (the other had seizures lasting less than 10 s). Localizing the focus was impossible in the remaining two youngest children (under 2 years of age and with history of infantile spasms) but SPECT disclosed a clear temporal focus. SPECT permitted the discovery of a subtle cortical lesion on MRI in two cases. SPECT subtraction images were concordant with electrocorticography in two/two cases and validated by the cessation of seizures after surgery in the three patients operated on (6–22 months of follow-up). Ictal SPECT and particularly ictal-interictal subtraction SPECT images co-registered to MRI seems to be a helpful technique for non-invasively localizing the onset of seizures and guiding intracranial recording in temporal lobe epilepsies of children.

Introduction

Children with refractory epilepsy are increasingly referred for epilepsy surgery. Post-surgical outcome is tightly linked to the accurate localization of the epileptogenic focus, which is specially difficult in infantile epilepsy. Temporal lobe epilepsy is much less frequent in the paediatric population than in adults, and semiology of seizures may be more difficult at this age. Definitely localizing the epileptogenic focus, and delineating the epileptogenic region of cortex to be resected, often requires invasive EEG recordings, contrary to adults (Holmes et al., 1996; Wyllie, 1996). Non-invasive functional neuroimaging techniques using positron emission tomography (PET) and single-photon emission computed tomography (SPECT) have proven to be very helpful in localizing temporal epileptic foci in adults, ictal SPECT reaching the impressive sensitivity of 0.97 (Devous et al., 1998). Both techniques have been adapted in children but PET experience remains restricted to a few centres, and SPECT studies have been mostly interictal. The first reports of ictal SPECT in temporal epilepsy showed a sensitivity of at least 0.90 (Harvey et al., 1993; Cross et al., 1995; Menzel et al., 1996; Packard et al., 1996; O'Brien et al., 1998) but they are still too few to compare ictal SPECT with other methods in this population. SPECT images usually demonstrate hypoperfusion interictally and hyperperfusion ictally, and are traditionally visually analysed. Most authors point out the importance of combining the visual analysis of ictal and interictal imaging to improve sensitivity (Devous et al., 1998). The first attempts to calculate difference images from ictal to interictal SPECT scans increased the localizing value in temporal and extra-temporal lobe seizures (Zubal et al., 1995; O'Brien et al., 1998). The present study selected the patients with temporal lobe epilepsy among a larger population of refractory partial epilepsy, in order to evaluate the interest of ictal SPECT in presurgical evaluation when using a particular image processing, ictal-interictal scans co-registered to MRI. Results are preliminary since some patients of the series are still waiting for surgery, or surgical follow-up is too short to draw any definite conclusions.

Patients

Forty-four children with refractory partial epilepsy underwent together ictal SPECT, interictal SPECT, and MRI. Among them, the ten having temporal lobe epilepsy were selected. They were aged from 18 months to 16 years (mean 8.7 years), had a drug-resistant epilepsy and were investigated after obtaining informed consent from the parents. MRI disclosed a cerebral lesion in nine cases, two left and eight right, three mesial and six lateral, supposedly focal cortical dysplasia in five, hippocampal sclerosis in two and dysembrio-neuroepithelial tumours in two, according to MRI signs. To date, two patients underwent intracranial EEG recording (with both grids for electrocorticography and some stereo-EEG electrodes), and three have been operated on. They all were seizure free at follow-up ranging from 6 to 22 months.

Temporal onset of seizures was evident from ictal semiology in three patients (Group 1): one experienced fear, chewing movements, and hands automatisms (#1), the two others had epigastric aura (#2 #3) followed by staring, orofacial automatisms and contralateral dystonia in one (#3). Temporal ictal discharge was present in all three and temporal lesion in two of them (#1 #3). Temporal localization of the focus was more difficult from electroclinical semiology in the other five patients (Group 2): three had very brief seizures (lasting less than 10 s in #4) with staring immediately followed by tonic extension of both arms (#4 #5 #6) and a frontal or temporo-frontal discharge, one had staring with swallowing and rapid generalization initiated by temporal flattening on EEG and with temporo-insular lesion on MRI (#7), the last one had staring, unilateral eyelid clonia and ipsilateral temporo-parietal EEG discharge but no lesion detected on MRI before SPECT (#8) (Fig. 1). In the last two patients (Group 3), both aged less than two years and having experienced infantile spasms during the first year of life, temporal origin of seizures was not suspected before SPECT: one experienced eyelid jerks in clusters

Chapter 22 Ictal SPECT in temporal lobe seizures in children

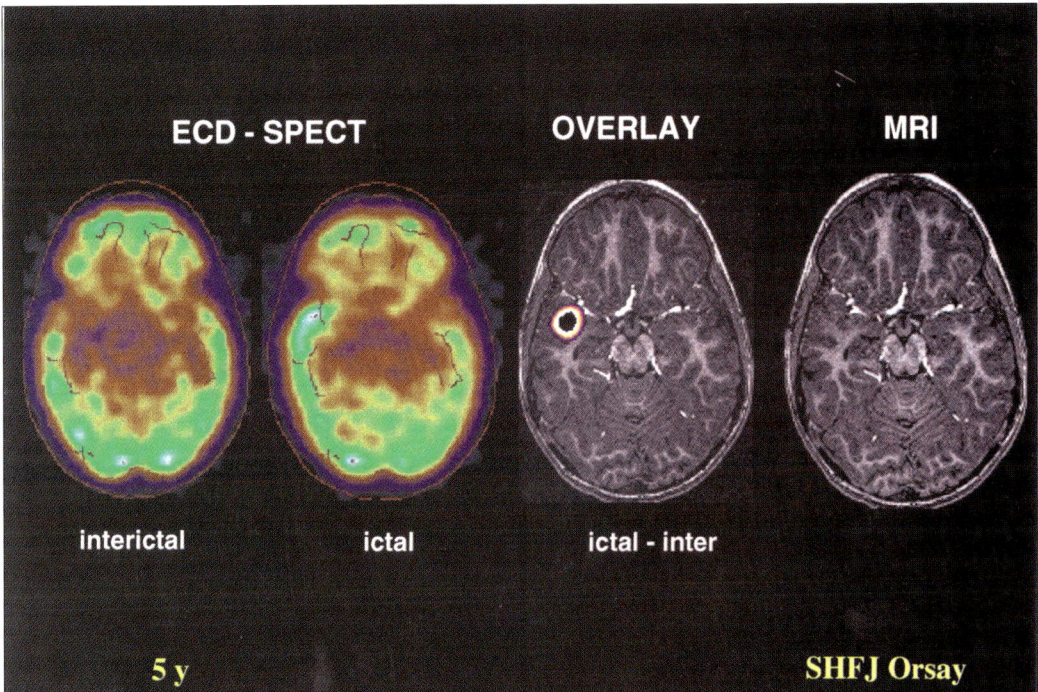

Fig. 1. In this 5-year-old girl (#8), interictal SPECT shows a left temporal hypoperfusion which is replaced by a hyperperfusion at ictal SPECT. Subtraction image (ictal–interictal) superimposed on MRI (overlay image) clearly shows the increase of cerebral blood flow in the right temporal lobe during the seizure. This focus corresponds to a probable dysplastic lesion, which has been discovered on MRI after having analysed ictal SPECT and is caracterized by a lack of the delineation of grey and white matter in the right temporal lobe.

without any EEG focus (#9), the other seemed to be frightened, covering her eyes when experiencing an hemispheric discharge and had a history of an ipsilateral focus at the time of spasms (#10), and none of them had any detectable lesion on MRI before 2 years.

Methods

All children had ictal and interictal perfusion scans 48 h later, both performed 1 h after intravenous injections of 740 MBq (20 mCi) of ^{99m}Tc-ECD for 1.73m^2, with a double head rotating gamma-camera (DST, SMVi) equipped with ultra-high resolution fan-beam collimators. Ictal injections were performed during video-EEG documented seizures. Patients under 6 years or being non-cooperative were sedated by intra-rectal pentobarbital (5 mg/kg) administered after ECD injection. MR images were obtained just after the interictal SPECT using a 1.5 Tesla MRI imager (Signa, General Electric), and T1 weighted 1 mm thick axial slices.

The interictal and ictal perfusion scans of each children were registered to the children's MRI scans using a local computer 3D-registration programme. For each child, extracted MRI boundaries were co-registered to the interictal and ictal perfusion scans to verify the accuracy of co-registration. Then, the co-registered ictal and interictal perfusion scans were normalized according to the mean pixel counts in the brain and interictal scans were subtracted from ictal ones to obtain subtraction images showing increases during ictus compared to interictal. Subtraction images were smoothed with a 3D-Deriche filter. Then the image representing 30 per cent of the maximum of the smoothed subtraction images was superimposed on MRI scans.

Results

Using ictal-interictal scans co-registered to MRI (overlay images), eight/ten patients exhibited at least one image in temporal lobe. That was hyperperfusion in seven of them, who received EDC injection at a mean time of 15 s (5–30 s) after seizure onset, and hypoperfusion in the eighth who was injected postictally. Among the two remaining patients who did not exhibit any temporal image on subtraction SPECT, the first experienced seizures lasting less than 10 s and the second had received the injection very early during a seizure lasting 60 s, precisely during the epigastric aura.

Other foci of hyperperfusion were found in six/eight patients, involving cortex in three (two frontal and one insular), homolateral striatum in five, and contralateral cerebellum in three. One patient exhibited the so called 'temporal pattern' described by Duncan *et al.* (1993) as associating hyperperfusion in temporal lobe, frontal lobe and striatum homolaterally and in cerebellum contralaterally. Using classic visual analysis of interictal and ictal SPECT separately, other foci of hyperperfusion were detected only in four/eight patients and temporal focus was missed in one more. Hyperperfusion was observed in striatum in only three cases and in cerebellum in two.

In Group 1, we found one case with temporal hyperperfusion (#1), the case with postictal hypoperfusion (#2) (Fig. 2), and the patient without any image and injected during aura (#3). In the first case, a temporal lesion supposed to be a dysplasia had been missed on MRI and discovered '*a posteriori*' after having seen SPECT images. The second patient had no lesion detectable on MRI. The last patient underwent intracranial recording which showed ictal discharges coming from the mesio-temporal lesion and the pole. Surgical exeresis involved both regions, the lesion was proved to be dysplastic and seizures have disappeared for 22 months.

In Group 2, all patients but one had a temporal hyperperfusion on SPECT. The patient with no hyperperfused focus (#4) had very brief seizures and EEG discharges with flattening in mesial cortex and temporal pole on intracranial EEG. There was a rapid propagation to orbitofrontal and posterior temporal cortex. Surgical exeresis involved mesial and polar temporal cortex and the child became seizure free with 6 month follow-up. Two other patients disclosed temporal and frontal hyperperfusion well corresponding to a frontal propagation with tonic semiology (#5 #6). Both had large temporal lesions on MRI. One was operated on, without any intracranial EEG recording, and has remained seizure free for 1 year after an anterior lobectomy which removed a DNET. The fourth patient had temporal and insular hyperperfusion and temporo-insular lesion on MRI (#7). Ictal semiology with hypersalivation suggested that insula was involved in seizure propagation. The last patient had temporal hyperperfusion but homolateral eyelid clonia and SPECT revealed a temporal lesion which was initially missed on MRI (#8) (Fig. 1).

In Group 3, the two patients (#9 #10) had temporal hyperperfusion although no clinical feature permitted us to suspect the temporal onset of seizures. In the two cases, the temporal lesion was discovered after the SPECT on an MRI initially considered as normal.

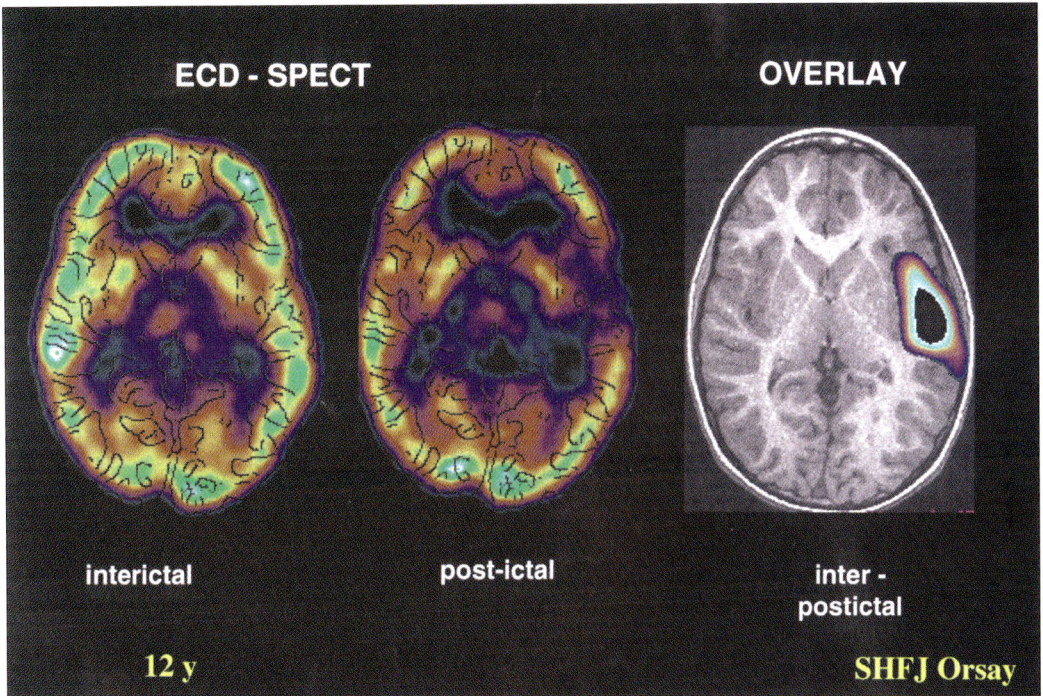

Fig. 2. In this 12-year-old girl (#2) with cryptogenic epilepsy (normal MRI), interictal SPECT shows a slight hypoperfusion in the anterior part of left temporal lobe as well as in the posterior part of the right temporal lobe. Perfusion was also slightly decreased in the left basal ganglia. Immediately postictal SPECT shows a significant hypoperfusion in the left anterior temporal lobe. Subtraction image (interictal – postictal) discloses the decrease of cerebral blood flow in this area in the immediate postictal period.

Discussion

This study confirms that ictal SPECT is a useful technique to localize the epileptogenic focus non-invasively in childhood temporal epilepsy planned for surgery. Moreover, our series is among the first examinations performed in very young children and shows that the co-registration of ictal, interictal and MRI scans is a more sensitive procedure that the classical analysis in paediatric population. Ictal-interictal SPECT subtraction images coregistered with MRI disclose the temporal focus and sometimes other cortical foci in agreement with the propagation of the seizures, as suggested by ictal semiology and confirmed by intracranial EEG recordings. In one third of the patients, a previously missed lesion was identified on MRI resulting from the analysis of SPECT images. In infants, ictal SPECT can disclose a clear temporal focus although the clinical features are most often non localizing. Therefore, ictal SPECT with coregistration image processing improves the ability of localizing foci in children with presurgical temporal epilepsy.

Temporal lobe epilepsy is not as frequent in children as in adults. In our series of refractory partial epilepsies planned for surgery, only 23 per cent were temporal. In children aged more than 10 years, ictal semiology is similar to that of adults and temporal onset relatively easily suspected. In younger children or in mentally retarded patients, 'temporal semiology' may be more difficult to assess or may become rapidly modified by the propagation of the discharge.

The development of non-invasive localizing techniques such as SPECT is potentially the most useful in this population.

Ictal SPECT is now proven to be the most sensitive imaging technique to localize the epileptogenic focus non-invasively in temporal lobe epilepsy in adults. Meta-analytic sensitivity raises from 0.44 to 0.75 and 0.97 for interictal to postictal and ictal SPECT, in accordance with standard evaluation and/or surgical outcome (Devous *et al.*, 1998) whereas interictal FDG-PET or MRI alone reaches a sensitivity about 0.70 (Spencer, 1994; Mauguière & Ryvlin, 1996). Studies are still limited in paediatric population, and therefore sensitivity cannot be established on a large series. Preliminary reports nevertheless revealed a hyperperfused focus consistent with the epileptogenic area in more than 90 per cent of the patients (Harvey *et al.*, 1993; Kuzniecki *et al.*, 1993; Cross *et al.*, 1995; Menzel *et al.*, 1996; Packard *et al.*, 1996; O'Brien *et al.*, 1998) compared to 25 per cent to 80 per cent using interictal SPECT. These series also include extratemporal epilepsies, the most frequent in children, contrary to adults. In a study dedicated to temporal epilepsy in children aged from 7 to 14 years, Harvey *et al.* (1993) showed that ictal SPECT was informative in 14 of 15 patients, disclosing a unilateral temporal hyperperfusion concordant with ictal EEG, MRI and pathology, and provided additional localizing information in four cases. Regarding young children, data are very scarce since less than 10 isolated cases concern infants aged less than four years (Bye *et al.*, 1993; Green & Buchhalter, 1993; Alfonso *et al.*, 1997; Koc *et al.*, 1997).

Regarding the localization of the focus in adults, visually comparing ictal and interictal cerebral perfusion images is superior to either analysing ictal or interictal ones (Devous *et al.*, 1998) and coregistering ictal, interictal and MRI images superior to visually comparing scans (Zubal *et al.*, 1995; O'Brien *et al.*, 1998). The latter procedure increases sensitivity from 39 per cent to 88 per cent in a large series of extratemporal and bitemporal adult epilepsies (O'Brien *et al.*, 1998). It was first performed in a series of 17 children with mainly extratemporal epilepsy and showed a sensitivity of 94 per cent. It also provides specific localizing information in 92 per cent of the 38 patients investigated at the Mayo Clinic (O'Brien *et al.*, 1998). In our personal series, such image processing improves the ability to detect and localize a hyperperfused focus from 74 per cent to 93 per cent (Véra *et al.*, 1999). In the present temporal epilepsy study, subtraction images increase the ability to detect a temporal focus from 70 per cent to 80 per cent and to assess to probable foci of propagation from 50 per cent to 75 per cent.

Conclusion

Our results confirm that ictal SPECT in children with refractory temporal lobe epilepsy is, as in adults, a useful non-invasive technique to localize the epileptogenic focus, and to guide the intracranial recording. Sensitivity of ictal SPECT is improved by coregistering images with interictal SPECT and MRI. The perfusion changes are concordant with clinical, EEG and MRI findings. Ictal SPECT may provide useful information about propagation of the seizure and even the only localizing sign for temporal lobe in very young children.

Acknowledgements: This work was supported by a grant from the 'Programme Hospitalier de Recherche Clinique', Assistance Publique – Hôpitaux de Paris (IDF94001).

References

Alfonso, I., Harvey, S., Acuna, A., Velez, E., Papazian, O., Litt, R. & Gainey, M. (1997): Interictal and ictal SPECT in a neonate with hemimegalencephaly. *Clin. Nucl. Med.* **22**, 323–324.

Bye, A.M., Parle, J. & Haindl, W. (1993): Single photon emission computed tomography in intractable infantile seizures. *Clin. Exp. Neurol.* **30**, 117–123.

Cross, J.H., Gordon, I., Jackson, G.D., Boyd, S.G., Todd-Prokopek, A., Anderson, P.J. & Neville, B. (1995): Children with intractable focal epilepsy: ictal and interictal ^{99m}Tc HMPAO single photon emission computed tomography. *Dev. Med. Child Neurol.* **37**, 673–681.

Devous, M.D., Thisted, R.A., Morgan, G.F., Leroy, R.F. & Rowe, C.C. (1998): SPECT brain imaging in epilepsy: a meta-analysis. *J. Nucl. Med.* **39**, 285–293.

Duncan, R., Patterson, J., Roberts, R., Hadley, D.M. & Bone, I. (1993): Ictal/postical SPECT in the presurgical localisation of complex partial seizures. *J. Neurol. Neurosurg. Psych.* **56**, 141–148.

Green, C. & Buchhalter, J.R. (1993): Ictal SPECT in a 16-day old infant. *Clin. Nucl. Med.* **18**, 768–770.

Harvey, A.S., Bowe, A.S., Hopkins, I.J., Shield, L.K., Cook, D.J. & Berkovic, S.F. (1993): Ictal ^{99m}Tc-HMPAO single photon emission computed tomography in children with temporal lobe epilepsy. *Epilepsia* **34**, 869–877.

Holmes, M.D., Dodrill, C.B., Ojemann, L.M. & Ojemann, G.A. (1996): Five-year outcome after epilepsy surgery in nonmonitored and monitored surgical candidates. *Epilepsia* **37**, 748–752.

Koc, E., Serdaroglu, A., Kapucu, O., Atalay, Y., Gucuyener, K. & Atasever, T. (1997): Ictal and interictal SPECT in a newborn infant with intractable seizures. *Acta Pediatr.* **86**, 1379–1381.

Kuzniecki, R., Mountz, J.M., Wheatley, G. & Morawetz, R. (1993): Ictal single-photon emission computed tomography localized epileptogenesis in cortical dysplasia. *Ann. Neurol.* **34**, 627–631.

Mauguière, F. & Ryvlin, P. (1996): Morphological and functional neuro-imaging of surgical partial epilepsies in adults. *Rev. Neurol.* **152**, 501–516.

Menzel, C., Steidele, S., Grunwald, F., Hufnagel, A., Pavics, L., Elger, C.E. & Biersack, H.J. (1996): Evaluation of technetium-99m-ECD in childhood epilepsy. *J. Nucl. Med.* **37**, 1106–1112.

O'Brien, T.J., So, E.L., Mullan, B.P., Hauser, M.F., Brinkmann, B.H., Bohnen, N.I., Hanson, D., Cascino, G.D., Jack, C.R. & Sharbrough, F.W. (1998): Subtraction ictal SPECT co-registered to MRI improves clinical usefulness of SPECT in localizing the surgical seizure focus. *Neurology* **50**, 445–454.

O'Brien, T.J., Zupanc, M.L., Mullan, B.P., O'Connor, M.K., Brinkmann, B.H., Cicora, K.M. & So, E.L. (1998): The practical utility of performing peri-ictal SPECT in the evaluation of children with partial epilepsy. *Pediatr. Neurol.* **19**, 15–22.

Packard, A.B., Roach, P.J., Davis, R.T., Riviello, J., Holmes, G., Barnes, P.D., O'Tuama, L. A., Bjornson, B. & Treves, S.T. (1996): Ictal and interictal technetium-^{99m}-bicisate brain SPECT in children with refractory epilepsy. *J. Nucl. Med.* **37**, 1101–1106.

Spencer, S.S. (1994): The relative contribution of MRI, SPECT, and PET imaging in epilepsy. *Epilepsia* **35**, S72-S89.

Véra, P., Kaminska, A., Cieuta, C., Hollo, A., Stievenart, J.L., Gardin, I., Ville, D., Mangin, J.F., Plouin, P., Dulac, O. & Chiron, C. (1999): Optimizing the localization of seizure foci in children using subtraction ictal SPECT co-registered to MRI. *J. Nucl. Med.* **40**, 786–792.

Wyllie, E. (1996): Epilepsy surgery in infants. In: *The treatment of epilepsy: principles and practice*, ed. E. Wyllie, pp. 1087–1096. Baltimore: Williams and Wilkins.

Zubal, I.G., Spencer, S.S., Imam, K., Seibyl, J., Smith, E.O., Wisniewski, G. & Hoffer, P.B. (1995): Difference images calculated from ictal and interictal technetium–^{99m}-HMPAO SPECT scans of epilepsy. *J. Nucl. Med.* **36**, 684–689.

Chapter 23

MRI in limbic structures in the epileptic and non-epileptic child

Ludovico D'Incerti

Department of Neuroradiology, Istituto Nazionale Neurologico 'C.Besta', via Celoria 11, 20133 Milan, Italy

Summary

Modern MRI techniques allow highly detailed demonstration of the anatomy of the limbic system. MRI demonstration of the developmental changes of hippocampal formation in embryos has also been obtained. Knowledge of developmental steps and of the normal anatomy of the limbic structures allows us to understand the morphologic features of malformative pictures.

MRI has proved to be highly sensitive in the demonstration of hippocampal sclerosis. Hippocampal sclerosis is rarely reported at paediatric age: no definite data about its incidence and development are at present available. Herpes encephalitis is finally mentioned among the causes of epilepsy at paediatric age for its characterisic location to the limbic structures.

Since the introduction of magnetic resonance imaging (MRI) in clinical practice, an increasing number of MRI studies has focused on the anatomy of the temporal lobe and the limbic system (Naidich *et al.*, 1987). Modern MRI techniques provide a highly detailed demonstration of the normal anatomy of the limbic system.

Parts of the limbic structures, such as cingulate gyrus or the hypothalamic mammillary bodies, their connection with the thalamus and with the different segments of the fornix are recognizable on standard MRI studies (Fig. 1).

High-resolution MRI is required for demonstration of the internal structures of the hippocampus: the digitations of the head, the dentate gyrus and the Ammon's horn are easily distiguished from the alveus and from the fimbria (Fig. 2).

MRI has been recently employed also in embryos to study the development of the limbic stuctures (Kier *et al.*, 1995). Knowledge of the developmental changes of hippocampal formation results in a better understanding of the complex morphologic aspects and functional connections of these structures, and to explain its morphologic features in different malformative pictures such as agenesis of the corpus callosum or neuronal migration disorders.

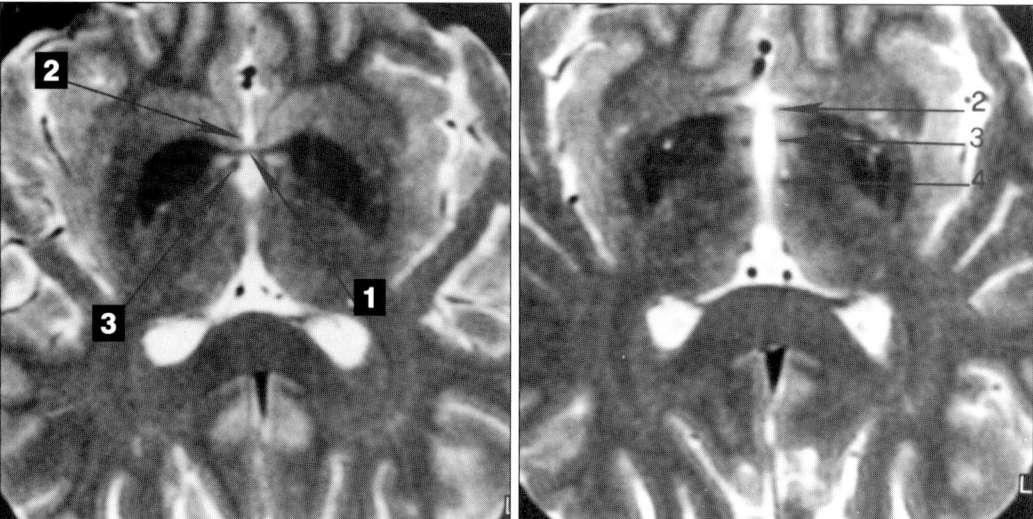

Fig. 1. a(left) – b(right): Axial T2-weighted images.
1. anterior commissure; 2. pre-commissural fibres of the fornix;
3. columnae fornicis; 4. mammillo-thalamic tract.

The foetal appearance of the hippocampal formation consists in its incomplete evertion; on MRI coronal sections globoid shape and vertical rotation of its transversal axis are seen.

This feature is more frequently observed in callosal agenesis and in extended cortical dysplasias (Fig. 3).

Hippocampal developmental abnormalities may be observed in association with malformative pictures of different extension. They may be part of severe neuronal migration disorders involving large parts of the cerebral hemispheres (open lip schizencephaly or pachygiria), or may be associated with cortical dysplasias involving the temporal lobe.

Hippocampal dysgenesis may be the only malformative feature in the absence of any other brain abnormality (Baulac,1998).

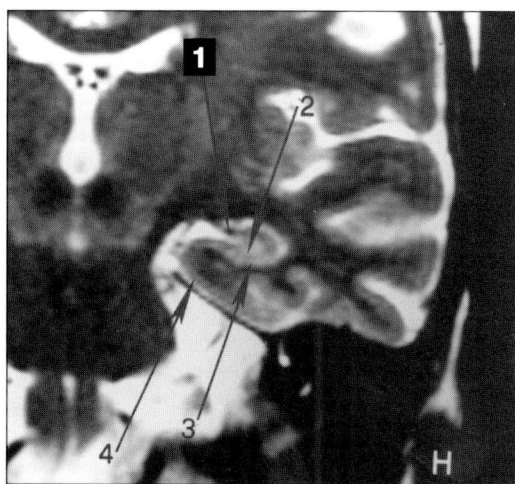

Fig. 2. Coronal T2-weighted image through the hippocampal body.
1. fimbria;
2. alveus;
3. dentate gyrus;
4. parahippocampal gyrus.

Minor intra- and extrahippocampal developmental abnormalities are more frequently observed in brain MRI studies for epilepsy. Small cyst remnants of the hippocampal sulcus are frequently seen in coronal sections. Due to the frequency of this finding, it is important to be aware of its existence and of the mechanism of its formation, in order to avoid erroneous attributions of pathological significance (Sasaki et al., 1993).

Small arachnoid cysts within the choroid fissure, sometimes exerting slight mass effect upon the hippocampal body, should not be confused with tumours.

MRI is highly sensitive in demonstrating hippocampal sclerosis (HS): the well-known radiologic features of size reduction and T2-hyperintensity correspond to the pathological data of atrophy and gliosis.

MRI features of hippocampal sclerosis are easily demonstrated in thin dual-echo and T1-w.i. coronal sections of the hippocampi. Different sequences (FLAIR and Myelin suppression) may be employed in association with conventional spin-echo acquisition in order to show hippocampal hyperintensity.

Choice of the appropriate technique is crucial to demonstrate radiological features of HS; nevertheless an appropriate training in neuroimaging of epilepsy is equally essential for the neuroradiologist.

HS may be quantified by volumetric measurements: although useful for statistic purposes, quantitative evaluation of hippocampal atrophy is not necessary for diagnosis of HS. Qualitative evaluation, if performed by an experienced neuroradiologist, has proved to be equally or more effective (Cheon et al., 1998).

HS may be bilateral. Radiological diagnosis of HS is always done by comparison of the normal appearance of the healthy hippocampus with the contralateral one. Knowledge of the normal and pathological anatomy allows recognition of HS features also in cases in which comparison is not possible.

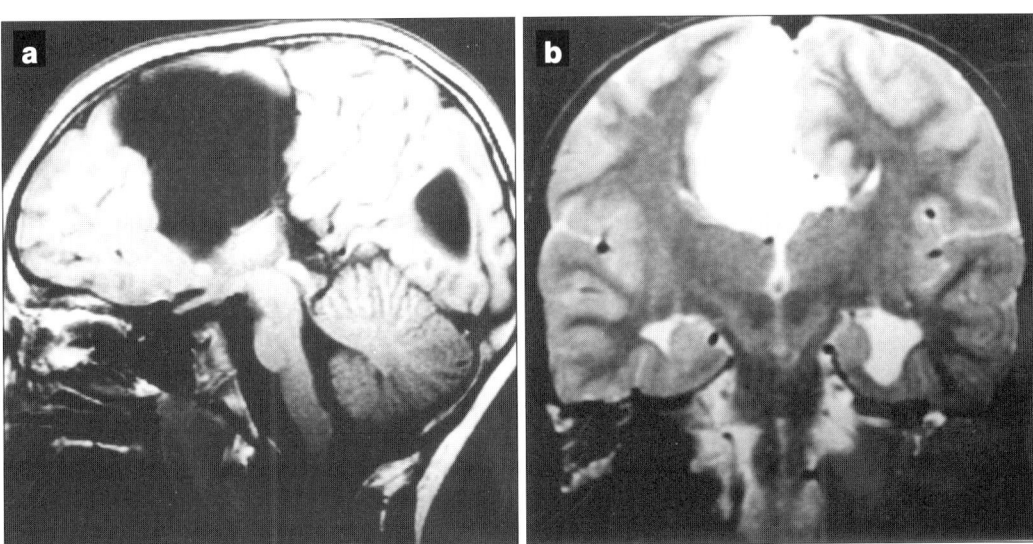

Fig. 3. Callosal agenesis.
(a, left): Sagittal T1-weighted image. Absence of the whole corpus callosum
(b, right): Coronal T2-weghted image. Globoid shape of the incompletely everted hippocampi.

HS is much more rarely observed at paediatric than at adult age and is reported only in a few papers. Although association of HS with febrile convulsions is well known, at present there are no definite data regarding the incidence of hippocampal sclerosis in children.

Moreover, two major questions are still waiting to be answered: whether HS is the cause of, or is caused by epilepsy, and how much time is needed for development of HS after the onset of the febrile seizures.

In a recent report by Van Landingham *et al.* (1998), hippocampal atrophy is described in two of 15 patients 9 months after the onset of febrile complex focal seizures. This paper confirms that HS may be observed in children and demonstrates that it may become evident to MRI a few months after the onset of epilepsy. On the other hand, the number of patients reported cannot answer the question about the time of development of HS.

Several factors may influence the development of HS: the number of seizures, their duration, and the presence of status epilepticus.

The observation of hippocampal signal abnormalities on MRI does not always mean HS: T2 hyperintensity in a swollen hippocampus may reflect oedema caused by seizures. Swelling may revert, generally in a few days or weeks, but no definite data are available to assess the evolution in atrophy (Tien & Felsberg, 1993).

Difficulties in assessing the incidence of hippocampal abnormalities at paediatric age are due to the very rare longitudinal MRI studies of children with febrile convulsion.

MRI is mandatory to assess the prognosis of epileptic patients. This is confirmed, for instance, in a recent paper by Harvey *et al.* (1997) in which among a large group of epileptic patients the risk of intractable seizures is greater in the patients with severe antecedents and with positive MRI.

Finally, HS may be associated with different developmental intra- or extrahippocampal abnormalities (so called dual pathology).

In these cases the epileptogenicity of the affected hippocampus and the relation of HS with the origin of the seizures is even more controversial (Kuzniecky & Jackson, 1995). Due to its characteristic location to the temporal area and to limbic structures, herpes encephalitis is mentioned among the causes of epilepsy at paediatric age.

Herpes virus infection is frequent at all ages and rarely involves the CNS. Encephalitis from herpes simplex more frequently occurs at paediatric age.

On the basis of serology two types of virus are recognized. Type 1 herpes virus (HSV1) causes orofacial infections and is associated with herpes virus encephalitis in patients aged more than 6 months. Type 2 herpes virus (HSV2) is related to genital infections and causes most of the congenital or perinatally acquired infections. With either serotype, cerebritis may develop from a primary infection or from reactivation of a pre-existing infection.

Herpes simplex encephalitis consists of an acute necrotizing meningoencephalitis that usually begins in the temporal lobes and tends to involve the insular cortex and the limbic structures, particularly the cyngulate gyrus. MRI demonstrates white matter T2 hyperintensity, with later involvement of the cortex. A haemorrhagic component is frequently observed and, together with the temporal location, may be the clue for radiological diagnosis (Fig. 4).

The location to temporal lobes, typical of HSV 1 encephalitis, may be recognized also in type 2

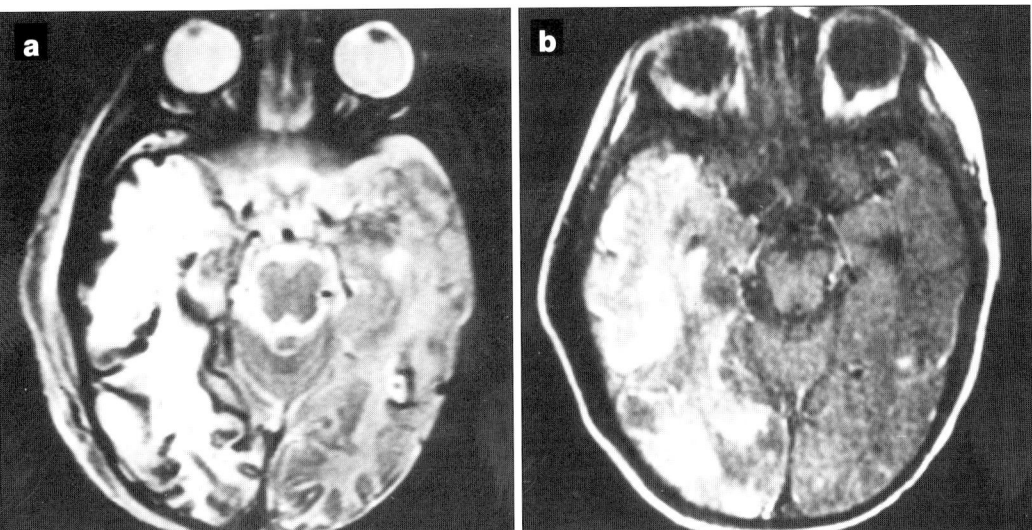

Fig. 4. Herpes encephalitis from HSV2 in a one month-infant.
(a, left): Axial T2-weighted image. Extended areas of signal hyperintensity are preferentially located in the right temporal lobe.
(b, right): Axial T1-weighted image. Signal hyperintensity is consistent with haemorrhagic component of the lesion.

infections, more frequent in children, in which a diffuse involvement of the whole brain is usually present.

Prognosis, expecially for the early infancy infections, is poor. In survivors MRI demonstrates severe encephalomalacia with loss and gliosis of the white matter and with thinning of the cortex (Barkovich, 1995).

References

Barkovich, A.J. (1995): *Pediatric neuroimaging*, 2nd edn. New York: Raven Press.

Baulac, M., De Grissac, N., Hasboun, D., Oppenheim, C., Adam, C., Arzimanoglou, A., Semah, F. & Lehéricy, S. (1998): Hippocampal developmental changes in patients with partial epilepsy: magnetic resonance imaging and clinical apsects. *Ann. Neurol.* **44**, 223–233.

Cheon, J.E., Chang, K.H., Kim, H.D. & Han, M.H. (1998): MR of hippocampal sclerosis: comparison of qualitative and quantitative assessments. *AJNR* **19**, 465–468.

Harvey, A.S., Berkovich, S.F., Wrennal, J.A. & Hopkins, I.J. (1997): Temporal lobe epilepsy in childhood: clinical, EEG, and syndrome classification in a cohort with new-onset seizures. *Neurology* **49**, 960–968.

Kier, E.L., Fulbright, R.K. & Bronen, R.A. (1995): Limbic lobe embryology and anatomy: dissection and MR of the medial surface of the fetal cerebral hemisphere. *AJNR* **16**, 1847–1853.

Kuzniecky, R.I. & Jackson, G.D. (1995): *Magnetic resonance in epilepsy*. New York: Raven Press.

Naidich, T.P., Daniels, D.L. & Haughton, V.M. (1987): Hippocampal formation and related structures of the limbic lobe: anatomic-MR correlation. Part 1: Surface features and coronal section. *Radiology* **162**, 747–754.

Sasaki, M., Sone, M., Ehara, S. & Tamakawa, Y. (1993): Hippocampal sulcus remnant: potential cause of change in signal intensity in the hippocampus. *Radiology* **188**, 743–747.

Tien, R.D. & Felsberg, G.J. (1993): The hippocampus in status epilepticus: demonstration of signal intensity and morphologic changes with sequential fast spin-echo MR imaging. *Radiology* **194,** 249–256.

Van Landingham, K.E., Heinz, E.R. & Cavazos, J.E. (1998): Magnetic resonance imaging evidence of hippocampal injury after prolonged focal febrile convulsions. *Ann. Neurol.* **43**, 413–426.

Chapter 24

The medical therapy of limbic seizures in children

Paola Costa, Andrea Van Lierde[*] and Laura Mira[†]

Divisione di Neuropsichiatria Infantile, Istituto per l'infanzia Burlo Garofolo, via dell'Istria 65/1, 34137 Trieste, Italy; [*] *II Cattedra di Clinica Pediatrica dell'Università di Milano, via Commenda 9, 20122 Milan, Italy;* [†] *Fondazione Pierfranco e Luisa Mariani, viale Bianca Maria 28, 20129 Milan, Italy*

Summary

There are no invariant rules in the choice of the therapy of limbic seizures in children. However, some considerations can be made. For instance there is evidence pointing to a progressive course of temporal epilepsy, with the appearance of drug resistance, behavioural and psychiatric disturbances and impairment of cognitive functions. Prolonged febrile seizures and epileptic status in infancy are considered risk factors for the development of this type of epilepsy. These considerations raise the question of whether to attempt prevention of prolonged febrile seizures and status epilepticus and whether to initiate treatment after the first seizure. Moreover, the role of interictal discharges must be considered and drugs affecting interictal discharges, and not only the spread of the discharge, should be preferred. On the other hand, the physician must consider the long term effects of therapy on a developing brain and the fact that the immature brain reacts differently from the mature one to seizure-related damage and adverse effect of antiepileptic drugs (AEDs) on behaviour and cognition. Single drug therapy prevents the combined adverse effects of different AEDs. In drug resistant patients a better seizure control is achieved with two- and three-drug therapy. A small proportion of patients are eligible for surgery.

The medical therapy of limbic seizures in children

Limbic seizures are the manifestation of early onset, mostly symptomatic epilepsies. For some of them, as demonstrated elsewhere by Aicardi, the pathogenetic role of prolonged febrile seizures and epileptic status in infancy has been claimed, raising questions about the prevention of such episodes in young children.

The aim of the therapy is twofold: first, to prevent the recurrence and self maintenance of seizures through the characteristic mechanisms we have shown in Chapter 16 of this book; second, to prevent the cognitive, behavioural and psychiatric disturbances associated with intractable temporal epilepsies and described by Wieser, Dravet and Riva (Chapters 17, 18 & 19).

A major problem in the treatment of children with epilepsy is that the long term effects of such a therapy on a developing brain are not known (Devinsky et al., 1994), nor even if there is an age-specific vulnerability. All we know is that the immature brain is a constantly developing structure, where the balance between excitation and inhibition varies according to age. The immature brain is more liable to seizures due to both increased excitability (consequent to the richness of postsynaptic excitatory potentials and of excitatory synapses localized in the dendritic layers of pyramidal neurons in CA3 and increased density of NMDA sites) and reduced inhibition (consequent to low GABA levels and reduced concentration of GABA receptors). It reacts to seizure-related damage and adverse effects of antiepileptic drugs differently from the mature brain (Holmes, 1997; Moshé, 1993). Pharmacodynamics and pharmacokinetics also differ between adults and children, and drugs effects cannot be reliably predicted from data gathered in adults or animals. Despite these differences, no attempts to develop age-specific therapies have been made so far, at least to our knowledge, and drugs are largely, if not only, tested and developed in adults.

In the course of developing a new experimental drug, the first phase on animals is followed by a controlled trial in adults with drug-resistant epilepsies as combination therapy together with one or more traditional drugs: therefore, the drug is tested in an adult who has already had a heavy history of epilepsy and antiepileptic therapies. Theoretically, trials should instead be carried out in newly diagnosed patients, well selected for seizure type or epileptic syndromes, by double-blind randomized studies comparing the new drug with old therapies, both in adults and children. The efficacy of the drug on the natural history of epilepsy could then be reliably evaluated, but ethical problems subsist.

Nowadays a wide range of drugs for the therapy of partial epilepsies are available.

Phenobarbital was put on the market in the first decade of the century. It was soon followed by phenytoin, primidone and carbamazepine. Carbamazepine, which is highly effective, relatively free of side effects and easy to handle, soon became the first-choice drug for the therapy of children's partial seizures. Sodium valproate was introduced many years later and its use as first-choice drug in the therapy of partial seizures began in the mid-eighties. A multicentric prospective trial comparing valproate and carbamazepine in 260 children with partial or generalized epilepsy (Verity et al., 1995) demonstrated that the two drugs are equally effective in controlling partial seizures with secondary generalization and in generalized tonic–clonic seizures. De Silva et al. (1989) came to the same conclusion comparing phenobarbital, valproate and carbamazepine in children. Camfield et al. (1997) compared the effect of carbamazepine, phenobarbital and phenytoin in 417 children with complex partial seizures with secondary generalization and generalized tonic–clonic seizures and concluded that carbamazepine was more effective than the other drugs in partial complex seizures.

On the other hand, the choice of antiepileptic therapy is influenced not only by the expected efficacy of the drug in controlling seizures, but also by the efficacy/side effects trade-off and, further, by pharmacokinetic properties and cost. Tolerability differs widely from one drug to the other and this has led to limited use of phenobarbital, primidone and phenytoin in children, at least in Italy, while in other European countries phenobarbital and phenytoin are still widely used. Carbamazepine had variable fortunes in the USA, mostly related to economical rather than medical reasons.

Much has been said about the adverse effects of phenobarbital on cognitive development of children, especially with pre-existent mental retardation (Holmes, 1997; Chen et al., 1996).

According to recent reports, it would seem that at least some of these adverse effects persist even after withdrawal of therapy (Holmes, 1997). The subacute and chronic reversible toxicity of phenytoin on intellectual functions and memory of children, especially those with pre-existing neurological damage, is well known (Reynolds, 1983; Trimble, 1987). On the contrary, the possible effects of VPA on cognitive functions have been less investigated (Legarda *et al.*, 1996). However, we know that temporal lobe epilepsies can be associated with more or less selective cognitive disturbances and hyperkinetic behaviour with attention deficits, features which could be enhanced by the therapy.

Recently, new antiepileptic agents have been devised in the attempt to reduce side effects and achieve a better control of seizures. With the introduction of new drugs we come back to a combined drug regimen approach, in order to identify therapeutical associations with favourable pharmacodynamic interactions. Addition of vigabatrin, lamotrigine, felbamate and topiramate improved control of seizures by 10–15 per cent in patients with drug-resistant epilepsy (Marson *et al.*, 1996).

So far only a few studies have compared these new agents, either as single or combined drug therapy. From a meta-analysis of 28 randomized, controlled trials in drug-resistant patients treated with gabapentin, lamotrigine, tiagabide, topiramate, vigabatrin and zonisamide in combination, it appears that all these drugs are equally effective in partial seizures (Marson). However, none of these studies compared one drug with the other directly and none considered the dose-efficacy relationship. Moreover, on statistical grounds, it is likely that if a continuous variable (seizure frequency) were changed into a binary variable (reduction of seizure frequency by 50 per cent) differences would become less evident. The mechanisms of action of the new drugs are different and in many cases multiple, therefore it is possible that these drugs may act differently on different drug-resistant partial epilepsies.

From a double-blind controlled study in adults and adolescents with focal epilepsies and drug resistant partial complex seizures, it would seem that addition of vigabatrin, even at high doses, does not interfere with cognitive functions (Dodrill, 1995). However, since it has been reported to cause psychiatric disturbances when given at high doses in susceptible subjects, its use in children with temporal lobe epilepsy is questionable (and requires great caution). As Wieser points out elsewhere in this book, learning disorders, hyperactivity, rage attacks and aggressiveness occur more frequently in children with drug-resistant temporal epilepsies than in other resistant epilepsies. However, triggering of psychiatric disturbances could also be caused by prolonged discharges.

Some papers have recently reported persistent bilateral concentric visual field constriction associated with the use of vigabatrin (Eke *et al.*, 1997). This side effect may be symptomatic or, more commonly, asymptomatic and is currently under investigation. It could be attributed to impairment of retinal GABAergic mechanisms (Baulac, 1998). Obviously, risk/benefit trade-off for such therapy must be evaluated in individual patients and, if GABA-mimetic antiepileptic agents such as vigabatrin (but also others as tiagabine) are administered, visual field assessment must be performed periodically.

Since we have limited experience with the new drugs in children with newly diagnosed epilepsies and still know little about long term side effects or rare but potentially severe adverse reactions, and since they are very expensive, the new drugs are not considered first-choice in children's epilepsies. There is no conclusive evidence that they are more effective than traditional drugs in newly diagnosed epilepsies.

From two recent randomized prospective studies comparing the efficacy of lamotrigine and carbamazepine (Brodie *et al.*, 1995) and of lamotrigine and phenytoin (Marson *et al.*, 1996) as single drug therapy in newly diagnosed partial or generalized tonic–clonic seizures it appears that lamotrigine is not more effective than carbamazepine or phenytoin. A similar study was carried out with vigabatrin and carbamazepine (Kalviainen *et al.*, 1995) and with carbamazepine and oxcarbamazepine.

These studies are flawed by having taken into account seizure types rather than epileptic syndromes. In children's epilepsy (with the possible exception of infantile spasms and Lennox–Gastaut syndrome) very little is known about the effect of different epileptic drugs in the different syndromes, although in children's temporal lobe epilepsies we treat in a different way the partial seizures with affective symptomatology described by Dalla Bernardina or the partial complex seizures of infancy described by Watanabe *et al.* (1989), with respect to the cryptogenic or symptomatic temporal lobe seizures.

It has been pointed out that prolonged febrile seizures and status epilepticus in infancy are major predisposing factors for temporal lobe epilepsy and mesial temporal sclerosis in the presence of a pre-existing pre- or perinatal damage (Cendes *et al.*, 1993). This raises the question of whether it is helpful to attempt prevention of prolonged febrile seizures and status epilepticus. In the last consensus on febrile seizures (Consensus, 1992) all participants agreed that children who are at risk for developing epilepsy are those with complex, repeated and prolonged (30 min) febrile seizures and that febrile status epilepticus causes a damage which is responsible for the subsequent epilepsy, although the risk is limited to children with pre-existing brain damage. However a *continuous* prophylaxis with PB or VPA was not recommended since the potential risk of these drugs is higher than their potential benefit (i.e. the prevention of recurrences). Intermittent prophylaxis, according to the doctor's judgement, was recommended. The issue is still unsettled. A recent meta-analysis by Rantala *et al.* (1997) of 28 studies on febrile seizures prophylaxis shows (with all the drawbacks of such a procedure) that the only effective prophylaxis is continuous prophylaxis with PB or VPA, while intermittent prophylaxis with oral or rectal DZP does not differ significantly from placebo. A systematic prophylaxis of febrile seizures does not appear to be justified, but according to the authors it could be recommended in subjects at high risk of recurrences, i.e. those presenting partial febrile seizures and/or seizures longer than 15 min, early age seizures or pre-existing neurological abnormalities and/or developmental retardation.

A progressive course of temporal lobe epilepsy has been suggested in this work (though the relevance of the epileptic mechanisms induced by seizures is still to be confirmed by prospective controlled studies in humans): seizures, initially well controlled by AEDs, would later become drug-resistant and frequently associated with behavioural and psychiatric disturbances and impairment of cognitive functions. If, as Wieser and Aicardi observed, these disturbances are worsened not only by seizures and drugs, but also by interictal discharges, drugs such as CBZ and PHT, which have been shown to prevent the diffusion of the discharge but not to affect focal spikes, should theoretically be less advisable for these subjects.

Lastly, we must discuss the therapeutic approach to first seizures: if it is true, as Wyllie states, that partial complex seizures are at higher risk of recurrence (from 80 to 90 per cent, Wyllie, 1996), and, as Camfield observed (Camfield *et al.*, 1997), that partial complex seizures in children are more difficult to treat than secondarily generalized seizures, would it not be better to start treatment immediately after the first seizure in these cases?

In conclusion, there are no invariant rules in the choice of therapy. Single drug therapy prevents the combined adverse effects of different AEDs. In drug resistant patients, two-drug therapy with traditional AEDs would give an additional 11 per cent benefit in seizure control (Mattson *et al.*, 1985) and therapy with new drugs would add another 10 per cent. In these patients, the question of surgical treatment also arises. However, as in other epilepsies, temporal lobe epilepsies, especially if cryptogenetic (but also when symptomatic) can respond well to medical therapy and patients who are eligible for surgery are only a small part of them.

References

Baulac, M., Nordmann, J.P. & Lanoe, Y. (1998): Severe filed constriction and side-effects of GABA-mimetic antiepileptic agents. *Lancet* **352**, 15; 546.

Brodie, M.J., Richens, A. & Yuen, A.W.C. (1995): Double-blind comparison of lamotrigine and carbamazepine in newly diagnosed epilepsy. *Lancet* **345**, 476–479.

Camfield, P.R., Camfield, C.S., Gordon, K. & Dooley, J.M. (1997): If a first anti-epileptic drug fails to control a child's epilepsy, what are the chances of success with the next drug? *J. Pediat.* **131**, 821–824.

Cendes, F., Andermann, F., Gloor, P., Lopes-Cendes, I., Andermann, E., Melanson, D., Jones Gotman, M., Robitaille, Y., Evans, A. & Peters, T. (1993): Atrophy of mesial structures in patients with temporal lobe epilepsy: cause or consequence of repeated seizures? *Ann. Neurol.* **34**, 95–801.

Chen, Y.J., Kang, W.M. & So, W.C (1996): Comparison of antiepileptic drugs on cognitive function in newly diagnosed epileptic children: a psychometric and neurophysiological study. *Epilepsia* **37**, 81–86.

Consensus Conference: Il bambino con convulsioni febbrili. Milano, 22.02.1991 (1992): *Boll. Lega Ital. Epil.* **77**, 23–26.

De Silva, M., McArdle, B., McGowan, M., Neville, B.G.R., Johnson, A.I. & Reynolds, E.H. (1989): *A prospective, randomised comparative monotherapy clinical trial in childhood epilepsy*. Proceedings of the Fourth International Symposium on Sodium Valproate and Epilepsy, pp. 81–86. London: Royal Society of Medecine.

Devinsky, O., Vazquez, B. & Luciano, D. (1994): New antiepileptic drugs for children: felbamate, gabapentin, lamotrigine, and vigabatrin. *J. Child. Neurol.* **9** (Suppl. 1), 33–45.

Dodrill, C.B., Arnett, J.L., Sommerville, K.W. & Sussman, N.M. (1995): Effects of differing dosages of vigabatrin (Sabril) on cognitive abilities and quality of life in epilepsy. *Epilepsia* **36** (2), 164–173.

Eke, T., Talbot, J.F. & Lawden, M.C. (1997): Severe persistent visual field constriction associated with vigabatrin. *BMJ* **314**, 180–181.

Holmes, G.L. (1997): Epilepsy in the developing brain: lessons from the laboratory and clinic. *Epilepsia* **38**, 12–30.

Kalviainen, R., Aikia, M., Saukkonen, A.M., Mervaala, E. & Riekkinnen, P.J. (1995): Vigabatrin *vs.* carbamazepine monotherapy in patients with newly diagnosed epilepsy. A randomized controlled study. *Arch. Neurol.* **52**, 589–996.

Legarda, S.B., Booth, M.P., Fennel, E.B. & Maria, B.L. (1996): Altered cognitive functioning in children with idiopathic epilepsy receiving valproate monotherapy. *J. Child. Neurol.* **11**, 321–330.

Marson, A.G., Kadir, Z.A. & Chadwick, D.W. (1996): New antiepileptic drugs: a systematic review of their efficacy and tolerability. *BMJ* **313**, 1169–1174.

Mattson, R.H., Cramer, J.A., Collins, J.F., Smith, D.B., Delgado-Escueta, A.V., Browne, T.R. et al. (1985): Comparison of carbamazepine, phenobarbital, phenytoin and primidone in partial and secondarily generalized tonic–clonic seizures. *N. Engl. J. Med.* **313**, 145–151.

Moshé, S. (1993): Seizures in the developing brain. *Neurology* **43** (Suppl. 5), S3–S7.

Rantala, H., Tarrka, R. & Uhari, M. (1997): A meta-analytic review of the preventive treatment of recurrences of febrile seizures. *J. Pediatr.* **131**, 922–925.

Reynolds, E.H. (1983): Mental effects of antiepileptic medication: a review. *Epilepsia* **24** (Suppl. 2), S85–S95.

Trimble, M.R. (1987): Anticonvulsant drugs and cognitive function: a review of the literature. *Epilepsia* **28** (Suppl. 3), S37–S45.

Verity, C.M., Hosking, G. & Easter, D.J. (1995): On behalf of the Paediatric EPITEG collaborative group. A multicentre comparative trial of sodium valproate and carbamazepine in paediatric epilepsy. *Dev. Med. Child Neurol.* **37,** 97–108.

Watanabe, K., Yamamoto, N., Negoro, T. *et al.* (1989): Benign complex partial epilepsies in infancy. *Pediatr. Neurol.* **3,** 201–211.

Wyllie, E. (1996): Surgery for catastrophic localization-related epilepsies in infants. *Epilepsia* **37** (Suppl. 1), S22–S25.

Chapter 25

Surgical treatment of 'limbic' seizures in children: methodological aspects and strategies

Claudio Munari*†, Lorella Minotti‡, Giorgio Lo Russo*, Laura Tassi*, Roberto Mai*, Stefano Francione*, Emilia Berta*, Dominique Hoffmann‡, Francesco Cardinale*, Massimo Cossu† and Philippe Kahane‡

*Centro Regionale per la Chirurgia dell'Epilessia, Ospedale Niguarda Ca' Granda, Milan, Italy;
†Istituto di Clinica Neurochirurgica Università degli Studi di Genova, Italy;
‡Neurophysiopathologie de l'épilepsie, CHU, Grenoble, France

Literature data concerning surgical treatment of severe partial epilepsies in children are dyshomogeneous and puzzling. The first problem is the definition of patients considered as 'children': their age can cover a very large range, from a few months to over 20 years. Presurgical diagnostic strategies appear to be related to the possibilities of each surgical team, much more than to the individual characteristics of each single patient. Selection criteria are disparate: by type of the surgical intervention, by type of the epileptogenic lesion, by age at intervention. Even the definition of 'limbic' seizures does not seem to be established on very clear criteria.

Moreover, the term 'limbic' is too often used as synonymous with mesial temporal, ignoring the fact that mesial temporal lobe structures are only a part of the 'limbic' system, as has been stressed by Bancaud and his co-workers, in 1965, when they proposed the term of 'mediobasal limbic seizures' as a relatively homogeneous type of seizures.

The attempt to identify the clinical patterns of 'limbic' seizures in children is particularly difficult since this diagnosis requires:

- the demonstration that the ictal discharges really start in one or several 'limbic' structures only;
- the analysis of the clinical manifestations occurring when the ictal discharge is still limited to these areas;
- the differential diagnosis between these signs and symptoms, and those occurring after the spread of the discharge to other (limbic and/or extra-limbic) cortical areas.

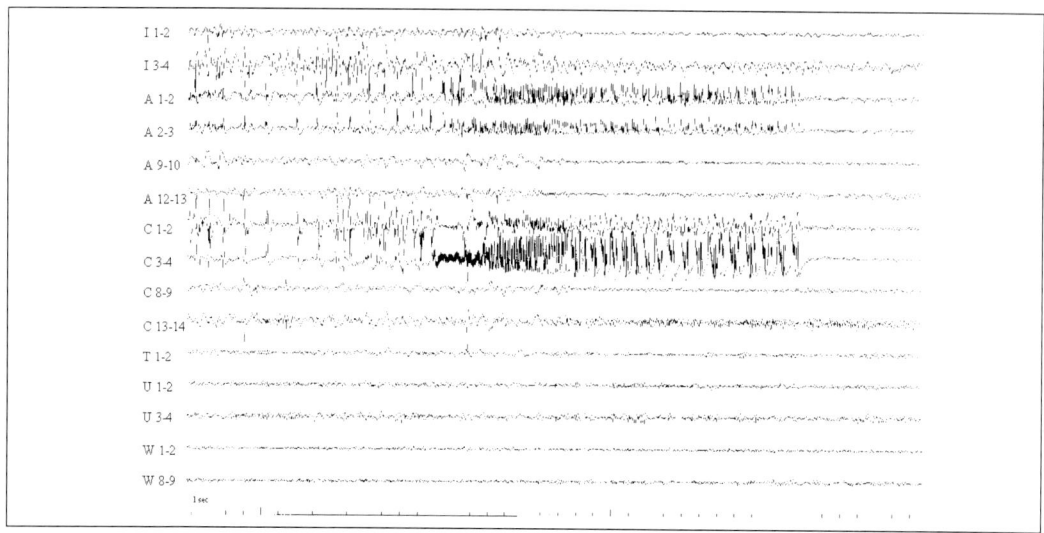

Fig. 1. Spontaneous seizure recorded in a patient with right temporal epilepsy during video-stereo-EEG monitoring. Clinically the patient reports his initial subjective manifestation (rising epigastric sensation without impairment of consciousness) only when questioned by the observer. Ictal initial discharge appears, like a mid-amplitude fast activity, on posterior hippocampus (C 1–2 and 3–4) and, with a slower frequency, on amygdala (A 1–2 and 2–3); note the secondary involvement of mesial temporal pole (I 1–2) and the minimal involvement (only an arrest reaction) of temporal neocortex (A 9–10 and 12–13; C 8–9 and 13–14). For placement of electrodes see Figs. 1a and 1b.

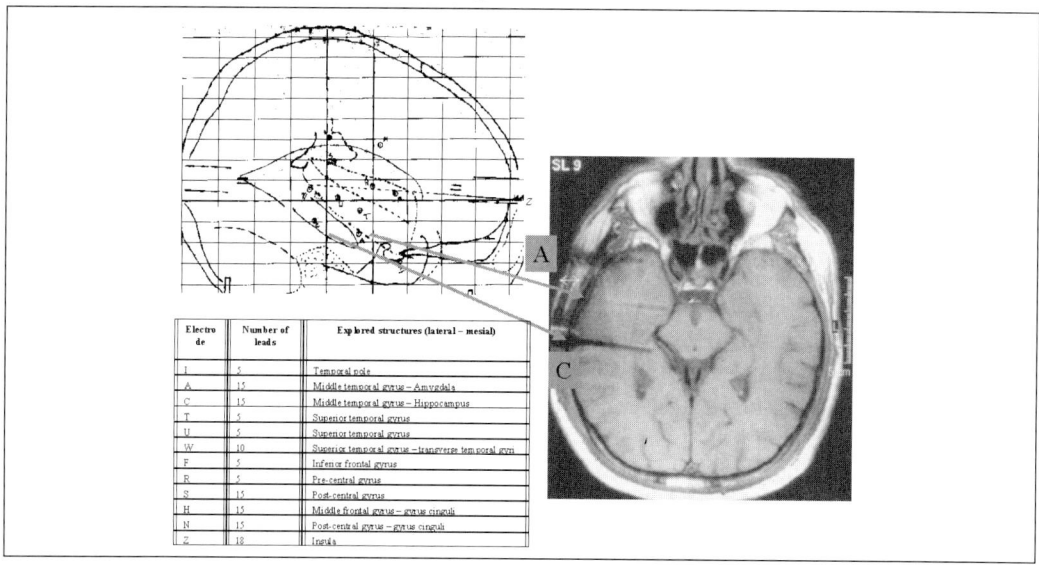

Fig. 1a. Temporo-perisylvian stereo-EEG study in a patient suffering from a cryptogenic partial epilepsy; right exploration by means of 11 sterotactically implanted electrodes; lateral view of the skull in the upper left corner with the complete plan of exploration and axial RM image in the lower right hand side, showing the intracerebral placement of three electrodes:
(A): Exploring amygdala with mesial contacts and the anterior portion of second temporal convolution (neocortex) with lateral contacts; (C): Exploring posterior hippocampus with mesial contacts and the posterior portion of second temporal convolution (neocortex) with lateral contacts.

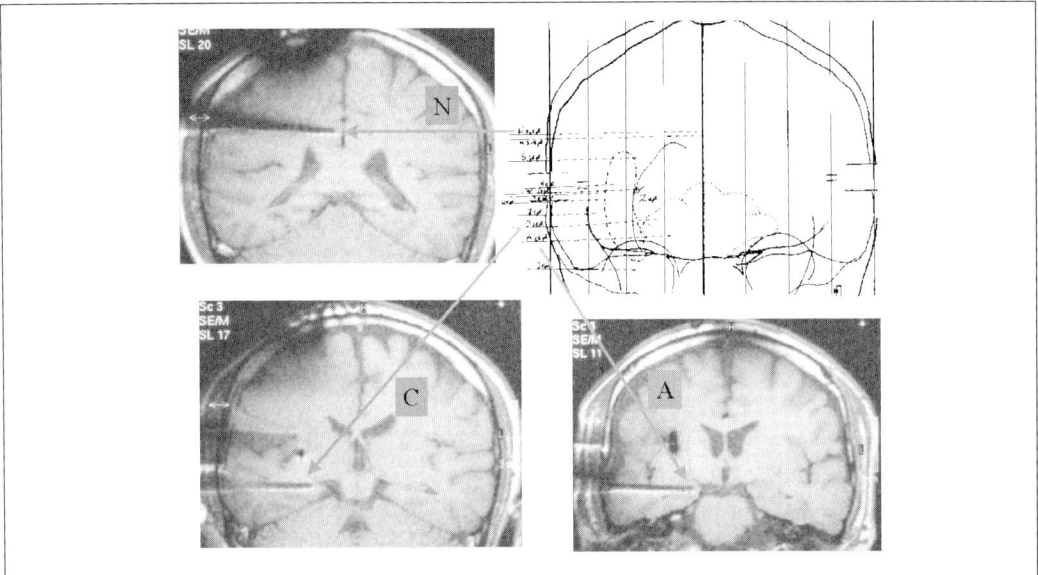

Fig. 1b. Temporo-perisylvian stereo-EEG study in a patient suffering from a cryptogenic partial epilepsy; right exploration by means of 11 sterotactically implanted electrodes; coronal view of the skull in the upper right corner with the complete plan of exploration and three coronal RM images showing the intracerebral placement of three electrodes:
(N) (upper left corner): Exploring gyrus cinguli with mesial contacts and parietal operculum with lateral contacts; (C) (lower left corner): Exploring posterior hippocampus with mesial contacts and the posterior portion of second temporal convolution (neocortex) with lateral contacts; (A) (lower right corner): Exploring amygdala with mesial contacts and the anterior portion of second temporal convolution (neocortex) with lateral contacts.

During the last 8 years, we progressively reduced the indications for the utilization of stereo-EEG investigations, mostly in children: this invasive procedure was used in 24 per cent of children with a symptomatic (but in all the children with a cryptogenic) temporal lobe epilepsy.

For this study we selected 23 consecutive children (age: 18 months – 16 years; mean: 10.5 years), in whom both temporal and extra-temporal limbic areas were simultaneously investigated, as well as other extra limbic cortical areas.

The small number of subjects, as well as the variety of the epileptogenic lesions, and the different topography and extent of the epileptogenic area(s), prevent any statistical evaluation. However, some results can be discussed:

- ictal discharges, only limited to temporal limbic structures, are rare, as was previously demonstrated in adults; during such limited discharges, the contact is not impaired (Fig. 1);
- the associated clinical semiology varies according to the type of the discharge: the more it is 'tonic', the more it is symptomatogenic (Figs. 1 and 2);
- the temporal neocortex is also, very often, simultaneously implicated: in these cases the symptomatology is more 'complex';
- the parietal cingulate gyrus is strictly physiologically connected with the posterior

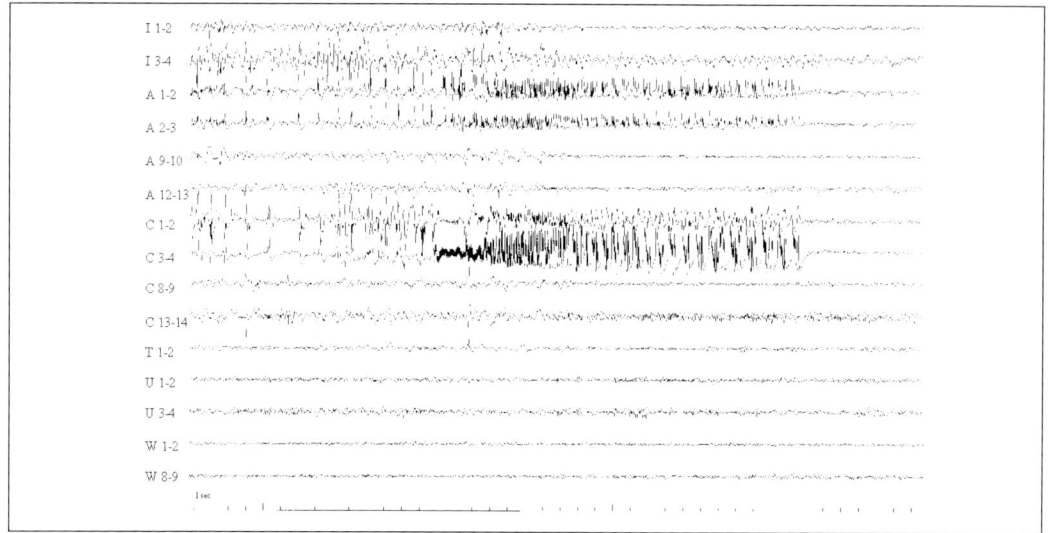

Fig. 2. Spontaneous seizure during video-stereo-EEG monitoring, in the same patient as Fig. 1. Clinically on this occasion the patient himself called the observer reporting his rising epigastric sensation. In fact, even with the same initial location of the previous discharge (see Fig. 1a), this ictal discharge appears more tonic on posterior hippocampus (C 1–2 and mainly 3–4) and on amygdala (A 1-2 and 2-3). This 'major intensity' of the discharge probably influences both clinical features and the 'propagation' of the discharge to all the leads exploring the temporal neocortex (A 9–10 and 12–13, C 8–9 and 13–14) and to the parietal cingylate gyrus (N 1–2) with no involvement of frontal cingulate gyrus (H 1–2). For placement of electrodes see Figs.1a and 1b.

hippocampus (but not with the anterior hippocampus), during the interictal periods, as well as during seizures (Fig. 2);

– the electrical activities of different parts of the cingulate gyrus are very often apparently independent;

– the anterior part of the cingulate gyrus (24 area) is strictly connected with the SMA, more than with the other components of the 'limbic' system;

– when ictal discharges, originating in the amygdalo-hippocampal areas, spread to the anterior part of the cingulate gyrus, both the temporal pole and the lateral temporal neocortex are previously involved by the discharge.

These preliminary data suggest that:

– the expression 'limbic seizures' includes several, very variegated, anatomo-electroclinical entities;

– this apparently clear expression should be proscribed;

– it is difficult to discuss the surgical treatment of 'limbic' seizures (and its results) without a previous and clear (whenever possible) differentiation among the different anatomo-electroclinical patterns.

Possible intra-individual variations, when several seizures are recorded in the same patient, do not simplify the decision about the extent of the surgical removal.

Chapter 26

Is there a benign limbic epilepsy in children?

Bernardo Dalla Bernardina*, Francesca Darra*, Elena Fontana* and Anne Beaumanoir[†]

*Servizio di Neuropsichiatria Infantile, Università di Verona, Italy;
[†]Fondazione Pierfranco e Luisa Mariani, viale Bianca Maria 28, 20129 Milan, Italy

Summary

The existence of a well-defined benign limbic epilepsy is far from being documented in spite of the presence in the literature of some observations that could permit the hypothesis of its existence. The approach to the problem is difficult because of the important dishomogeneity of diagnostic criteria, the incorrect tendency to confuse seizures with epilepsy, the unclear use of terms like 'complex partial seizures', 'psychomotor epilepsy' and 'temporal epilepsy', and finally the ambiguity in the use of the terms 'benign', 'idiopathic', 'genetic' and 'familial'.

If benign refers to an epilepsy likely to benefit from a spontaneous recovery, the rare cases observed in the literature are reported as cases of benign complex epilepsy or psychomotor epilepsy or benign partial epilepsy with affective symptoms. The more or less direct or indirect involvement of the temporal lobe in these cases is highly probable, but a well defined and unique involvement of the limbic system has not yet been proved.

Moreover, the cases reported as familial benign partial epilepsy with partial complex seizures or as familial temporal lobe epilepsy are characterized by an electroclinical picture and an evolutive polymorphism that preclude defining them as true benign epilepsies.

Looking to the actual contributions of the literature, it is only possible to observe and hypothesize that they exist during two periods of life, infancy and preschool age, in several cases of children suffering from frequent seizures with partial complex symptomatology, strongly represented by the expression of fear or terror (affective symptomatology) corresponding to a true benign epilepsy.

This hypothesis seems to be supported even by the significant variability of the interictal EEG paroxysms in functional and benign cases. The possible existence of a third, older form seems suggested by some clinical observations.

In these cases, anyway, the evolution is not really benign and there is again a clear ambiguity between the terms 'familial-idiopathic' and 'benign', which cannot be considered synonymous.

The authors report the electroclinical features in common between the cases with a real benign evolution and stress the importance of considering not only anamnestic, clinical, genetic and neuroradiological data but also interictal and ictal EEG patterns, in order to reach a correct diagnosis.

In the literature there are numerous cases underlining the possible existence, both in infancy and childhood, of epilepsies with complex partial seizures destined supposedly to a spontaneous definitive recovery.

In several of these cases the involvement of the temporal lobe seems to be predominant and in some it could be exclusive.

In spite of these observations the existence of a well-defined benign limbic epilepsy is far from being documented at any age.

Is it because a benign limbic epilepsy does not exist? or because it is difficult to recognize?

The approach to the problem is quite difficult for many reasons:

- because of the important dishomogeneity of the diagnostic criteria, population selection and follow-up periods;
- because of the frequent incorrect tendency to confuse seizures with epilepsy;
- because of the often unclear use of some terms like 'psychomotor epilepsy' and especially the persistent erroneous assumption of the equivalence between complex partial seizures and temporal lobe epilepsy (Holmes, 1997).

The main reason is finally represented by the great ambiguity in the conceptual and practical use of the terms 'benign' and 'idiopathic' as stressed by Genton & Guerrini (1994) and in some ways even of the terms 'genetic' and 'familial'.

If the term benign is used for defining epilepsies characterized by a more or less rapid and complete control of seizures, it appears that this possibility can be observed in different cases of partial epilepsy with partial complex seizures and of ascertained temporal lobe epilepsy, mainly cryptogenic but also symptomatic (Chao et al., 1962; Currie et al., 1971; Dravet et al., 1989; Lindsay et al., 1979; Takahashi et al., 1990; Kubota et al., 1990; Papazian et al., 1990; Pratap & Gururaj, 1989; Bourgeois, 1998).

The opposite is the case if benign refers to an epilepsy destined to have spontaneous and definite recovery, the rare cases observed in the literature are reported as cases of benign psychomotor epilepsy or benign partial epilepsy with affective symptoms in childhood (Cavazzuti et al., 1986; Plouin et al., 1980; Dulac & Arthuis 1980; Dalla Bernardina et al., 1980, 1984, 1992; Capella et al., 1971; Wakai et al., 1994; Loiseau et al., 1991) or as cases of benign partial epilepsy in infancy, benign partial epilepsy with complex partial seizures in infancy (Watanabe et al., 1987, 1990, 1993; Yamamoto et al., 1987; Okumura et al., 1996; Capovilla et al., 1998), or benign infantile familial convulsions (Vigevano et al., 1992).

Looking firstly at the childhood group, the predominant seizure symptoms are sudden fright or terror expressed by screaming, hiding, hiding head in hands, clinging to the closest person. A loss of contact and an absolute amnesia of the attack are invariably present.

The affective symptomatology can be associated with either chewing or swallowing movements, salivation and obvious vegetative manifestations like redness, pallor and sweating or assumed by the child's behaviour like abdominal pain (the child touches his abdomen and yells 'It hurts me, it hurts me ...').

In some cases rhythmic eyelids or peribuccal jerks can occur and in other cases independent brief orofacial seizures are observed in the absence of generalized seizures or other kinds of seizures.

The seizures lasting 1–2 min occur abruptly several times per day both whilst awake and during sleep, without postictal deficits even if some cases show a significant interictal behavioural disturbance that disappears through evolution. Invariably they are promptly stopped by clobazam or phenobarbital treatment without relapse throughout the evolution.

Referring to the 26 subjects reported by Dalla Bernardina et al. (1992), 16 aged between 15 and 28 years had been for a long time treatment- and seizure-free, whereas three subjects never received treatment and had recovered anyway. Still referring to the same subjects the EEG picture was as follows.

Background activity was normal in all cases and the organization of sleep was also normal in all cases, even during the periods with frequent seizures. The most frequent interictal abnormalities (73 per cent) were characterized by ample slow spike/slow waves (looking like the rolandic spikes of benign epilepsy with centro-temporal spikes – BECT) involving the fronto-temporal or parieto-temporal areas of one or both hemispheres. These abnormalities had a great tendency to appear and disappear throughout the course and were always activated by sleep, without changing morphology.

In more than half of the cases the only paroxysmal abnormalities, at least during the first months of evolution, were characterized by rhythmic sharp waves in the fronto-temporal or in the parieto-temporal areas of one hemisphere. In a similar proportion of cases, it was possible to observe the appearance of brief bursts of generalized spike waves, alone or in association with one of two types of focal abnormalities described above. These generalized spike waves could appear during drowsiness but never increased in frequency during slow sleep.

In 19 cases one or several seizures were recorded whilst awake and/or during sleep. In 15 instances the seizure discharges were clearly localized in the fronto-temporal, the centro-temporal or the parietal areas, whereas in four instances they were more diffuse from the onset and it was therefore difficult to recognize a localized onset. The polygraphic recordings showed that the attacks were associated with various movements but never with a tonic or clonic component. Furthermore they showed that in the same child the ictal pattern was relatively stereotyped both during wakefulness and sleep.

In these cases a significant involvement of the temporal lobe is highly probable especially if we consider the frequency with which the affective symptoms and especially fear are induced by the involvement of the temporal lobe (Gloor, 1972, 1992; Fish et al., 1993; Bancaud, 1987; Cendes et al., 1994). The EEG ictal pattern remains nevertheless ambiguous in order to show a temporal localization in the majority of the cases.

Looking at the cases reported as suffering from an infantile benign partial epilepsy we can observe that the predominant clinical symptoms are:

- a normal neuropsychological development;
- a significant incidence of familial antecedents of epilepsy;
- an onset under 12–18 months of life;
- an abrupt appearance of frequent/day relatively brief (1–3 min) partial complex seizures in clusters recurring both during wake and sleep without significant neurological impairment between seizures;
- an ictal semiology characterized by impairment of consciousness, motion arrest, and

vegetative manifestations, often with an expression of fear with or without secondary generalization;
- excellent response to treatment;
- a brief history of epilepsy without relapse even if the treatment is stopped a few years after its onset.

From the EEG point of view the peculiar findings are:
- normal background activity with normal organization during wake and sleep;
- absence of paroxysmal abnormalities;
- ictal events characterized by a rhythmic monomorphic discharge involving a temporal or a central area spreading to the other hemisphere or involving asynchronously both hemispheres. The hemisphere involved at onset often changes during the following seizures. In several cases during a seizure started in one hemisphere it is possible to observe the beginning of an important ictal discharge on the contralateral hemisphere;
- absence of postictal EEG sufferance.

In spite of the opinion of some authors (Dulac et al., 1989) these cases seem to document the existence of partial benign epilepsies in infancy.

Considering both the clinical and the EEG ictal findings, the more or less direct or indirect involvement of the temporal lobe, at least in some of these cases, is highly probable as stressed by Watanabe et al. (1990), but again a well defined and unique involvement of the limbic system is not yet demonstrated.

Considering the two reported forms (of infancy and childhood), both can be classified as idiopathic considering the clinical EEG and neuroradiological picture.

This is not considered anyway synonymous of benign because it is known that at least in some generalized forms like, for example, Janz syndrome (Wolf, 1992) even if the response to therapy is excellent a definitive recovery represents an exception.

Analogously in the two forms, the incidence of familial antecedents for epilepsy is significantly high and some cases are familial (Vigevano et al., 1992) but again familial is not synonymous with benign.

The possible existence of a familial form or temporal lobe epilepsy with adult onset has been suggested by Ciarmatori et al. (1989) and stressed as being characterized by a benign course by Berkovic et al. (1994).

According to Berkovic et al. (1994) the essential findings are:
- Mildly affected relatives often undiagnosed;
- Normal neurological picture;
- Onset usually in early adult life;
- Simple partial seizures suggestive of temporal lobe origin;
- Rare complex partial and generalized seizures;
- Non specific EEG abnormalities;

— Good response to treatment.

In these familial cases, anyway, the evolution is not always benign, as outlined by Cendes *et al.* (1994), confirming that familial and benign are not synonymous.

Even if a precise temporal focality remains difficult to ascertain in the youngest subjects as stressed by many authors (Wyllie *et al.*, 1993; Jayakar & Duchowny, 1990; Brockhaus & Elger, 1995), looking at all the contributions available in the literature, it is possible to hypothesize the existence during two periods of life, infancy and preschool age, of several cases of children suffering from an age dependent epilepsy characterized by the abrupt appearance and recurrence of partial complex seizures, strongly suggesting a temporal lobe involvement with a significant or predominant affective ictal component, of idiopathic nature, destined to have spontaneous recovery and therefore truly benign.

A familial predisposition of epilepsy probably plays a significant role and sometimes constitutes a familial form of epilepsy.

The common features are:

- a significant incidence of familial antecedents for epilepsy;
- a normal development;
- an abrupt onset of partial complex seizures, frequent and often recurring in clusters both during wake and sleep;
- the absence of clinical and EEG signs of cerebral sufferance between the seizures;
- the absence of obvious interictal EEG paroxysms, or the presence of paroxysms similar to those observed in the other benign partial epilepsies (rolandic and occipital);
- a frequent independent involvement of both hemispheres evoking something like a functional multifocal epilepsy;
- an immediate and complete response to treatment.

The complete and immediate response to treatment is necessary to the diagnosis but cannot alone guarantee the diagnosis. A positive family history of epilepsy is also a favourable element for diagnosis but does not guarantee it.

The diagnosis is more probable if the antecedents consist of an epilepsy recovered from before adolescence and in particular in infantile cases in the presence of very similar cases in the family (familial cases).

Contrarily to what characterizes benign epilepsy with rolandic spikes (Dalla Bernardina *et al.*, 1992) and more similarly to what can be observed in the early onset benign childhood occipital epilepsy of Panayiotopulous (1999a, b), both the infantile and childhood benign forms of partial epilepsy with partial complex seizures, or benign partial temporal lobe epilepsy, are characterized by a spontaneous short period of seizure recurrence and so they seem to represent, like benign neonatal convulsions, a true age-dependent epilepsy.

Considering this, if the brutality of onset can force the start of a drug therapy, a prolonged treatment in time would not be necessary and therefore an attempt to suspend the therapy at a relatively brief distance from the disappearance of the seizures (12 months) could not only be justified but might represent, in the absence of relapses, a further diagnostic confirmation.

References

Bancaud, J. (1987): Sémeiologie clinique des crises épileptiques d'origine temporale. *Rev. Neurol.* **143**, 392–400.

Berkovic, S.F., Howell, R.A. & Hopper, J.L. (1994): Familial temporal lobe epilepsy: a new syndrome with adolescent/adult onset and a benign course. In: *Epileptic seizures and syndromes*, ed. P. Wolf, pp. 257–263. London: John Libbey.

Bourgeois, B.F.D. (1998): Temporal lobe epilepsy in infants and children. *Brain Dev.* **20**, 135–141.

Brockhaus, A. & Elger, C.E. (1995): Complex partial seizures of temporal lobe origin in children of different age groups. *Epilepsia* **36**, 1173–1181.

Capella, L., Cavazzuti, G.B. & Nalin, A. (1971): Casi di epilessia psicomotoria insorti nel primo triennio. *Miner. Pediatric* **23**, 1359–1366.

Capovilla, G., Giordano, L., Tiberti, S., Valseriati, D. & Menegati, E. (1998): Benign partial epilepsy in infancy with complex partial seizures (Watanabe's syndrome): 12 non-Japanese new cases. *Brain Dev.* **20**, 105–111.

Cavazzuti, G.B., Ferrari, P., Finelli, T., Galli, V. & Ciccarone, V. (1986): Benign psychomotor epilepsy in childhood. *Pediatr. Med. Chir.* **8**, 787–795.

Cendes, F., Andermann, F., Gloor, P., Gambardella, A., Lopes-Cendes, I., Watson, C., Evans, A., Capenter, S. & Olivier, A. (1994): Relationship between atrophy of the amygdala and ictal fear in temporal lobe epilepsy. *Brain* **117**, 739–746.

Chao, D., Sexton, J.A. & Sautos Pardo, L. (1962): Temporal lobe epilepsy in children. *J. Pediatr.* **60**, 686–693.

Ciarmatori, C., Cardinaletti, L., Michelucci, R. & Tassinari, C.A. (1989): Sindrome epilettica benigna con crisi parziali complesse familiari: studio clinico-EEG di 3 famiglie. *Boll. Lega It. Epil.* **66/67**, 67–72

Currie, S., Heathfield, K.W.G., Henson, R.A. & Scott, D.F. (1971): Clinical course and prognosis of temporal lobe epilepsy: a survey of 666 patients. *Brain* **94**, 173–190.

Dalla Bernardina, B., Bureau, M., Dravet, C., Dulac, O., Tassinari, C.A. & Roger, J. (1980): Epilepsie bénigne de l'enfant avec crises à séméiologie affective. *Rev. EEG Neurophysiol.* **10**, 8–18.

Dalla Bernardina, B., Colamaria, V., Capovilla, G. & Bondavalli, S. (1984): Sleep and benign partial epilepsies of childhood. In: *Epilepsy, sleep and sleep deprivation*, eds. R. Degen & E. Niedermeyer, pp. 119–133. Amsterdam: Elsevier Science Publishers B.V.

Dalla Bernardina, B., Colamaria, V., Chiamenti, C., Capovilla, G., Trevisan, E. & Tassinari, C.A. (1992): Benign partial epilepsy with affective symptoms ('benign psychomotor epilepsy') In: *Epileptic syndromes in infancy, childhood and adolescence* (2nd edn), eds. J. Roger, M. Bureau, C. Dravet, F.E. Dreifuss, A. Perret & P. Wolf, pp. 219–223. London: John Libbey.

Dravet, C., Catani, M., Bureau, M. & Roger, J. (1989): Partial epilepsies in infancy: a study of 40 cases. *Epilepsia* **30**, 807–812.

Dulac, O. & Arthuis, M. (1980): Epilepsies psychomotrice bénigne de l'enfant. In: *Journées Parisiennes de pédiatrie*, pp. 211–220. Paris: Flammarion.

Dulac, O., Cusmai, R. & de Oliveira, K. (1989): Is there a partial benign epilepsy in infancy? *Epilepsia* **30**, 798–801.

Fish, D.R., Gloor, P., Quesney, F.L. & Olivier, A. (1993): Clinical responses to electrical brain stimulation of the temporal and frontal lobes in patients with epilepsy: pathophysiological implications. *Brain* **116**, 397–414.

Genton, P. & Guerrini, R. (1994): Idiopathic localization-related epilepsies: the non-rolandic types. In: *Epileptic seizures and syndromes*, ed. P. Wolf, pp. 241–256. London: John Libbey.

Gloor, P. (1972): Temporal lobe epilepsy: its possible contribution to the understanding of the functional significance of the amygdala and of its interaction with neocortical-temporal mechanism. In: *The neurobiology of the amygdala*, ed. B.E. Eleftheriou, pp. 423–457. New York: Plenum Press.

Gloor, P. (1992): Role of the amygdala in temporal lobe epilepsy. In: *The amygdala: neurobiological aspects of emotion, memory, and mental dysfunction*, ed. J.P. Appleton, pp. 505–538. New York: Wiley-Liss.

Holmes, G.L. (1997): Temporal lobe epilepsy in childhood. In: *Paediatric epilepsy syndromes and their surgical treatment,* eds. I. Tuxhorn, H. Holthausen & H. Boenigk, pp. 251–260. London: John Libbey.

Jayakar, P. & Duchowny, M.S. (1990): Complex partial seizures of temporal lobe origin in early childhood. *J. Epilepsy* **3,** 41–45.

Kubota, H., Fujikawa, Y., Fujiwara, T., Yagi, K. & Seino, M. (1990): Long-term seizure outcome of children with complex partial seizures. *Brain Dev.* **12,** 631.

Lindsay, J., Ounsted, C. & Richards, P. (1979): Long-term outcome in children with temporal lobe seizures. I: Social outcome and childhood factors. *Dev. Med. Child Neurol.* **21,** 285–298.

Loiseau, P., Duché, B. & Loiseau, J. (1991): Classification of epilepsies and epileptic syndromes in two different samples of patients. *Epilepsia* **32,** 303–309.

Okumura, A., Hayakawa, F., Kuno, K. & Watanabe, K. (1996): Benign partial epilepsy in infancy. *Arch. Dis. Childhood* **74,** 19–21.

Panayiotopoulos, C.P. (1999a): Early-onset benign childhood occipital seizure susceptibility syndrome: a syndrome to recognize. *Epilepsia* **40,** 621–630.

Panayiotopoulos, C.P. (1999b): *Benign childhood partial seizures and related epileptic syndromes.* London: John Libbey.

Papazian, O., Resnick, T.J., Cullen, R.F., Jr, Jayakar, P., Duenas, A., Alfonso, I., Alvarez, L., Duchowny, M. & Deray, M. (1990): Natural history of cryptogenic partial complex epilepsy of childhood. *Brain Dev.* **12,** 639.

Plouin, P., Lerique, A. & Dulac, O. (1980): Etude électroclinique et évolution dans 7 observations de crises partielles complexes dominées par un comportement de terreur chez l'enfant. *Boll. Lega Ital. Epil.* **29–30,** 139–143.

Pratap, R.C. & Gururaj, A.K. (1989): Clinical and electroencephalographic features of complex partial seizures in infants. *Acta Neurol. Scand.* **79,** 123–127.

Takahashi, I., Miura, K., Nomura, K., Furune, S., Maehara, M., Negoro, T. & Watanabe, K. (1990): Seizure prognosis and EEG evolution in complex partial seizures of childhood onset. *Brain Dev.* **12,** 498–502.

Vigevano, F., Fusco, L., Di Capua, M., Ricci, S., Sebastianelli, R. & Lucchini, P. (1992): Benign infantile familial convulsions. *Eur. J. Pediatr.* **151,** 608–612.

Wakai, S., Yoto, Y., Higashidate, Y., Tachi, N. & Chiba, S. (1994): Benign partial epilepsy with affective symptoms: hyperkinetic behaviour during interictal periods. *Epilepsia* **35,** 810–812.

Watanabe, K., Yamamoto, N., Negoro, T., Takaesu, E., Aso, K., Furune, S. & Takahashi, I. (1987): Benign complex partial epilepsies in infancy. *Pediatr. Neurol.* **3,** 208–211.

Watanabe, K., Yamamoto, N., Negoro, T., Takahashi, I., Aso, K. & Maehara, M. (1990): Benign infantile epilepsy with complex partial seizures. *J. Clin Neurophysiol.* **7,** 409–416.

Watanabe, K., Negoro, T. & Aso, K. (1993): Benign partial epilepsy with secondary generalized seizures in infancy. *Epilepsia* **34,** 635–638.

Wolf, P. (1992): Juvenile myoclonic epilepsy. In: *Epileptic syndromes in infancy, childhood and adolescence,* 2nd edn., eds. J. Roger, M. Bureau, C. Dravet, F.E. Dreifuss, A. Perret & P. Wolf, pp. 313–327. London: John Libbey.

Wyllie, E., Chee, M., Granström, M.L., Del Giudice, E., Estes, M., Comair, Y., Pizzi, M., Kotagal, P., Bourgeois, B. & Lüders, H. (1993): Temporal lobe epilepsy in early childhood. *Epilepsia* **34,** 859–868.

Yamamoto, N., Watanabe, K., Negro, T., *et al.* (1987): Complex partial seizures in children. Ictal manifestations and their relation to clinical course. *Neurology* **37,** 1379–1382.

Chapter 27

Synopsis

Giuliano Avanzini

Department of Experimental Research and Diagnosis, Istituto Nazionale Neurologico C. Besta, Via Celoria 11, 20133 Milano, Italy

The aim of the colloquium, from which this multi-author book originates, was to outline the specific expression of epilepsies involving the limbic structures in children and to establish a consensus on the evidence relevant to the clinical management of these epilepsies. This is by no means an easy task, as the reader can appreciate already from the first chapter, in which **Annette Beaumanoir & Joseph Roger**, authors of twin seminal papers on the 'épilepsie psychomotrice de l'enfant' published in 1954, review the evolution of terminology and concepts from Jackson's first description up to present-day views.

The different definitions that have been proposed reflect controversial opinions about pathophysiology, natural history and diagnostic criteria that are still unresolved.

In order to speak of a *limbic epilepsy*, we must be able to agree on the existence of a clinical entity unequivocally defined in terms of age of onset, type(s) of seizures, neurological and neuropsychological picture, time, course and prognosis. Once a consensus is reached about definition criteria, investigations on the pathophysiological basis, taking into account developmental aspects, might provide further measures for verification and point out the best strategies aimed at preventing the unfavourable evolution which is often observed. In addition, some typical risk factors should be outlined, which cannot reasonably be reduced to a unitary aetiology.

Typically, the pathological process leading to limbic epilepsies acts on the developing brain, and the general agreement among the contributors upon this point stresses the appropriateness of focusing this colloquium on childhood. When the clinical history can be traced back to early infancy with sufficient precision, an acute, usually convulsive and often febrile episode is often noticed, to be followed at a variable latency by recurring seizures, whose clinical symptomatology is consistent with the involvement of limbic structures. Their semiology is highly variable, ranging from short episodes of loss of contact to complex phenomenology including autonomic and emotional manifestations, illusions, hallucinations and automatisms, that can hardly be accounted for by a dysfunction of an individual structure.

Based on the anatomy and physiology of limbic structures reviewed by **Villani *et al.*** and **Avanzini**, and on the clinical and neurophysiological observations reported by **Mai *et al.*,**

Lüders, Biraben, Landré *et al.*, Kahane *et al.*, Isnard and **Tassi *et al.***, some anatomo-clinical correlations can be attempted.

According to the current classification of epileptic seizures (Commission on Classification and Terminology of the International League against Epilepsy, *Epilepsia* 22, 489, 1981) the impairment of consciousness is the hallmark of partial complex seizures whose generating discharge is assumed to involve limbic structures. This concept has been criticised from several points of view, its main weakness being the definition of consciousness itself, which presents too many philosophical implications to be a workable concept in epileptology (Gloor, *Epilepsia* 27, 514, 1986). Therefore this phenomenon is referred to as 'loss of contact' in **Francione *et al.*'s** paper, co-signed by **Munari,** in which the experience of the Niguarda Epilepsy Center (now named 'Claudio Munari' in honour of its founder) is reported. It is concluded that although this symptom is seldom observed during extra-limbic discharges, its localising value is limited and 'the impairment of contact appears to be related more to the extent, duration and/or modalities of the discharge rather than to the involvement of a precise anatomical structure'.

The alteration in the relationship to the environment is systematically reviewed by **Tassi *et al.*** (also co-authored by **Munari**). Illusions and hallucinations are often reported by patients with temporal or frontal lobe epilepsy; however, they may depend on a spread of discharge outside the limbic system. This is the case of auditory illusions or hallucinations, depending on the first temporal gyrus, while olfactory hallucinations, traditionally attributed to limbic temporal structures, are now referred to the orbital cortex and can therefore be considered either a limbic symptom or not, depending on whether this frontal area is included or not in the limbic system. Truly 'limbic' in origin are psychic symptoms of *déjà-vu*, *déjà-vécu* and dreamy state that express ictal alterations of memory-related hippocampal function, whereas forced thinking is considered a frontal symptom possibly unrelated to limbic structures. Also unrelated to the limbic system are language and/or speech alterations that according to **Lüders**'s report are frequently observed in patients with limbic seizures as a result of discharges spreading to the neocortical language areas. On the contrary, autonomic and emotional symptoms are primarily due to the involvement of the limbic system and can be considered as more or less stereotyped fragments of complex behavioural patterns aimed at maintaining homeostasis, individual survival (avoidance, fight and feeding reactions) or species preservation (sexual behaviour). Emotional reactions can be limited to changes in visual expression which **Landré *et al.*** have found to be the initial manifestation of mesial temporal seizures. Currently, the typical expression of the epileptic discharges arising in the hippocampus, parahippocampal gyrus and amygdalar nucleus is considered to be a sensation of epigastric heaviness often rising toward the throat, often associated with autonomic manifestations (tachycardia, polypnea, facial reddening). The issue is reviewed in **Isnard**'s chapter. Consciousness is preserved in the initial phase ('aura', from a few seconds to 1–2 min) and subsequently subsides, evolving toward a complete loss of contact. The initial symptoms may be less clearly reported (undefinable non-localised discomfort associated with motor arrest). Memory is usually impaired over the period of the seizure but also 1-2 minutes before seizure onset. Complex motor activities referred to as automatisms may occur during mesial temporal as well as other types of limbic seizures; they are analysed in **Biraben *et al.***'s chapter with reference to Loiseau and Jallon's definition (*Dictionnaire d'épileptologie clinique*, Paris: John Libbey Eurotext, 1990) as 'involuntary motor activity occurring during an epileptic seizure irrespective of the state of consciousness'.

In agreement with Munari *et al.*'s report (*Rev. EEG Neurophysiol.* 9, 236, 1979), chewing and oral movements were found to be associated with discharges arising in the amygdala and anterior Ammon's horn; they should be distinguished from viscero-vegetative movements such as deglutition: swallowing, spitting, lip licking, which imply the participation of suprasylvian regions. Simple gestural automatisms involving exploratory activities are said to originate in the temporal and orbito-frontal lobes, whereas complex automatisms such as pedalling, usually attributed to the activation of the medial orbito-frontal and medial frontal regions, are hypothetically related to a defective control of motor activity by the limbic system. Other types of motor symptoms such as postural changes depend on the spread of discharges outside the limbic system (**Landré** *et al.*). The issue of the preferential propagation pathways of limbic discharges is addressed on experimental and clinical grounds respectively in the chapters by **Chevassus-au-Louis** *et al.* and **Kahane** *et al.* Propagation of hippocampal discharges is age-dependent and tends to be restricted to the septum in the immature brain, whereas in later stages it involves both the septal and entorhinal areas, which are the main gates towards the neocortex. These pathways can be short-circuited by experimentally-induced hippocampal heterotopias in the rat, which can establish a bridge between the hippocampus and neocortex. The perisylvian cortex, namely the superior temporal gyrus and the suprasylvian opercular cortex, are most frequently involved in temporal lobe seizures; interestingly **Kahane** *et al.* found a hippocampal sclerosis in almost 40 per cent of patients with initial or early perisylvian involvement. Based on personal observations, **Isnard** maintains that critical discharges confined to the hippocampus may be completely asymptomatic and that the so called 'mesial temporal symptomatology' appears when the insular cortex is involved.

The information drawn from the above reviewed chapters stresses the limited localising value of individual signs and symptoms occurring during seizures involving the limbic structures if they are considered in isolation. To reconstruct the origin and propagation of a seizure discharge within and outside the limbic system, its dynamics must be carefully investigated through a chronological analysis of their ictal electroclinical phenomenology, to be correlated with all the available anatomical information. Such an analysis may be particularly difficult in children due to some peculiarities of seizure expression, and to the limitations in defining the subjective experience in infants. With reference to the anatomo-functional organisation of the limbic system reviewed in the chapters of **Villani** *et al.* (co-authored by **Spreafico**) and of **Avanzini**, fear and feeding automatisms can be ascribed to the involvement of amygdaloid nuclei, whereas autonomic reactions (changes in heart rate, blood pressure, pupillary diameter), whether or not associated with tremor or aggressive behaviour, are most frequently consequent to anterior cingulate activation. Nevertheless, it is difficult to establish a precise correlation between the symptoms and their sites of origin, even for the core structure of the limbic system, the hippocampus, whose functional significance is still elusive despite the impressive number of papers published on this subject. Substantial evidence supports the idea that due to their plastic properties, the hippocampal circuits are capable of recording and storing the traces of incoming information, thus constructing a cognitive map that is continuously updated on the basis of experience. This is consistent with the already mentioned ictal memory disturbances caused by discharges affecting the hippocampus, but does not resolve the controversial issue of the responsibility of the hippocampus in autonomic ictal symptoms. In general the available information on anatomo-clinical correlations does not allow to draw a systematic picture of the polymorphic symptomatology putatively attributed to the various limbic structures.

Much effort has been devoted to the identification of an unifying explanation of pathogenesis, at least for what is currently defined as mesial temporal lobe epilepsy (MTLE). The results of clinical, neuroradiological and experimental studies have led to elaborate some hypotheses about the pathogenetic processes that attempt to explain the typical biphasic natural history with seizures involving limbic structures. Typically, a potential early risk factor (often a febrile convulsion) occurring before the age of four years is followed after a latent period by recurring limbic seizures associated with discharges involving the mesial temporal structures. In adults, MTLE is frequently associated with mesial temporal sclerosis (MTS), defined as neuronal loss gliosis and evidence of synaptic reorganization. Results obtained in animal models of MTLE with MTS (e.g. kainic acid or pilocarpine rat models) support a pathogenetic role of the early acute risk factor in starting a process that develops during the latent period, leading to a MTS-associated synaptic reorganisation. This view is challenged by **Spencer et al.** who address here some relevant questions such as: do children of all ages have MTS ? Does it present all the pathological and clinical features of adults? The answer to the first question is yes, although the cell loss in children under age 12 is much more restricted than what is found in adults or adolescents. On the contrary the answer to the second question is negative, since in children under age 12 there is no evidence of reorganisation or sprouting. It is concluded that whereas cell loss and gliosis which are common across all age groups may have a pathogenic role in MTLE, the synaptic reorganisation is a secondary lesion, and its functional significance is still unknown. Febrile convulsions are confirmed as a frequent antecedent of MTLE by both **Spencer et al.** and **Van Lierde & Mira,** but their role as an aetiological factor is questioned. As an alternative it is suggested 'that hippocampal cell loss and structural hippocampal abnormality may be a pre-existing, genetically determined condition which facilitates febrile convulsions and underlies or contributes to the development of MTS' (**Spencer et al.**).

Are there any significant differences between the clinical presentation of epilepsies with limbic seizures in children with respect to adults? This question is addressed through the book, and especially in the chapters of **Landré et al., Isnard, Pachatz et al., Elger & Fernandez, Tassi et al., Franceschetti et al., Chiron et al.,** and **D'Incerti,** who review the clinical picture and the diagnostic criteria in children.

There is a general consensus on the similarity of limbic seizure phenomenology in adults and children after the age of 3, whereas during the first 3 years of life ictal phenomenology is usually subtle, fragmentary and often difficult to recognise (**Pachatz et al., Elger & Fernandez, Franceschetti et al.**). Moreover, whereas ictal low-voltage fast activity can be consistently localised on the temporal region, the topography of the interictal EEG abnormalities is much less defined in infants or children and often has a multifocal distribution (**Franceschetti et al.**). The stereo EEG recordings reviewed by **Tassi et al.** and **Isnard** in children aged more than 3 years confirm the experience of these groups on larger adults case series and support their warning about the risk of overestimating the responsibility of limbic structures (namely the mesial temporal ones) in patients in whom a systematic EEG exploration has not been carried out.

An interesting analysis on aetiology-based subgroups is reported by **Pachatz et al.** in the chapter co-signed by **Vigevano**: attention is called to the high probability of a tumoral origin of early-onset temporal lobe epiepsies.

Is there a benign limbic epilepsy in children? **Dalla Bernardina et al.** answer affirmatively in a chapter co-signed by **A. Beaumanoir** reporting the clinical characters and prognosis of both infantile and childhood benign temporal lobe epilepsy, although these forms are admittedly seldom encountered in clinical practice.

The diagnostic contribution of SPECT and MRI in children limbic epilepsies is discussed in two chapters by **Chiron** *et al.* and **D'Incerti** respectively. Both techniques are said to be as highly valuable in children as they are in adults. Ictal SPECT may provide useful information about seizure propagation, and even may be the only localising sign for temporal lobe involvement in very young children. As to MRI, it remains the first choice examination to detect MTS, although T_2- hyperintensity is found less frequently in children than in adults, possibly because sprouting and synaptic reorganisation are phenomena occurring relatively late in the course of MTLE (**Spencer** *et al.*). The contribution of MRI to the early detection of hippocampal dysgeneses, whether or not associated with MTS, is appropriately highlighted in **D'Incerti** chapter. The controversial issue of epilepsy-associated cognitive and behavioural disturbances is addressed in three chapters prepared by **Riva** *et al.*, **Dravet & Bureau** and **Wieser**. Although specific roles of cerebral damage, drug side-effects and of the negative environmental feedback can often be difficult to discriminate, there is a general consensus that early surgical treatment should be contemplated in children with intractable limbic epilepsies who fulfil the criteria for epilepsy surgery, in order to avoid the negative effects of psychosocial factors of seizures on psychological development.

The criteria for medical and surgical therapy of limbic seizures in children are reviewed in two contributions by **Costa** *et al.* and **Munari** *et al*. The medical therapy should be adjusted individually, taking into account the adverse effects of antiepileptic drugs on behaviour and cognition. Due to his terminal illness, Claudio Munari could not write this chapter; however, it seemed appropriate to select the abstract he had prepared for the Colloquium as the conclusion of this book. Munari's heritage will survive in his collaborators, who continue their work at the Claudio Munari Centre of Niguarda, and who are substantially represented in these proceedings. Munari's always bright, spirited, unique contribution to the life of the epileptologic community will be sadly missed and always remembered.

Index

A

affective brain	3
allocortex	13
alveus	15
Alzheimer's disease	24
Ammon's horn	89, 91, 94, 161
lesions	6
sclerosis	4, 5, 64
see also mesial temporal sclerosis	
amygdala	24–5
amygdalar nucleus	129, 130
amygdalo-hippocampic structures	129, 131
analytical semiology	65–9
anxiety disorder	181
automatic seizures	2
automatisms	143–4
complex	99–100
oro-alimentary	90–4
simple gesture	94–9
verbal	99
see also motor	
autonomic manifestations	61, 70–2
cardio-vascular	67–8, 74
digestive	66–7, 74
distinctive features	73–5
in epileptic seizures	62
genital	69
ocular	68, 74
pupillary	68
respiratory	68–9, 74
in temporal lobe seizures	62–70
thermo-regulatory	69
urinary	69
uro-genital	74

B

benign	
complex epilepsy	241
epilepsy with centro-temporal spikes	243
epilepsy with Rolandic spikes	245
partial epilepsy	241, 243–4, 245
partial temporal lobe epilepsy	245
Broca's area	84

C

Canada	207
catastrophic rages	177
Child Behavior Checklist	178, 179
Children's Depression Inventory	178
cingulate epilepsy	85
cingulate gyrus	25–6, 141
corpus callosum agenesis	225, 226
cortical	
dysgenesis	192, 195
focal	162
dysplasia	189, 191, 226
heterotopias	35–8
malformation	35
temporal gliosis	178
cryptogenic epilepsy	212
cryptogenic temporal lobe epilepsy	152

D

dorso-lateral cortex	142

E

emotional behaviour, intensification of	188

F

facial expression changes during temporo-limbic seizures	105–14
familial temporal lobe epilepsy	241
fascia dentata	21, 23, 27, 28
febrile status epilepticus	160
focal cortical dysgenesis	162
focal seizures	211–16
frontal lobe epilepsy	183
fronto-temporal epilepsy	183
frontopolar cortex	141

G

generalized	
absence seizures	62
seizures	160
tonic–clonic seizures	62, 182, 232, 234
Gerstman syndrome	84
gyration abnormalities	192

H

herpes virus	228
heterotopias	192
hippocampal	
atrophy	161, 162, 170–1, 228
dysgenesis	226
dysplasia	171
formation	13
sclerosis	152, 154, 161, 196, 227–8
neuropathological-clinical correlations	193–5
see also mesial temporal sclerosis	
seizure activity	35–8
seizure propagation	34–5
hyperkinetic syndrome	177–8

I

ictal	
activity	131–2, 204–5
discharges	119–21
EEG during limbic seizures	201–8
features	211–16
manifestations	139, 142–4
SPECT in temporal lobe seizures	217–22
idiopathic temporal epilepsy	5
in vivo data	34
infantile spasms	179, 234
intellectual disturbances see perceptual and intellectual disturbances	
intercritical activity	131
interictal abnormalities	204
interictal features	211–16
intermediate mesial core	141
isocortex	13

J

Janz syndrome	244
juvenile myoclonic epilepsy	181

K

kainate-induced seizures: *in vivo* data	34

L

lamina dissecans	13
language and speech disturbances	81–6
cingulate epilepsy	85
clinical significance	85–6
cortical language areas	81–2
language alterations	83–4
language deficits and 'conciousness' alterations	84–5
mechanisms for speech disturbances	79–81
Lennox–Gastaut syndrome	179, 211, 234
loss of contact	55–60
Luria-Nebraska Neuropsychological Test Battery – Children's Version	179

M

medical therapy	231–5
memory disturbances in early hippocampal pathology	167–72
mental defect	176–7
mesial temporal lobe epilepsy	1–3, 46–9, 64, 129–33, 148, 151
perceptual and intellectual disturbances	190, 192–3, 195–6
mesial temporal sclerosis	41–50, 159–63, 178, 203, 234
mesio-temporal seizures	129–35
clinical semiology	130–1
electroencephalographic semiology	131–3
partial seizure	129–30
temporal origin	133–5
mesocortex	13
mirror foci	4
MMPI clinical scales	180
mood disorders	188–9

motor automatisms	89–102
complex	99–100
definitions	90
oro-alimentary	90–4
simple gesture	94–9
verbal	99
motor manifestations	144
MRI in limbic structures	225–9

N

neocortex	35–8
neocortical propagation of hippocampal seizure activity by cortical heterotopias	35–8
neoplasia	192
neuro-vegetative manifestations in temporo-limbic seizures	61–75
autonomic manifestations	70–2
distinctive features	73–5
in epileptic seizures	62
in temporal lobe seizures	62–70
pathophysiological hypotheses	72–3
neuronal migration disorders	225, 226
neurotic symptoms	180
neurotransmitter systems and epileptogenesis	26–8

O

ontogenesis	17–20
of hippocampal seizure propagation	34–5
orbitary lobe	140

P

pararhinal sclerosis	162
parahippocampal cortex	21–4
pathophysiological hypotheses	72–3
perceptual and intellectual disturbances	187–96
Geschwind Syndrome	188–9
neurobehavioural, neuropsychological and psychiatric aspects of temporal lobe epilepsy	187–8
neuropathological-clinical correlations in hippocampal sclerosis	193–5
pre- and post-operative antiepileptic drug treatment in Zürich amygdalo-hippocampectomy series	190–3, 195
perisylvian cortex involvement and temporal lobe seizures	115–25
personality disorders	179, 180, 181
phylogenetic aspects	17
postictal aphasia	85–6
postural disturbances during temporo-limbic seizures	105–14
propagation of limbic seizures: experimental studies	33–8
neocortical propagation of hippocampal seizure activity by cortical heterotopias	35–8
ontogenesis of hippocampal seizure propagation	34–5
psychiatric disturbances	187–8, 190
psychic alterations in temporal lobe seizures	175–83
disturbances, types of and related factors	176–9
psychosis	179–80
psychic variant seizures	2
psychosis	179–80, 182, 188–9

R

Revised Children's Manifest Anxiety Scale	178
rhinencephalic seizures	2–4, 12

S

schizencephaly	192–3
schizophrenia	179, 180, 182, 188–9
semiological features	69–70
simple febrile convulsions	160, 162
simple gesture automatisms	94–9
spreading patterns	132–3
statum oriens	14
status epilepticus	187, 231, 234
febrile	160
stratum lacunosum-moleculare	14
stratum lucidum	14
stratum radiatum	14
superior temporal gyrus	115–21, 122–4
supplementary motor area	97, 141
supplementary sensorimotor area	85
suprasylvian opercular cortex	115–21, 123–4
surgical treatment	237–40
symptomatic epilepsy	212

T

temporal epilepsy	
idiopathic	5
intractable	231

automatisms	143–4	temporal lobe tumours	152–4
motor manifestations	144	*see also* mesial	
subjective disturbances	142–3	temporal lobe lesions	152, 156
temporal hyperfusion	220	temporal lobe seizures	2, 115–25
temporal lobe epilepsy	45, 151–7, 171, 242, 244	psychic alterations	175–83
		temporal lobe tumours	156, 189
benign partial	245	temporal partial epilepsy	134
cryptogenic	152, 155–6	temporal seizures	134
familial	241	temporo-mesial sclerosis	168, 171
febrile convulsions	159, 160, 161, 163	thermoregulation	74
focal seizures	211, 215	tonic seizures	62
ictal EEG	206–8	tuberous sclerosis	178, 179, 212
lesional	154–5		
medical therapy	233, 234, 235	**V**	
neurobehavioural aspects	187–8	visceral brain	3
neuropsychological aspects	187–8		
perceptual and intellectual disturbances	190, 195, 196	**W**	
perisylvian cortex involvement	115–25	Wernicke's language areas	83, 84, 86
psychiatric aspects	187–8	West syndrome	211
surgical treatment	239